USABILITY
Gaining a Competitive Edge

IFIP - The International Federation for Information Processing

IFIP was founded in 1960 under the auspices of UNESCO, following the First World Computer Congress held in Paris the previous year. An umbrella organization for societies working in information processing, IFIP's aim is two-fold: to support information processing within its member countries and to encourage technology transfer to developing nations. As its mission statement clearly states,

IFIP's mission is to be the leading, truly international, apolitical organization which encourages and assists in the development, exploitation and application of information technology for the benefit of all people.

IFIP is a non-profitmaking organization, run almost solely by 2500 volunteers. It operates through a number of technical committees, which organize events and publications. IFIP's events range from an international congress to local seminars, but the most important are:

- The IFIP World Computer Congress, held every second year;
- open conferences;
- working conferences.

The flagship event is the IFIP World Computer Congress, at which both invited and contributed papers are presented. Contributed papers are rigorously refereed and the rejection rate is high.

As with the Congress, participation in the open conferences is open to all and papers may be invited or submitted. Again, submitted papers are stringently refereed.

The working conferences are structured differently. They are usually run by a working group and attendance is small and by invitation only. Their purpose is to create an atmosphere conducive to innovation and development. Refereeing is less rigorous and papers are subjected to extensive group discussion.

Publications arising from IFIP events vary. The papers presented at the IFIP World Computer Congress and at open conferences are published as conference proceedings, while the results of the working conferences are often published as collections of selected and edited papers.

Any national society whose primary activity is in information may apply to become a full member of IFIP, although full membership is restricted to one society per country. Full members are entitled to vote at the annual General Assembly, National societies preferring a less committed involvement may apply for associate or corresponding membership. Associate members enjoy the same benefits as full members, but without voting rights. Corresponding members are not represented in IFIP bodies. Affiliated membership is open to non-national societies, and individual and honorary membership schemes are also offered.

USABILITY
Gaining a Competitive Edge

***IFIP 17th World Computer Congress —
TC13 Stream on Usability: Gaining a Competitive Edge
August 25-30, 2002, Montréal, Québec, Canada***

Edited by

Judy Hammond
*University of Technology, Sydney
Australia*

Tom Gross
*Johannes Kepler University of Linz
Austria*

Janet Wesson
*University of Port Elizabeth
Republic of South Africa*

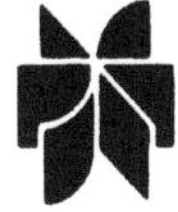

SPRINGER SCIENCE+BUSINESS MEDIA, LLC

Library of Congress Cataloging-in-Publication Data

IFIP World Computer Congress (17th : 2002 : Montréal, Québec)
Usability: gaining a competitive edge : IFIP 17th World Computer Congress—TC13 stream on usability: gaining a competitive edge, August 25-30, 2002, Montréal, Québec, Canada / edited by Judy Hammond, Tom Gross, Janet Wesson.
p. cm. — (International Federation for Information Processing ; 99)
Includes bibliographical references and index.

DOI 10.1007/978-0-387-35610-5

1. User interfaces (Computer systems)—Congresses. 2. Computer software—Development—Congresses. I. Hammond, Judy. II. Gross, Thomas, 1954– . III. Wesson, Janet. IV. Title. V. International Federation for Information Processing (Series) ; 99.

QA76.9.U83 I355 2002
005.4'37—dc21 2002073056

Printed on acid-free paper.

www.springer.com/mycopy

Contents

Frameworks for Usability

Usability: Who Cares?

Preface

Usability has become increasingly important as an essential part of the design and development of software and systems for all sectors of society, business, industry, government and education, as well as a topic of research. Today, we can safely say that, in many parts of the world, information technology and communications is or is becoming a central force in revolutionising the way that we all live and how our societies function. IFIP's mission states clearly that it "*encourages and assists in the development, exploitation and application of information technology for the benefit of all people*". The question that must be considered now is how much attention has been given to the usability of the IT-based systems that we use in our work and daily lives.

There is much evidence to indicate that the real interests and needs of people have not yet been embraced in a substantial way by IT decision-makers and when developing and implementing the IT systems that shape our lives, both as private individuals and at work. But some headway has been made. Three years ago, the IFIP Technical Committee on Human-Computer Interaction (IFIP TC13) gave the subject of usability its top priority for future work in advancing HCI within the international community. This Usability Stream of the IFIP World Computer Congress is a result of this initiative. It provides a showcase on usability involving some practical business solutions and experiences, and some research findings.

As interactive systems have become the norm and the variety of hardware and software has increased, the focus has shifted. It is no longer sufficient to just make the technology work in a functional and reliable manner. Now the usability of the technology for any given application or situation can be measured in terms of how easily, effectively and efficiently people can use it to accomplish their tasks and achieve their goals. Just as important as functionality, is whether and to what extent users of technology are satisfied with their experiences when using technology.

For many years, empirical research has provided ample evidence of numerous problems in human terms with the use of technology, that often result in people suffering from information overload, stress and other physical, mental and emotional disorders. These can no longer be ignored. New ways of design and development, incorporating usability, have been proposed and documented and many projects undertaken to explore how to improve and enhance the lives of people when using information technology and communication systems. Improving the design process and product quality benefits not only business and industry, but also the people who use the systems and products. These benefits can only be achieved today by integrating usability into the mainstream of the system development life cycle. We need to better understand the problems created by poorly designed and implemented software and systems and develop strategies and plans to incorporate usability processes, principles and guidelines into our daily practice.

This book adds to the literature on usability from both an industry and research perspective. The proceedings present contributions from practitioners and researchers from many countries that are involved in the field.

The keynote paper introduces the problems that industry faces today, and suggests usability solutions to these problems. The following sessions establish the user-centred design process as a powerful model for developing usable software. This is followed by three practically-oriented papers relating to the usability of mobile systems, and two papers on the very important subject of analysing and specifying user requirements in the early phase of the development life cycle.

Usability evaluation is often seen by practitioners as only needed once the product or system has been developed. The next papers discuss various aspects of the large topic of usability evaluation, explaining how it fits into the iterative design process within an industry and educational format.

Usability researchers have created usability frameworks, tools and techniques to assist developers. Several papers provide interesting views on large areas of concern, such as the problems that people with low vision have when viewing web sites, how to develop programming languages and environments for programmers whose home language is not English, and what to teach in usability courses at university.

Papers discussing various applications are also included in the proceedings, with a special focus on those concerned with web site design. The latter is a particularly important area for inclusion in this topic area. Web sites have a myriad of possibilities and problems associated with their development and maintenance. But it is the users of the web sites who choose to stay or revisit the site, depending upon their level of satisfaction with their experience. The final paper gives a 'reality check' for industry today, and suggests ways in which the various stakeholders in the whole organisation and development process can help to improve the level of awareness and inclusion of usability in their work.

There are many other topics to discuss in the vast area of usability. These proceedings give only a glimpse of this wealth of information, techniques, guidelines and practical experiences on the subject. International standards for usability and user-centred design, such as ISO9241 and ISO13407, are now available for people to use. Interpretation of these standards and examples of best practice are a subject for discussion at this conference and elsewhere and are very much needed. This conference and proceedings has made a start in developing IFIP TC13's interest and involvement in the area. Considerably more usability research needs to be done in providing best practice examples and experiences that will assist organisations in the years ahead.

Finally, we sincerely thank all those who have spent effort in developing their papers and making their presentations. All the papers submitted were blind reviewed by three international experts in the field and their names are recorded in this volume. The important role of the international reviewers is acknowledged, as their judgements made it possible for us to assemble papers on a range of topics and so enable the sharing of usability knowledge and research both at the conference and in the Proceedings.

With the three co-chairs of this Stream being geographically distributed, the organisation of the program was made possible by technology. Email and the World-Wide Web were employed at all stages and for most processes. We learned a lot about usability and technology during the time we worked together.

Judy Hammond, Tom Gross and Janet Wesson

Programme Chairs

Judy Hammond, University of Technology, Sydney, Australia
Tom Gross, Johannes Kepler University of Linz,, Austria
Janet Wesson, University of Port Elizabeth, South Africa

International Programme Committee

Julio Abascal, Euskal Herriko Univertsitatea, Spain
Sandrine Balbo, UK
Alan Colton, Surge Works, USA
Peter Gorny, University of Oldenburg, Germany
Darelle van Greunen, University of Port Elizabeth, South Africa
Elizabeth Grey, Brimstone Hill, Australia
Jan Gulliksen, Uppsala University, Sweden
Timo Jokela, Oulu University, Finland
Matt Jones, University of Waikato, NZ
Joaquim A Jorge, INESC, Portugal
John Karat, IBM, USA
Alistair Kilgour, UK
Paula Kotze, University of South Africa
Mary Frances Laughton, USA
Zhengjie Liu, Dalian Maritime University, China
Monique Noirhomme-Fraiture, Facultés Universitaires Notre-Dame de la Paix, Belgium
Julie Nowicki, USA
Philippe Palanque, Université Toulouse, France
Fabio Paternò, CNR, Italy
Annelise Mark Pejtersen, Riso National Laboratory, Denmark
Karen Renaud, University of Glasgow, UK
Brian Shackel, HUSAT, UK
Thomas Spyrou, University of the Aegean, Greece
Manfred Tscheligi, University of Vienna, Austria
Juergen Ziegler, Fraunhofer Institute, Germany

PART ONE

Keynote Speaker

Usability: Gaining a Competitive Edge
IFIP World Computer Congress 2002
J. Hammond, T. Gross, J. Wesson (Eds)
Published by Kluwer Academic Publishers

Deconstructing Silos:

The Business Value of Usability in the 21st Century

Gitte Lindgaard
Carleton Human Computer Interaction Institute
Carleton University
Ottawa, Ontario, Canada
gitte_lindgaard@carleton.ca

Abstract: This talk aims to show how traditional divisions of labour and responsibilities prevent businesses from adopting a customer focus, and, more importantly, the negative impact this has on their bottom line. I discuss how Human Computer Interaction (HCI) specialists can help to break down this silo structure and establish a user- or customer-centred focus. By applying HCI methods wisely, internal communication patterns can be revised to maximise the business value of a User-Centred Design (UCD) approach. Focusing first on the Systems Design & Development Process, I draw attention to certain points at which HCI can easily be integrated into the process, outlining some of the costs and the benefits an individual IT project stands to gain. Invariably, both of these sets of figures are surprisingly high. A brief discussion of the user- versus the customer experience aims to show their similarities and how they differ.

Key words: ROI, usability, task analysis, stakeholder

1. INTRODUCTION

Imagine a scenario like the following. Michael S, a 34-year old telco sales manager, has just installed a new super printer. Having tried every trick he knows, and having read all 189 pages of mostly uninterpretable instructions in the user manual, the printer still refuses to cooperate. Michael cannot get it to print. A thorough search finally leads him to the telephone number of 'Customer Support' on page 153 in the user manual, so he calls the company. Operator: "Good afternoon. This is SuperStarX. My name is Petra. Can I help you?" Customer: "Oh, excuse me, is this BestPrinter customer services?". "Yes it is, Sir. What can I do for you?". "Well, I bought a printer this morning. I have just installed it but it refuses to print." "Have you sent in the warranty card yet?" "No. I have only just unpacked the printer." "Ok, strictly speaking I am not allowed to help you until the warranty procedures have been completed, but seeing that you are on the line I will do so anyway. What version is your printer?" "Oh, I think it is called a CXP1800S or SX, but I am not sure. It doesn't say on the printer. It is a B&W laser printer. I have the user manual in front of me, though. It lists a whole range of printers, but there are no pictures, so I can't really tell." "Mmmm! what you are telling me can't be right. I will need you to turn the printer upside down and look in the far right corner. There should be a name just above the serial number."..... etc. etc. etc, until, after a 15-minute question-answer game in which the friendly operator works tirelessly and patiently to establish the source of the problem finally succeeds, saying something like "I am terribly sorry, Sir, but I can't help you with that. Yours is a technical problem. You will need to call Tech Support. Their number is 789 101 5566. Thank you for callling SuperStarX." .... Or, if the company is really customer-centred: "I am terribly sorry, Sir, but I can't help you with that. Yours is a technical problem. I will try to connect you to a Tech Support agent, but in case I lose you, their number is 789 101 5566. Thank you for calling SuperStarX. Please stay on the line while I connect you".

"So what?", I hear you think. "What has all this got to do with the IT Department?" After all, Customer Support, Help Desk, and Tech Support are not owned by the Product Development, the IT Section, the Systems Branch, or whatever the development arm is called in your company – it falls squarely under the auspices of Operations. Seen from inside a large organisation, yes, the problem of serving customers belongs to someone else. But think for a moment of yourself as wearing the customer's hat: in that role it does not matter to you who inside 'owns' 'your' problem. What does matter is that it be fixed as quickly, as effortlessly, and with as little fuss as possible. Unfortunately, companies all too often send customers on a wild goose chase from pillar to post to solve a problem that should not have occurred in the first place. Even worse, too often companies do not know (a) that this particular problem exists, (b) how frequently it occurs, (c) how much it is costing in customer service, or (d) how to extract the business value from customer feedback, including the calls customers make to the company's own help desk.

In this talk I aim to show how traditional divisions of labour and responsibilities prevent the business from adopting a customer focus, and, more importantly, the negative impact this has on its bottom line. I discuss how Human Computer Interaction (HCI) specialists can help to break down this silo structure and establish a user- or customer-centred focus. By applying HCI methods wisely, internal communication patterns can be revised to maximise the business value of a User Centred Design (UCD) approach. Focusing first on the Systems Design & Development Process, I draw attention to certain points at which HCI can and should be integrated into the process, outlining some of the costs and benefits an individual IT project stands to gain. A brief discussion of the user- versus the customer experience aims to show their similarities and how they differ. The main difference, I argue, is in the relative size of the 'experience' envelope. But first – what exactly are the problems with the above scenario?

2. INTERNAL COMMUNICATION BARRIERS: ORGANISATIONAL SILOS

In a typical organisation, a satisfactory solution to the problems in the above example could involve at least six different departments, depending on where the problem source is. Hardware designers decide where to place different kinds of information, including the name and version of the product. The ideal place is certainly not on the bottom of a product that should never be turned upside down once the print cartridge has been installed. Software designers are responsible for ensuring the correctness, completeness, and usability of the installation procedure, but Michael may have been unable to understand what to do from the information provided on the screen. Quality Assurance takes ownership of delivering fault free products, but it is possible that some aspect of the product was faulty. Technical writers own the user manual, but the instructions provided in the manual may have been unclear. At any rate, they were apparently well hidden, as indeed was the help desk telephone number. The training department ensures that help desk operators are equipped to diagnose and solve customers' problems efficiently. It is unclear whether Michael's problem was pointing to inadequate operator training or whether internal turf protection simply got in the way of providing the operator with the information necessary to solve the problem. Finally, customer services are responsible for help desk operations. It may have failed to notify the training department of the need to train operators adequately to deal with this particular problem as well as in the effective use of the telephone. If the company has developed its own help desk support system, the IT department may be responsible for providing correct and complete information for the help desk operator. Evidently, the operator's system was of little help in diagnosing, and of no help in solving the problem. The important lesson here is to note that no one department could take ownership of Michael's problem, and without ownership it is unlikely to be resolved. The customer service as a complete package could certainly do with a serious overhaul. To put it bluntly – the customer experience here sucks!

Because it is so difficult for people to communicate across the boundaries of departments in typical companies, it is unlikely that the information about Michael's inability to locate the printer name would ever get back to the hardware designers. Likewise, the inconvenience to the user of hiding the help desk telephone number towards the back of the user manual is unlikely ever to reach the technical writers. But without this feedback, how are hardware designers supposed to fix the problem or even to know what problem(s) to fix? How are technical writers expected to improve their documentation? Indeed, how is the business going to improve its products and services, and how can it possibly monitor progress without mining and integrating feedback from customers into all its business processes? Sales figures alone provide only one source of feedback, and no company can afford to release products into the market place with sales projections based on no firm data whatsoever. However, few of the data sources that ARE available and could assist in making business predictions are utilized to the full. This, I claim, is one area in which HCI experts can help.

One important factor in dysfunctional customer experiences is thus the way large organisations tend to be structured, in silos. Each department has its own turf, its well-defined responsibilities, budgets, boundaries, and accountabilities – it lives in its own silo. However, across the board, no one "owns" the customer experience as a whole in such organisations and so, no resources are devoted to tracking precisely that. Everyone owns one perspective and each of these represents a mere fraction of the total customer experience. Not surprisingly, efforts to repair it tend to amount to uncoordinated band aid treatment, with each department seeking to improve its contribution in isolation, often in a vacuum completely devoid of feedback from actual customers or from other departments. It is not a lack of organisational motivation that underlies a fractured customer experience. Each department is usually trying its very best to serve customers well from its own limited view of the world, but in the absence of a company wide coordinated customer focus the customer experience is likely to be confused and fragmented.

One major reason why companies have not yet embraced a customer-centred focus is that both the costs associated with poor, uncoordinated customer service, and the benefits that could accrue from adopting a holistic business perspective are largely invisible. However, case studies that outline costs and benefits associated with customers usually report such staggering figures that one has to admit that, as a profession, we have not yet communicated our message effectively. For example, in one case users had problems installing a printer driver, resulting in more than 50,000 calls to the help desk, the services of which amounted to roughly $500,000 per month, or a cool $6 million per year. The estimated cost of a help desk call lies between $12 and $250 (Wiklund, 1994). Translated into the printer driver problem, additional costs thus amounted to somewhere between $600,000 and $12,5 million. Apart from this cost, the manufacturer sent out letters of apology to all customers with a patch diskette costing $3 each, spending some $900,000 on fixing this simple, small problem (Donahue, 2001). In another case, the mere design and implementation of an internal documentation style guide and template in a large telecommunications company saved 50% of the documentation production costs which, at the time, amounted to roughly $140,000 per month, or $1.68 million per year. The cost of producing these tools was $40,000. The payback period was thus a mere 17 days (Lindgaard, 1995). Availability of the tools relieved the technical writers of many low level design decisions normally made for each individual document. Likewise, time-consuming negotiations with clients who owned the products for which the user manuals were being written were rendered unnecessary, saving valuable client time as well that was not included in the equation. Over time, the consistency across user manuals that the tools achieved helped to increase customer satisfaction for the business as a whole. Customers simply learned the 'geography' of the user manuals so that they knew what information to expect approximately where in any user documentation.

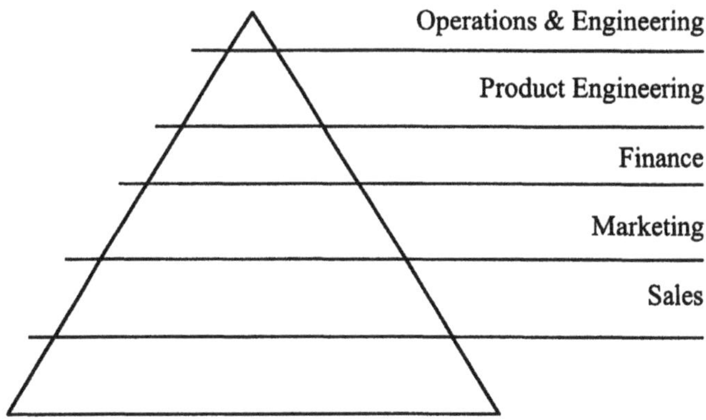

Figure 1: The spread of information in a silo-structured organisation

In order to focus on the end-to-end customer experience, we need to collect and coordinate data obtained from a variety of sources. A study just completed in our lab showed that knowledge of a high proportion of questions customers asked of the help desk personnel could benefit several departments. However, the information stayed in the help desk system, which was used to keep track of the status of problems until they had been resolved. Valuable customer feedback was thus lost to the business. For example, it is extremely useful for the CIO to know that, say, 5% of customers of a particular product have problems using a certain feature. The problem can then be resolved in the next run and avoided in all related products in the future.

It is virtually impossible to cross traditional organisational boundaries that characterise the silo model. In one part of a large case study aiming to facilitate access to large amounts of data (Fabris, 1999), the author asked 70 people to describe from whom they received documents and to whom they sent them. This information enabled him to track information flow through the company and hence to model the internal communication patterns and structure. He learned that company politics determined who gets to see what information when in the product life cycle. Secrecy was jealously guarded principally to keep competitors guessing the company's strategy. He learned that most projects followed a pattern in which the earliest stages were the most secretive. The conception and early development phases were driven by operations and engineering executives. Thereafter, product engineers would start the design. Eventually, finance, marketing, public relations and the sales departments would get involved. This way, as illustrated in Figure 1, more people became involved and saw the specifications after each milestone was reached. Access to information was contained strictly within projects so that a manager heading one project had no access to information about other ongoing projects.

Not only does this model prevent transfer of learning between concurrent projects, it also blocks learning between project teams over time as well as being a hindrance to incremental organisational learning. People do not have an opportunity to learn tips, tricks and pitfalls from each other, and errors occurring in one project are likely to raise their head in others. Consistency between products is extremely difficult to achieve under these circumstances, and it is impossible for a project to benefit from solutions developed in another. As a consequence, the proverbial wheel may well be reinvented many times over. To the customer buying, or thinking of buying, a company's products, there is little chance for transfer of learning from one generation of the product to the next, especially if the two were developed by different project teams. This is unimportant for many consumer products such as hair dryers or washing machines that perform basic and well-known functions, but it does become an issue when dealing with more complex products such as PDAs, photocopiers, or printers for that matter.

2.1 Integrating usability into systems development

In a recent paper, Rubin (2002) discusses what he calls the 'three waves of usability'. Rubin attributes the first wave to Human Factors research aiming to improve airplane cockpit design during the Second World War. Until then, knobs and dials were placed wherever they would fit in the very restricted environment without regard for the pilot, his physical and cognitive capabilities or limitations. The second usability wave, Rubin attributes to the arrival of computers, from mainframes to the later ubiquitous Personal Computer. During this second wave, Rubin argues, the objective was to improve the performance of computer users. Improvements were achieved largely through empirical testing of prototypes, an understanding of tasks and task flows, but there was no talk about the customer experience as a whole. He goes on to argue that the third usability wave focuses on the wider customer experience which expands beyond the sheer interaction between an individual user and a computer terminal to encompass the end-to-end interaction with a company.

It is true that the Internet is assuming an increasingly important role in most people's lives in the western world and that therefore, the end-to-end customer experience has risen in importance. However, Rubin's 'second usability wave' is still highly relevant to the design, development, implementation, use, and evaluation of traditional applications, many of which are developed for internal use. Furthermore, web-based Intranets and Extranets increasingly resemble the custom-tailored applications that evolved from the text-based systems - to GUI applications in the late eighties and early nineties for which we designed style guides and guidelines, and in the context of which usability evaluation methods emerged from a range of disciplines. While the application development time frames have been reduced dramatically compared with those of the mid-nineties, the need for usable and useful applications has not diminished. Quite the contrary! With increasing experience users have become much more discerning, more demanding and less tolerant of unforgiving, uncompromising and unusable applications. In the context of business-to-customer e-commerce, potential customers are likely to move on to the next company if they encounter usability problems.

Enough is known about how to achieve high levels of usability that there is no excuse for releasing cumbersome applications or web sites. Yet, according to some researchers, a sobering 65% of potential online shoppers give up before completing a transaction (Souza, 2001). At the same time, ease of use is seen as the most important element in web site design (Souza, 2001). However, a survey of Fortune 1000 companies showed that these spend an average of $1.5 million to $2.1 million per year on site redesigns without knowing whether the redesign makes the site easier to use (Kalin, 1999). One widespread misunderstanding is that usability is 'soft' and cannot be measured. Therefore, many companies set 'soft' redesign goals that tell them precisely nothing about Return Of Investment (ROI). A goal, for example, to "improve the site", "update the look and feel", or "make the site simpler" (Souza, 2001) is useless, impossible to measure, and holds nobody accountable. Without quantifiable usability and business goals there is no way of knowing if usability improvements have been achieved. It is much like saying that "a business must make a profit". HCI does have methods, processes, and metrics that are readily integrated into the systems design and development lifecycle (Lindgaard, 1994; Vredenburg et al., 2001). Let us therefore look at a number of ways that HCI can contribute to improving applications.

2.1.1 Usability in the requirements capture phase

Software engineers have long known that if the cost of fixing a problem during the requirements capture phase is one unit, this increases to 10 units if fixed during the development phase and to 100+ if coming to the fore after an application has been released (Pressman, 1992). Likewise, it is well known that 80% of service costs are spent on unforeseen user requirements that have been neglected during the design phase (Karat, 1997). Indeed, 80% of software problems only emerge once the application has been released, and of these, 80% could have been avoided if a complete User Needs Analysis (UNA) (Lindgaard, 1994) had been performed during requirements capture. In outlining a set of HCI methods and findings in the discussion below I will assume redesign of an existing application for internal use.

HCI objectives during the requirements capture phase are first to facilitate a shared and realistic vision for the application among all stakeholders. Second, task analysis facilitates a detailed understanding of the tasks users perform. Task analysis highlights problems with the task procedure and the tools, it yields a concrete basis for setting usability goals, and it helps to identify how and where improvements may be made to all of these. Knowledge gleaned from the task analysis forms the basis for designing future tasks, for shaping the future tool/application, and for predicting future task performance.

2.1.1.1 Stakeholder analysis

The objective of the stakeholder analysis is to develop a shared vision of the future application and to agree on the role it will fulfil as well as decide on the features it will contain. If marketing wants to promote certain features in the future product, IT needs to assess the technical feasibility of including those features in the planned software version, and whether it has the expertise to make firm promises given the restricted time lines and budget it works under. Finance must be involved to ensure that the cost of the features will be covered. The training department needs to assess the cost of its commitment to train users. If the product is intended for clients outside the organisation, questions such as how much training will add to the customers' expense need to be asked. How these features relate to the company's strategic plans, the life cycle of the product, and its relationship with other, similar products in its range are also issues to be discussed, as is the business goal with the product – is the company to be first to bring the product to market? Is it intended to increase market share? To enter into a new market sector? Or are the features to be provided because the competitors are bringing out the same features?

No doubt compromises will need to be made – give a little here, take a little there, but bringing all the stakeholders together to discuss and eventually agree on the business goal helps everyone to set realistic and achievable goals. The stakeholder analysis follows a structured approach with a number of questions to be answered (e.g. Maguire, 1997).

2.1.1.2 Task analysis/task projection

Deriving a detailed understanding of the users' tasks is seen by many as a waste of time because, it is argued, "we are designing for the future here - no point recreating the present". True, but what this viewpoint misses is that without knowing how, why, when, and where the present application fails to support the users' tasks, there is little chance of eliminating those stumbling blocks. Similarly, rather than redesigning the way these tasks will be performed in a vacuum, it makes sense to understand what works well and what causes problems for users.

Alternatively, it is often believed that 'someone', for example, the business analysts, systems analysts, marketing, sales personnel, or whoever already has that information at hand. Not so! The level of detail we need to improve the processes and tasks to be supported is not contained in any other document or indeed in anyone's head. If it were we would not find that 80% of problems revealed after release point to problems in the requirements capture phase. In one case, in which a task analysis was performed the sign-on procedure in an application used by several thousand people was found to be more cumbersome than necessary. The company spent $20,700 on usability work to improve it. The resulting improvement saved the company $41,700 on the first day the new procedure was used (Karat, 1990).

In a task analysis of telco customer service operators mentioned earlier my research team found that each operator spent 85 minutes per day on unnecessary activities during customer calls. Activities labeled unnecessary were those for which the information needed in the transaction should have been displayed on the screen but were not, and where the customer was put hold during the transaction to obtain the information. For example, the need to call the organisation 18 times a day to book a technician to visit a customer could have been avoided if operators had had access to the technicians' schedules. The communication bill to cover this activity alone amounted to $1.6 million per annum, not including the 34 seconds these calls took on average, involving both the operator and another person in the organisation.

Of these 85 minutes wasted per day per operator, over half could be reduced dramatically if not entirely eliminated with relatively little effort on behalf of the project team, by simply providing the needed information during the transaction. Since these figures provide valuable information that can be employed in project usability goals, it is worth discussing just one of these activities in some detail. Let me focus on one such activity occurring when connecting a new line. The operator must find and allocate a phone number. Vacant numbers were kept in a hardcopy "Vacant Number File" (VNF) floating around somewhere in the open-plan office shared by some 35 operators. The customer was put on hold while the operator located the VNF which was never in the place it was supposed to be kept; operators tended to bring it to their desk so as to cross out the number they had just selected. Once the VNF had been found, the operator would write down several numbers in her hand and race back to her desk. Next, she would try ringing the first number on her list to ensure it had not already taken, in which case she would hear a ringing tone. If the number had been taken, she would try the next on her list and so on until a vacant line could be found. At this point she would pick up the customer again, enter the number in her file and complete the transaction. Upon completion of the call, the operator was expected to locate the VNF again and cross out the number she had just allocated. Having timed several hundred calls in this category, an event diagram was produced showing the average time spent on each activity including this one in the average 12-minute call. No one knew that this or any of the many other problems revealed by the study existed in the six types of transaction these operators performed. Clearly, the solution was to present the VNF online and remove phone numbers as they were taken, a mere cut and paste operation which should take maximum 5 seconds. Even allowing a generous 10 seconds for the operator to call up the list and select a number, this still represented a saving of 4 minutes and 20 seconds per transaction (Lindgaard, 1992). With an average of six such transactions per day per operator and a total of 2,500 operators across the country earning an average of $25,000 per annum, the cost of the VNF procedure is easy to calculate:

Operator costs before redesign:

Annual salary per operator per year	$ 25,000.00
Salary per day, counting 215 working days per annum	$ 116.28
Salary per minute, counting 450 working minutes per day	$ 0.26
Salary per call @ 4 minutes 30 seconds	$ 1.16
Salary for 6 calls per day per operator	$ 6.97
Salary for 6 calls/day and 215 days per operator	$ 1,496.40
and for 2,500 operators per year	**$3,741,000.00**

Operator costs after redesign:

Salary for 10 seconds per call per operator per year	$ 55.90
and for 2,500 operators per year	**$ 139 749.89**

Savings:

Costs before redesign	$3,741,000.00
less costs after redesign	$ 139 749.89
Total savings per year	**$3,601,250.11**

Thus, merely by making the VNF available online, the company would save over $3 million per year, and this was not the only place or the only transaction in which savings could be made with comparatively little effort (Lindgaard, 1992).

The important point to note is that, in addition to the sheer dollar value for the business, figures such as these also feed directly into setting quantifiable usability goals. In this transaction and from the above data alone, our data clearly showed that 4 minutes and 20 seconds would be saved per call, or 93 hours 10 minutes per operator per year – more than two full working weeks! Even if nothing else were changed in the user interface or in the way the transaction was to be performed in the redesign, this saving was a concrete, risk-free business goal that the project team knew it could make by letting the task analysis data tell their story. The trick is, of course, to know what transactions are to be supported in the new application and what activities these involve. It is impossible and meaningless to measure everything an operator does. Therefore, the stakeholder analysis helps to focus on those tasks that will continue to be supported and in which it quickly becomes obvious that business value is to be gained relatively easily.

2.1.1.3 Shortcomings of the existing application

Ok, so task analysis data should help the analyst identify how and where in the transactions there is scope for tangible, quantifiable improvements. The application itself has, however, not been absolved yet. An HCI audit involves a thorough going over of all screens and transactions using standards and guidelines for information design as well as observing users in action to identify stumbling blocks. Information & Screen Design Standards are based on principles of human information processing, psychophysics, human memory, social norms and other human capabilities and limitations. Our research on telco operators revealed that the screen design principles employed in the application were highly problematic. When interacting with a customer on the phone, for example, operators tend to request personal details in a certain order, following the social norms of their particular culture. Upon requesting their surname, they naturally ask for a first name, then initial. Next comes the address – Street number, Street name, Suburb or Town, and so on. Our observations showed that operators invariably followed these social norms instead of the form layout on the screen. This forced them to jump all over the screen, as data belonging together were separated in what seemed a random fashion. Apart from rendering the interaction cumbersome, this also had a severe impact on the accuracy of operator performance. One in every five operations had to be repeated to locate a missing entry,which added significantly to the transaction time. However, the application refused to accept an incomplete transaction, forcing the operator to walk through up to 15 screens to find the culprit. Even so, 30% of transactions accepted by the application were later refused, causing a delay in the delivery of whatever service the customer had requested as well as providing full time work to another 35 people elsewhere in the organisation. As with the previous example, many of the problems could easily be rectified by rearranging the data entry forms in accordance with social norms and telephone manners.

Again, simply by observing how much the design blocks the interaction and by applying a model much as described above it is possible and easy to estimate the cost of these as well as the value of improvements. Likewise, these observations help to identify benchmark tasks on which to assess the magnitude of improvements in the redesign. In that sense, the field observations provide baseline data against which usability goals are set and measured in the redesign.

2.1.1.4 Usability goals, benchmark tasks, and task scenarios

Armed with analyses of the critical tasks and realistic improvement indicators to be employed in the redesign, the stakeholders can now meet again to set usability goals and select benchmark tasks. Usability goals are concrete and quantifiable, stated in business terms, and they are based on the observations made in the task analysis and application audit. Tasks that are critical for the business are likely to be known already, in which case much of the task analysis effort concentrates on collecting data that point to opportunities for improvements to these. The task analysis may reveal frequently performed, but problematic, tasks with severe stumbling blocks that should be included in the benchmarks as well.

The purpose of the stakeholder discussion at this point in the procedure is to agree on a set of realistic usability goals and the level of usability that should be attained. For example, 'connecting a new line' was a critical task. The usability goal could be expressed as "At least 95% of test users must be able to work through the transaction in less than five minutes, committing maximum one error. If an error is committed, the operator must be able to recover in a single attempt." This criterion may turn out to be too ambitious, so it is set as the 'ideal'. A lower criterion, say 90% of test users and allowing two errors and two trials to recover, may represent an 'acceptable' goal, and finally a yet lower one may determine the 'minimum acceptable' level of usability for the application to 'pass' the final usability test on this task. Because a shared vision has evolved for the product, and since the usability goals are set in accordance with business goals and based on actual data, the risk of failing to attain them is very low.

Task scenarios are stories that serve to guide both the user interface designers and usability test users by providing a conceptual hatrack. Scenarios are written for all the benchmark tasks, and users from the field help us write them to ensure face validity and that no details have been left out. A task scenario provides an end-to-end detailed walkthrough of the task. When designing the user interface, scenarios enable the designers to check that all information appears in the right place and the right time in the transaction, and in the format that best suits the particular users for whom the application is designed. In the usability test, it provides all data the user will need to perform the task.

All the facts, figures, observations, business and usability goals, scenarios, and benchmark tasks are now stored in the stakeholder report, which is signed off by the key stakeholders.

2.1.1.5 High-level user interface design

As every good software engineer knows, testing is done just before the application is shipped. Not so in HCI! Not surprisingly, this cultural difference causes a lot of irritation at times – none of us would like some smart charlies to tell us how to do our expert job, especially if they tell us to change our ways. In our HCI world, the earlier we test the emerging user interface, the more problems we can iron out before coding even begins. So, delaying tests till the end is bad, bad news for us! Therefore, as we approach the end of the UNA we design the user interface at a high level to accommodate at least the benchmark tasks. The very first user interface draft is actually a series of drafts. In this early phase the objective is to generate as many presentation ideas as possible in rapid succession and without critique. Next, we sort the wheat from the chaff, throwing out the least appealing examples and those that will not work, and we hang on to the best features of the sample just generated. Eventually, we select the design we want to take further. This draft, still in paper form, is then expanded to accommodate the benchmark tasks. Believe it or not, but testing is actually very valuable at this point, before the next version is created using standard rapid prototyping tools, even just Visual Basic or PowerPoint. This cycle of design, test, revision, test is continued until it is evident that the usability goals can be reached and the design does not overstep the boundaries of the technology to be employed. This is the point at which coding the user interface can begin.

2.1.2 The development phase

Testing continues during the development phase, according to the Test & Evaluation Plan and as modules become available. The skilled HCI specialist will have designed the tests so that data obtained in one test can be directly compared with those arising from the next. That is, the measures and the conditions under which they are collected are held constant. It is this consistency between tests that enables us to map our progress towards accomplishing the usability goals. If it turns out that even the 'minimum acceptable' usability goal cannot be accomplished for a given task, the stakeholders are called back as soon as this is obvious. The goals are then either renegotiated or more resources are devoted to the project, depending on the flexibility of the business goals.

In this phase the HCI folks coordinate their activities with the technical writers and the training people to ensure consistency throughout. Just like usability goals are set for the application proper, so goals are also set for documentation usability and for the adequacy of the evolving training program.

The implementation, or roll-out, plan is now designed, and the impact on users can be assessed more accurately. This activity is performed together with human resources, and with the Occupational Health & Safety personnel to ensure the job design is updated and acceptable to users and their union. It is also necessary to estimate the time for the system to be 'run in' and to allocate additional resources in the work place during this period. Unfortunately, it is often the case in Anglo-Saxon and Anglo-American companies that massive savings achieved with a new application in terms of staff time are translated into down-sizing the staff. Contrast that with the large Swedish insurance company that, upon streamlining its internal computer systems, entrusted the front line operators with client portfolios to ascertain how the company could save its customers money by rearranging their existing insurance, going through these one by one (Edvinsson & Malone, 1997). Rather than dismissing the people who could now have been regarded as superfluous, the company maximised the value of its human capital by adopting this pro-active procedure. Human capital is defined as the "sum total of all knowledge, experience and human performance capability on organisation processes that can be applied to create wealth" (Stolovitch & Maurice, 2001). Not only did the change in operator jobs in the Scandinavian company result in higher satisfaction levels among the staff, it also increased the business by several hundred percent in the first two years.

2.1.3 The implementation and 'in use' phase

It makes sense for HCI people to 'hang out' in the work place during implementation of the application simply because a lot can be learned about what is going well and what is amiss immediately after the system has been implemented. Special attention is paid to issues like what must be done differently next time, what can be avoided, and how the process can be handled better.

Post-implementation field studies are invaluable for collecting the kinds of data I outlined in the requirements capture phase, but field studies are unfortunately rarely performed. New projects come along, resources are scarce, life moves on. However, if performance were monitored even through regular spot checks, much time would be saved in the planning and requirements capture phase of the next version of the same or a similar application.

2.2 User experience vis à vis customer experience

For those of you who are involved in developing consumer products, web sites and the like, I hear your sighs. Yes, so far I have talked about the development of applications for internal use. However, the procedures involved in these are not so different from those in which we design for consumers. The relationship between these is shown in Figure 2.

The point of the Figure is to show how the customer experience differs from that of internal employees. Customers see the product later in its lifecycle, but employees are involved throughout the development as well.

The lower part of the Figure shows the feedback loops in a typical consumer product. During development, the main phases of which are shown in the enclosed large box, information flows between the IT and other departments in iterative cycles. The IT department as such is unlikely to be directly involved in feasibility studies, but information from these flows into it. Likewise, IT usually has little say in the product lifecycle in terms of when it is phased out. This is driven partly by the strategic business goals and partly by customers.

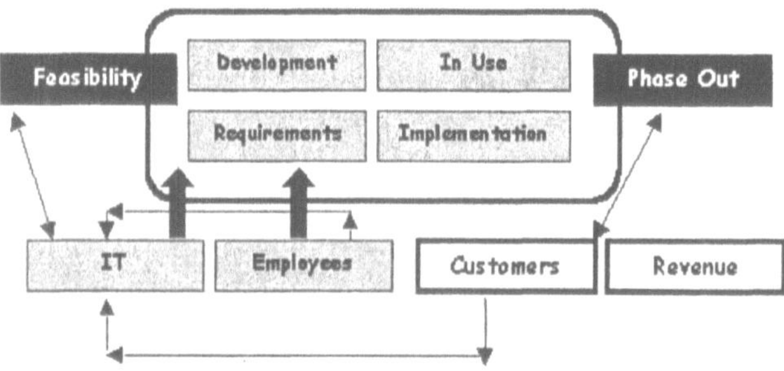

Figure 2: The relationship between IT design/development processes and the consumer business model

Employees usually have little say in whether or not a given product is purchased, developed, redeveloped or phased out, but customers must be persuaded to buy your company's products instead of selecting competitors' wares. The entire marketing and sales machinery comes into play, and issues from packaging to advertising, from usability to aesthetic appeal and your company's reputation all play a role in the success of the product. Thus, the 'customer experience' envelope is much broader than that of the internal user. Space does not allow a detailed discussion of the customer experience here. Suffice it to say that, although it offers many more opportunities for success or failure than the internal product or application, the role of the latter should not be disregarded. Flaws in the tools, tasks, or in the environment in which employees work can be extremely costly in both human and ROI terms. By focusing on users, HCI offers methods, tools and techniques that can improve both substantially.

2.3 The cost of usability

Oh, I hear you say, but all this usability stuff delays our development schedules. HCI folks impose a lot more work on us, this soft fluff is impossible to incorporate into our development methodology, and they cost a lot of money too. No, no, and no! Earlier I alluded with a glimpse to just one example of the benefits a thorough UNA can bring. In that same study, the total cost to the business of the various flaws to the system, its procedures, and the impact on work processes around the business amounted to an annual loss of $30 million. The substantiating data showed clearly that nearly half of this loss could be avoided before the application was even touched (Lindgaard, 1995). The HCI costs of this comprehensive ergonomic review were $90,000. The user-centred approach takes into consideration the wider business context rather than focusing exclusively on the application. Yet, it benefits both. It is estimated that the return for every dollar invested in usability is somewhere between $10 and $100 and that a lack of usability input to the design translates into 80% of service costs on unforeseen user requirements further down the line (IBM, 2001). Evidence supporting these figures is mounting in the literature.

2.4 Silo replacements

The model shown in Figure 2 suggests that information is flowing freely between 'employees', a group that amorphously includes everyone in the organisation, and the IT department. Unfortunately, that is usually not the case – companies are still predominantly organised into silos. The biggest hindrance for a business to become truly customer centred is this traditional parallel positioning of people who will never know how much they have in common or how much sharing information could benefit their jobs and the business as a whole. Our reward structures are designed to reward individuals for contributions that amount to fragments of the customer experience rather than rewarding whole teams who take collective responsibility for the success of the company's products and the end-to-end customer experience. Breaking down these barriers to free up communication lines and allowing people access to information that focuses on the higher level business goals while keeping an eye on the details is the only way business can evolve into becoming user and customer-centred. This paper is an attempt to demonstrate how HCI folks can help achieve this goal.

3. REFERENCES

Donahue, G.M. (2001). Usability and the Bottom Line, *IEEE Software*, January/February.

Edvinsson, L. & Malone, M.S. (1997). *Intellectual capital: Realizing your company's true value by finding its hidden brain power*, HarperBusiness, New York, N.Y.

Fabris, P. (1999). You think tomaytoes I think tomahtoes, *WebBusiness Magazine*, April 1.

http://www.cio.com/archive/webbusiness/040199/_nort.html

IBM (2001). Cost justifying ease of use: Complex solutions are problems. http://www.3ibm.co/ibm/easy/eou_ext.nsf/Publish/23

Kalin, S. (1999). Mazed and confused, *WebBusiness Magazine*, April 1. http://www.cio.com/archive/webbusiness/040199/_use.html

Karat, C.M. (1997). cost-justifying usability engineering in the software life cycle, in T. Landauer & P. Prabhu (Eds), *Handbook of Human-Computer Interaction*, Elsevier Science, Amsterdam.

Karat, C.M. (1990). Cost-benefit analysis of usability engineering techniques, *Proceedings of the Human Factors Society 34th. Annual Meeting*, Volume 2, Orlando.

Lindgaard, G. (1992). Evaluating user interfaces in context: The ecological value of time-and-motion studies, *Applied Ergonomics*, 23, (2),105-114.

Lindgaard, G. (1994). *Usability testing and system evaluation: A guide for designing useful computer systems*, Chapman & Hall, London.

Lindgaard, G. (1995). Cementing human factors into product design: Moving beyond policies, *Proc. 15th. International Symposium on Human Factors in Telecommunications*, Melbourne, 361-371.

Maguire, M. (1997). *RESPECT: User Requirements Framework Handbook*, HUSAT Research Institute.

Pressman, R. S. (1992). *Software Engineering:A Practitioner's Approach*, McGraw Hill, New York.

Rubin, J. (2002). What business are you in? The strategic role of usability professionals in the "New Economy" world, *User Experience*, Winter, 4-11.

Souza, R. (2001). Get ROI from design, *The Forrester Report*, June. Available from http://www.forrester.com

Stolovitch, H.D. & Maurice, J.-G.(2001). Calculating your ROI: *Calculating Return On Investment in human performance interventions and the increased value of human capital*, http://www.creativityatwork.com

Vredenburg, K., Isensee, S., Righi, C., (2001). *User-Centered Design: an Integrated Appraoch*, Prentice Hall PTR, Upper Saddle River, NJ.

Wiklund, M.E.,(1994). *Usability In Practice: How Companies Develop User-Friendly Products*, Academic Press, Boston.

PART TWO

Technical Sessions

Usability: Gaining a Competitive Edge
IFIP World Computer Congress 2002
J. Hammond, T. Gross, J. Wesson (Eds)
Published by Kluwer Academic Publishers

A Method-Independent Process Model of User-Centred Design

Timo Jokela
University of Oulu, Finland

Abstract: We propose a method-independent process model of user-centred design (UCD). It is based on recognised sources and its structure was developed in a set of assessments in industrial settings. The result is a process model that identifies six main processes of UCD. Each of these is defined through a set of outcomes. The model makes tangible the interface between the usability engineering and design processes. The model has provided a practical basis for the assessment of UCD processes, which was the original scope of the model. In addition, we have found the model as a useful asset in training UCD and in planning UCD activities in projects.

Key words: user-centred design, UCD, usability methods, usability engineering, process model, assessments, training

1. INTRODUCTION

We propose a method-independent process model of user-centred design (UCD). The background of the model is in the assessment of UCD processes where a process model is a key asset. We also have found the model effective in other uses, such as training and project planning.

The purpose of an assessment is to identify the strengths and weaknesses of UCD in a product or software development organisation, for the purpose of providing a basis for process improvement. During an assessment, the existing UCD practices of a development organisation are mapped against a process model of UCD. The process model should represent an ideal UCD process. It also should be method-independent: it should state 'what', not 'how'. For example, a process model may state that 'current user tasks should be analysed' but should not insist a specific method (e.g. 'contextual inquiry') to be used for that. The assessment result is typically a quantitative statement about the extent to which the development practices meet the requirements of a process model.

There exist a number of methods for the assessment of UCD processes. During the 1990's, methods such as Trillium (Coallier et al., 1994), IBM (Flanagan, 1995), Philips (Taylor et al., 1998), and INUSE (Earthy, 1998), (Earthy, 1997) were proposed. The most recent developments are ISO 18529 (ISO/IEC, 2000) and Human-System Life Cycle Processes (ISO/IEC, 2001).

We carried out a set of assessments of UCD processes. We used ISO (International Organization for Standardization) 18529 as a hypothesis process model. Throughout the experiments, we tried to understand what kind of process model makes sense and is effective. For that, we gathered data about how the development staff perceived the models presented using questionnaires and interviews. In addition, each member of the assessment team made observations, which were shared and discussed jointly in sessions after the assessments. Step by step, the structure of the UCD process model evolved. The scope of this paper is to describe the evolvement and the main features of the model. Also the assessment approach as a whole changed to a one that we call *KESSU*, as described in Jokela et al. (2001).

In the next section, we justify the selection of our hypothesis model and our experiments with it. Thereafter, we describe how the process model evolved during the subsequent experiments. We then describe the new process model, and finally in the last section summarise the results and examine limitations, implications and further research topic.

2. THE EXPERIMENTS WITH THE HYPOTHESIS MODEL

UCD principles, activities and methods are described in many books. The main reference is the book *Usability Engineering* by Nielsen (Nielsen, 1993). Later books have been published, such as *Developing User Interfaces: Ensuring Usability Through Product & Process* (Hix and Hartson, 1993), *Contextual Design* by (Beyer and Holtzblatt, 1998), *The UCD Lifecycle* (Mayhew, 1999), *Software for Use* (Constantine and Lockwood, 1999). All of these describe well the UCD processes. They, however, are all more or less method-oriented (at least partially they propose 'how-to-do' rather than 'what-to-do'), and thereby cannot be used as reference models in assessments.

We regard ISO 13407, *Human-Centred Design Processes for Interactive Systems*, (ISO/IEC, 1999) as an appropriate general reference model of UCD. It contains the core substance of UCD in a concise and understandable way. The four key UCD activities (processes) of ISO 13407 are illustrated in Figure 1. The processes are described in an informal way, with 1 to 2 pages of text for each process. The processes can be briefly described as follows:

- *Understand and Specify Context of Use.* Know the user, the environment of use, and for what tasks he or she uses the product.
- *Specify the User and Organisational Requirements.* Determine the success criteria of usability for the product in terms of user tasks, e.g. how quickly a typical user should be able to complete a task with the product. Determine the design guidelines and constraints.
- *Produce Design Solutions.* Develop design solutions incorporating HCI (human-computer interaction) knowledge, including visual design, interaction design, and usability.
- *Evaluate Designs against Requirements.* The usability of designs is evaluated against requirements.

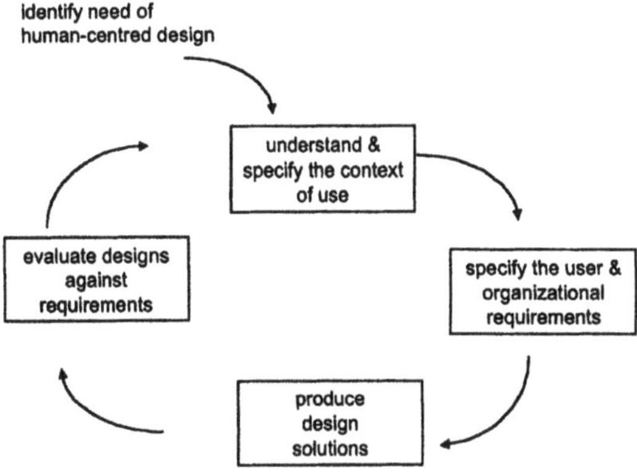

Figure 1. Processes of UCD as defined in ISO 13407

2.1 ISO 18529 - Human-Centred Lifecycle Process Descriptions

A subsequent activity following on from ISO 13407 was the creation of ISO 18529 (ISO/IEC, 2000), which defines the processes more precisely than does ISO 13407. The objective was to meet the formality of process definitions required by the process assessment standard ISO 15504 (ISO/IEC, 1998). ISO 18529 identifies the same core processes of UCD, as does ISO 13407, Figure 1. One can say that the essential substance in these two sources is the same – the difference is in the format of presentation.

Our rather natural selection for the hypothesis model for the assessments was ISO 18529. It is developed for assessment purposes, and its background is in a recognised UCD standard.

In ISO 18529, each process is defined with a *purpose statement* and a set of *base practices*. The purpose of the process is 'typically achieved' by implementing the base practices. Assessments are normally carried out through analysing the extent to which the base practices are implemented. The purpose statement is 2 to 3 lines of text, and a list of outcomes. The number of base practices per process varies between 5 and 8. For example, the process *Specify The User and Organisational Requirements* is defined as follows:

"The purpose of the process is to establish the requirements of the organisation and other interested parties for the system. This process takes full account of the needs, competencies and working environment of each relevant stakeholder in the system. As a result of successful implementation of the process, the following will be defined:

- Required performance of new system against operational and functional objectives
- Relevant statutory or legislative requirements
- Co-operation and communication between users and other relevant parties
- The users' jobs (including the allocation of tasks, users' comfort, safety, health and motivation)
- Task performance of the user when supported by the system
- Work design, and organisational practices and structure
- Feasibility of operation and maintenance
- Objectives for the operation and/or use of the software and hardware components of the system.

The purpose is typically achieved by the performance of the following practices:

- Clarify and document system goals
- Analyse stakeholders
- Assess risk to stakeholders
- Define the use of the system
- Generate the stakeholder and organisational requirements
- Set quality in use objectives."

The definitions of base practices include some further notes. The other three processes are defined in an analogous way.

2.2 The experiments with ISO 18529

We used the ISO 18529 model as the process reference model in the first two assessments. In the first assessment the customer representatives - most of whom were neither usability nor process assessment professionals - encountered difficulties in understanding the process model. For example, the usability specialist for the company reported afterwards in an interview "the model was not understood here". Some of the staff had a perception that the assessment was "academic stuff driven by the interests of the university". In addition, the assessment team found it difficult to agree on the ratings of the capability of the processes. Specifically, it was difficult to determine whether the base practices (see the example in the previous section) were truly performed or not.

Our conclusion from the assessment was that the basic process structure of ISO 18529 seems to make sense to people but we need more precise and unambiguous interpretations of the process definitions. This was rather a surprise: ISO 18529 was chosen as our hypothesis model because its definitions are formalised.

Even if we met some problems with ISO 18529, the reference model was the same for the second assessment in another company. In the latter case, the main reason for this was that the lead assessor was from a different organisation. The feedback from this assessment indicated similar problems as we had in the previous assessment. The staff perceived the models of the assessment difficult to understand, and the results not concrete enough. Another problem was – again - in the interpretation of the process definitions. The interpretations caused even more disputes within the assessment team than in the earlier case because now there were members from two organisations in the team.

An example will illustrate our interpretation problem. The process *Specify The User and Organisational Requirements* (see previous section) has a base practice 'Analyse stakeholders'. In an assessment, one should determine the extent to which this base practice is performed using the scale 'none, partially, largely, fully'. First, we found it difficult to determine what kind of activities the 'analysis of stakeholders' should incorporate. A second problem was related to the quality of performing a practice: what does it mean if a practice is performed but in an inappropriate way? A third problem was in the exploitation of the results of a practice: what does it mean if a practice is performed but its results are ignored in the development process?

Our main conclusion from these experiments was that we need to have a precise and understandable interpretation of ISO 18529 for the following assessment.

3. ITERATION STEPS

We distinguish two major steps in the evolvement of the process model. In the first step, we changed the way of defining processes and split the 'Produce design solutions' process into two separate processes. In the second one, we added one new process and did some changes to the contents of processes.

3.1 The first iteration step

We decided to try a modified process model in the third assessment. It had two different characteristics compared with ISO 18529: (1) definition of processes through outcomes, and (2) structuring the UCD activities into five processes (rather than four).

(1) We decided to define the processes through concrete *outcomes* of processes. In the previous assessments, we had problems with the interpretation of the base practices. We first tried to create 'unambiguous interpretations' of those practices but found it difficult. Therefore we decided to try an alternative approach: defining processes through outcomes. In contrast with the outcome definitions of processes in ISO 18529 (the purpose definitions contain also outcomes, see the example in the last section), we limited the outcomes to *concrete deliverables*.

For example, we defined the process *Specify The User and Organisational Requirements* with two outcomes: *Usability Requirements*, and *UI Design Requirements*, *Figure 2* (compare with the definition shown in the previous section). We also gave a simpler name to the process: *User Requirements*. We worked analogously with other processes, and identified the relevant outcomes of each of the processes.

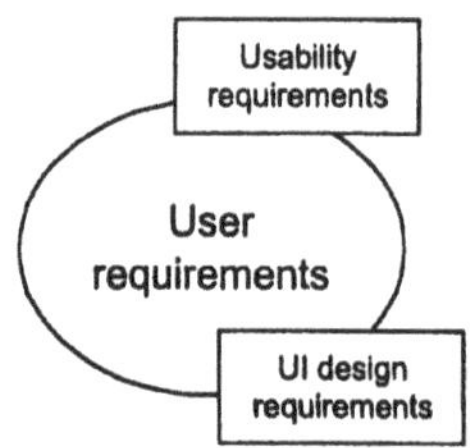

Figure 2. Illustrating the outcomes: User requirements process

(2) We split the *Produce Design Solutions* process into two processes. We found this solution sensible because we find two different scopes in

design: user task design, and user interaction design. These two scopes are significantly different from the viewpoint of UCD. User task design is a characteristic activity of UCD while user interaction design is always performed as user-interface elements are developed – even if there is no user-centredness in the development process. In summary, we now had five main processes: *Context of Use* process, *User Requirements* process, *User Tasks Design* process, *Produce User Interaction Designs* process, and *Usability Evaluation* process. The processes with outcomes are illustrated in *Figure 3*.

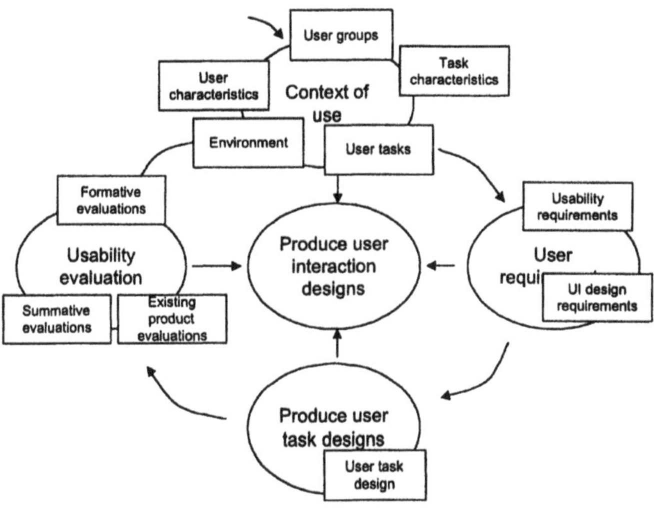

Figure 3. The modified UCD process model: the first iteration

We got better responses from this model than from the one we used earlier. One project manager stated immediately after an assessment workshop that she "already started to challenge herself on how to implement improvements in user requirements". The development staff reported that the revised UCD process model made a lot of sense: "The process model pointed out many issues to consider in the following projects"; "Now we know that task analysis is important. We also need to work on usability requirements". The usability specialists of the company received the process model as a useful reference on how UCD processes should be developed.

All those members of the assessment team who had attended the previous assessments found this assessment more successful and sensible than the earlier ones. One illustrative comment from an assistant assessor was, "Interview by interview, the model became clearer. This is the way we should have done from the beginning: to make a clear interpretation of our own about the process models".

Our clear feeling after the assessment was that we wanted to try this kind of process model again.

3.2 The second iteration step

In the next assessment, we found that the process model generally worked well but not in all respects. We faced challenges especially with the *Context of Use* (CoU) process. The product that was under development is a new product type. Our earlier interpretation of the CoU process was 'to know the user and his/her work and work environment as it is now'. In this case, however, the environment where the new product is used is partly very different from the earlier environment: a mobile environment ('anywhere') instead of office or home environment. A new product also means some new user tasks.

Our conclusion was that one should discuss separately the outcomes related to the user tasks already in use and user tasks of the future (with the new product that is to be developed). Our solution was to define two different parts: *Context of Use of Old System*, and *Context of Use of Future System* in the CoU process, *Figure 4*.

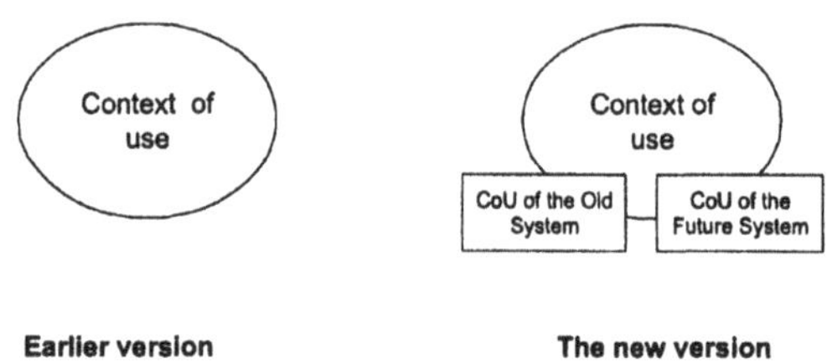

Figure 4. Changes in the Context of Use process

Another challenge during the assessment was that we wanted to elegantly describe and rate a situation where the product under development obviously has several user groups but the project team has identified and analysed only one user group. Our solution was to split the *Context of Use* process into two processes: *Identification of User Groups* and *Context of Use of User Group 'N'*. We found that with this kind of structure we were able to explain the situation more concretely and elegantly.

Another refinement of the model was about the *Usability Evaluation* process. We removed the sub-process *Existing Products Evaluation*. The reason was that we started to consider this activity as a *method* that actually should belong to the User requirements process: existing products are evaluated in order to know where to set the usability goals with the future product. Because our goal was a method-independent model, we removed this activity.

As a result, we identified a total of six processes of UCD as illustrated in Figure 5. One should note that *Context of Use* process has more than one instance, one for each user group.

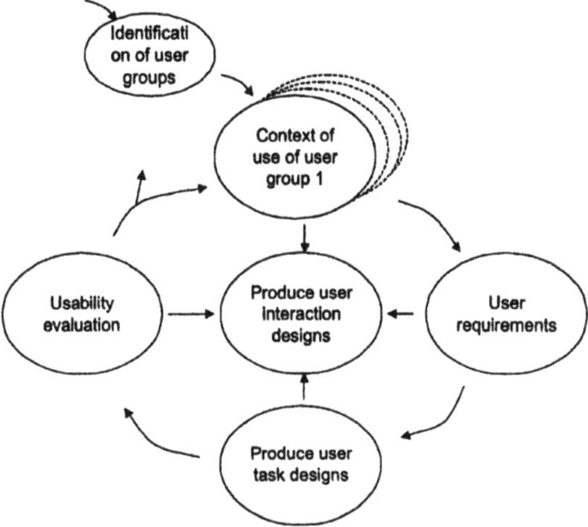

Figure 5. The six processes of UCD after the second step

4. THE PROPOSED PROCESS MODEL

After the experiments described above, we have a UCD process model of six processes. In the following, we give the definitions of each of the processes. The model is illustrated in *Figure 6.*

4.1 Process: Identification of User Groups

The purpose of the Identification of User Groups process is to identify the different user groups: who are potential users of the product or system. The substance of this process is not explicitly included in ISO 13407 or ISO 18529.

The outcomes of the process are:

- *User Groups Definitions*. The intended user groups of the system are identified. Typically a characteristic name is given to each user group, and the sizes (how many users) of the groups are also determined.

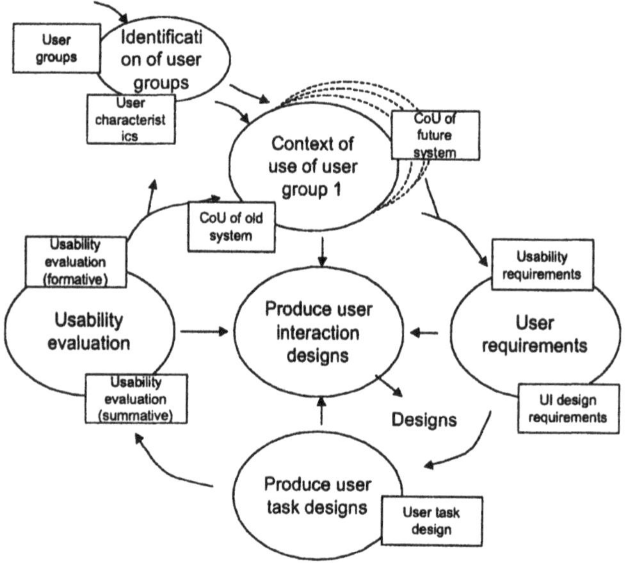

Figure 6. Outcomes of the latest version of the process model

- *User Characteristics*: The characteristics of the users of the user group are documented. These may include knowledge, language, physical capabilities, anthropometrics, psychosocial issues, motivations in using the system, priorities, etc.

4.2 Process: Context of Use of User Group 'N'

The purpose of the Context of Use of User Group 'N' process is to identify the characteristics of the users, their tasks and the technical, organisational and the physical environment in which the product system will operate.

A new product or system will always replace an existing one. The existing product may be close to the new one, e.g. a new version of a product will replace an old one. The new product may also be very different from the old one. For example, a fixed location application may be replaced with a mobile one.

This process needs to have an instance for each user group identified by the *Identification of Users Groups* process.

The outcomes of the process are:

- *Context of Use of the Old System:* The context of use of the old system is about describing the use of the existing system as relevant for designing the new one. The outcome has the following parts:

a) The user accomplishments related to the old product are identified and documented. The accomplishments should be described in terms of user and organisational activities, not in terms of equipment functions or features of the product

b) The user tasks that users perform to achieve the accomplishments are described and documented.

c) The real operational environment of the product, including the factors that affect the performance of users, is described.

d) The non-functional attributes of tasks should be identified and documented. The attributes may be for example: frequency, duration of performance, criticality for errors, identification of problems and risks that users meet when performing their tasks.

- *Context of Use of the Future System:* The context of use of the future system is about describing the context of use of the product under development. It is described to the extent that the context of use is different contrasted with current context of use. The outcome has the following parts:

a) The user accomplishments related to the product are identified and documented. Especially the differences compared with the existing context of use are identified.

b) The real operational environment of the product, including the factors that affect the performance of users, is described.

c) The non-functional attributes of tasks should be identified and documented. The attributes may be for example: frequency, duration of performance, criticality for errors, identification of problems and risks that users meet when performing their tasks.

NOTE. This sub-process is essential for systems that are 'totally' new.

4.3 Process: User Requirements

The purpose of the user requirements process is to define usability and user interface design requirements for the product. The main input for this process is the context of use information and business goals of the project. While business goals should drive all the processes of the UCD capability area, they especially should drive the user requirements process.

One should understand that usability requirements may contradict with other requirements. Resolution between conflicting requirements should be performed in this process.

The outcomes of the process are:

- *Usability Requirements:* The usability requirements are determined and documented. With usability requirements, we mean the required performance of the product *against the context of use.* Usability requirements typically are given in terms of effectiveness, efficiency, and satisfaction in the specific context of use (ISO/IEC, 1999).

NOTE. The requirements should integrate requirements of things that have impact on the total user-experience: not software only but also user documentation, user training, and in packaging the product.

- *UI Design Requirements:* The guidelines and restrictions that should be considered when the UI is designed should be identified and documented. Typically these include general user interface design heuristics, style guides, or company or project standards.

4.4 Process: User Task Design

The purpose of the user task design process is to design how users would carry out their tasks with the new product being developed.

This is the design phase where 'the work of the users' is designed: what are the accomplishments that their product will support, and what are the scenarios of steps for how these accomplishments are to be reached. This phase is not yet design of user interface elements.

The outcomes of the process are:

- *User Task Descriptions:* The tasks relating to how a user plans to use the product to achieve the goals are described and documented. The tasks should also be designed in relation to such tasks as user documentation and user training,

NOTE. Special emphasis should be paid to the tasks on which explicit requirements are set in the User requirements process.

4.5 Process: Produce User Interaction Designs

The purpose of the produce user interaction design process is to design those elements of the product that users interact with. These elements include interaction and graphical design of user interfaces, user documentation, user training and user support.

This process has a specific role among all the processes: this process produces the concrete designs while all other processes have a supporting role. Another specific feature of this process is that the different outcomes should be produced in parallel. People from different departments (user interface development, user documentation, customer training) typically work together.

The outcomes of the process are:

- *User Interface:* The user interface (interactions, visual design) is produced.
- *User Documentation:* The user documentation is produced.
- *User Training:* The user training material and concepts are produced.
- *Other relevant outputs:* Other relevant outputs are generated, for example packaging, user support procedures etc.

4.6 Process: Usability Evaluation

The purpose of this process is to evaluate the product (including user documentation, user training etc.) against the requirements in terms of the context of use.

This process addresses on usability only from the task performance aspect. Those activities that evaluate the generic, non-task driven issues (for example, heuristic evaluations, or adherence to style guides etc.) are activities relating to the produce user interaction solutions process.

The outcomes of the process are:

- *Formative Usability Evaluation Results:* The purpose of the Formative usability evaluation process is to collect qualitative feedback on the usability of the product under development.

NOTE. The outcome of this process is typically an iterative set of evaluation results. The outcome is extensively produced if the designs are evaluated against all major user tasks.

- *Summative Usability Evaluation Results:* The purpose of the Summative usability evaluation process is to evaluate to what extent the product meets the defined usability requirements. The outcome of this process is typically an evaluation result report. The outcome is extensively produced if the designs are evaluated against all major user tasks defined in by the user requirements process.

5. SUMMARISING THE RESULTS

Our target was to create a method-independent process model that clearly describes the essentials of UCD. We started with a recognised model, and ended up with a structure that contains six UCD processes and definition of the processes through outcomes.

The model makes clear the integration challenge between usability processes and the design processes. Product designs are produced by visual, software and hardware designers. Others but usability specialists typically produce interaction designs. The challenge of usability specialists is to integrate their work to the central process carried out by the designers. As widely recognised, this is a true challenge in many cases.

The model does not require the use of any specific methods. However, in order to produce valid outcomes, one should use valid methods in a professional way. Therefore, it is in an assessment one should examine not only whether outcomes are produced but also the validity of the methods used. This is done by the professional judgement of the assessors.

Although our main use for the process model has been the assessments, we have identified other uses for it, too. When communicating the assessment model and results to the development staff, our observation has been that the model seems to be an effective asset in training the essence of UCD. Feedback from the experiments indicate that focusing on 'what needs to be produced' rather than on methods seems to communicate well (especially in assessment situations where the past practice of the staff is mapped against the model). We have seen that many practitioners have learned UCD only through methods. People have reported that discussing UCD without methods has 'opened their eyes'.

The model also seems to be a useful teamwork asset when planning UCD activities for a development project. At the first stage, one discusses at the level of outcomes: what usability deliverables are essential, and where to put efforts. This discussion can be carried out together with development staff. The method issues (how the outcomes are produced) are a separate issue that is discussed later within the usability group.

6. DISCUSSION AND CONCLUSIONS

We propose a method-independent process model of UCD. It is based on recognised sources and its structure was developed in a set of assessments in industrial settings. The result is a process model that identifies six main processes of UCD. Each of these is defined through a set of outcomes. The model makes tangible the interface between usability engineering and design processes. The model has provided a practical basis for the assessment of UCD processes, which was the original scope of the model. In addition, we have found the model as a useful asset in training UCD and in planning UCD activities in projects.

One should understand that the model has evolved from one experiment to another, and is still subject to refinements. Our goal is to have a communicative and elegant model. New experiments and situations may reveal need for further refinements.

While the key thing in the model is its structure, we have been forced to make some interpretations of the substance of UCD. It may well be that all do not agree with us about all those interpretations.

We want to emphasise that the process model is a complementary one to our starting point, ISO 13407 and ISO 18529. If formal process assessment is desired, it is important that the process model is a recognised and widely approved one, such as ISO 18529.

This kind of process model could possibly be used for other purposes, too. The research focus in UCD methods is still generally usability evaluation method focused. A process model like these may help identifying other areas where new effective methods are required. For example, our experience is that definition of usability requirements is perceived difficult. New methods in this area are required.

In our future research, we will carry out further experiments where we plan and implement improvements in UCD together with our partner companies. In these different efforts – whether they are assessments, training, or planning and implementation of usability activities – we will further evaluate the model and make refinements as needed.

7. REFERENCES

Beyer, H. and Holtzblatt, K. (1998), *Contextual Design: Defining Customer-Centered Systems,* Morgan Kaufmann Publishers, San Francisco.

Coallier, F., McKenzie, R., Wilson, J. and Hatz, J. (1994), *Trillium Model for Telecom Product Development & Support Process Capability*, Release 3.0. Internet edition, Bell Canada.

Constantine, L. L. and Lockwood, L. A. D. (1999), *Software for Use,* Addison-Wesley, New York.

Earthy, J. (1997), *Usability Maturity Model: Processes. INUSE/D5.1.4(p), EC INUSE (IE 2016) final deliverable (version 0.2),* Lloyd's Register, London.

Earthy, J. (1998), *Usability Maturity Model: Human Centredness Scale. INUSE Project deliverable D5.1.4(s). Version 1.2.,* Lloyd's Register of Shipping, London.

Flanagan, G. A. (1995), Usability Leadership Maturity Model (Self-assessment Version). Delivered in a Special Interest Group session, In *CHI '95: Human Factors in Computing Systems* (Eds, Katz, I., Mack, R., Marks, L., Rosson, M. B. and Nielsen, J.) Denver, USA.

Hix and Hartson (1993), *Developing User Interfaces: Ensuring Usability Through Product & Process,* John Wiley & Sons.

ISO/IEC (1998), *15504-2 Software Process Assessment - Part 2: A reference model for processes and process capability,* ISO/IEC TR 15504-2: 1998 (E).

ISO/IEC (1999), *13407 Human-Centred Design Processes for Interactive Systems,* ISO/IEC 13407: 1999 (E).

ISO/IEC (2000), *18529 Human-centred Lifecycle Process Descriptions,* ISO/IEC TR 18529: 2000 (E).

ISO/IEC (2001), *Ergonomics - Human system interface - Human-system life cycle processes,* ISO/IEC TC 159 / SC 4 / WG 6. Version 1.0, committee draft: HSL-Og (E).

Jokela, T., Iivari, N., Nieminen, M. and Nevakivi, K. (2001), Developing A Usability Capability Assessment Approach through Experiments in Industrial Settings, In *Joint Proceedings of HCI 2001 and IHM 2001* (Eds, Blandford, A., Vanderdonckt, J. and Gray, P.) Springer, London, pp. 193-209.

Mayhew, D. J. (1999), *The Usability Engineering Lifecycle,* Morgan Kaufman, San Francisco.

Nielsen, J. (1993), *Usability Engineering,* Academic Press, Inc., San Diego.

Taylor, B., Gupta, A., Hefley, W., McLelland, I. and Van Gelderen, T. (1998) ,HumanWare Process Improvement - institutionalising the principles of UCD, In Tutorial PM14 H Human-centred processes and their impact, In *Human-Computer Interaction Conference on People and Computers XIII,* Sheffield, Hallam University, England.

Usability: Gaining a Competitive Edge
IFIP World Computer Congress 2002
J. Hammond, T. Gross, J. Wesson (Eds)
Published by Kluwer Academic Publishers

Use and Reuse of HCI Knowledge in the Software Development Lifecycle

Existing Approaches and what Developers Think

Eduard Metzker[1] and Harald Reiterer[2]

[1] DaimlerChrysler Research and Technology Centre, Software Technology Lab, HCI Research Group, P.O.Box 2360, D-89011 Ulm, Germany, eduard.metzker@daimlerchrysler.com, [2] University of Konstanz, Department of Computer and Information Science, P.O.Box D 73, D 78457 Konstanz, Germany, harald.reiterer@uni-konstanz.de

Abstract: In this paper we give an overview of existing approaches for capturing HCD(Human-Centred Design) process and design knowledge. We present an alternative approach that aims at fostering the integration of UE (Usability Engineering) activities and artifacts into existing software development processes. The approach is based on six claims that are derived from an analysis of existing UE process models and requirements of software developers. Our approach is embeddable in existing process improvement frameworks such as the UMM (Usability Maturity Model) and is supported by a web-based tool. An explorative study that we have conducted with software developers from various software development organizations confirms the potential of our approach. However the study indicates that our approach is more strongly preferred by developers with experience in user interface design.

Key words: usability maturity, process improvement, human-centred design methods, computer-aided usability engineering environment

1. INTRODUCTION

The relevance of usability as a quality factor is continually increasing for software engineering organizations: usability and user acceptance are about to become the ultimate measurement for the quality of today's telematics applications, e-commerce web sites, mobile services and tomorrow's proactive assistance technology. Taking these circumstances into account, human-centered design (HCD) methods for developing interactive systems are changing from a last minute add-on to a crucial part of the software engineering lifecycle.

It is well accepted both among software practitioners and in the human-computer interaction research community that structured approaches are required to build interactive systems with high usability. On the other hand specific knowledge about exactly how to most efficiently and smoothly integrate HCD methods into established software development processes is still missing (Mayhew, 1999). While approaches such as the usability maturity model (UMM) (Earthy, 1999) provide means to assess an organization's capability to perform HCD processes they lack guidance on how to actually implement process improvement in HCD. It often remains unclear to users of HCD methods if and why certain tools and methods are better suited in a certain development context than others (Welie, 1999). We need strategies and tools that support engineering organizations in evolving and selecting an optimal set of HCD methods for a given development context and perform systematic process improvement in HCD. Little research has been done on integrating methods and tools of HCD in the development process and on gathering knowledge about HCD activities in a form that can capture relationships between specific development contexts, applicable methods and tools and their impact on the engineering process (Henninger, 2000).

2. EXISTING HCD PROCESS MODELS: THEORY AND PRACTICE

A review of existing literature and case studies of some of the HCD approaches most applied revealed a number of organizational obstacles encountered in establishing HCD methods in mainstream software development processes (Metzker and Offergeld, 2001a). We summarized these problems in the following three claims.

Claim 1 *Existing HCD process models are decoupled from the overall software development process.*

One common concern relating to HCD approaches is that they are regarded by software project managers as being somehow decoupled from the software development process practiced by the development teams. It appears to project managers that they have to control two separate processes: the overall system development process and the HCD process for the interactive components. As it remains unclear how to integrate and manage both perspectives, the HCD activities have often been regarded as dispensable and have been skipped in case of tight schedules (Mayhew, 1999).

Claim 2 *Most of the HCD approaches do not cover a strategy of how to perform HCD methods and process models depending on the usability maturity of the software development organization.*

Most approaches assume that the usability maturity of the development organization is high.

One typical assumption is that experienced human factors specialists are available throughout the development team and therefore HCD methods can be performed ad hoc. However, recent research shows that even highly interactive systems are often developed without the help of in-house human factors specialists or external usability consultants (Metzker and Offergeld, 2001b). Therefore HCD methods often can not be utilized because the necessary knowledge is not available within the development teams (Earthy, 1999, Mayhew, 1999).

Another point that is also ignored by the approaches described is that development organizations with a low usability maturity are often overwhelmed by the sheer complexity of the proposed HCD process models. The models lack a defined procedure for tailoring the development process and methods for specific project constraints such as system domain, team size, experience of the development team or the system development process already practiced by the organization.

Claim 3 *Integrating Usability Engineering (UE) Methods into mainstream software development process must be understood as an organisational learning task..*

Almost all approaches do not account for the fact that turning technology-centered development processes into human-centered development processes must be seen as a continuous process improvement task (Norman, 1998). A strategy for supporting a long-lasting establishment of HCD knowledge, methods, and tools within development organizations is still missing. A model is needed that guides the introduction, establishment and continuous improvement of UE methods in mainstream software development processes.

To learn more about the way that HCD methods are actually used in software development organizations we conducted a study with software developers who are working on the design of interactive systems in a variety of domains (DaimlerChrysler Aerospace (DASA) Ulm, Sony Fellbach,

Grundig Fuerth and DaimlerChrysler Sindelfingen. All sites are located in Germany.) (Metzker and Offergeld, 2001b). The study revealed that the organizations examined are practicing highly diverse individual development processes. However none of the UE development models proposed by (Mayhew, 1999, Nielsen, 1994, Constantine and Lockwood, 1999, Beyer and Holtzblatt, 1998) are actually used. Furthermore, the persons who are entrusted with the ergonomic analysis and evaluation of interactive systems are primarily the developers of the products. External usability or human factors experts or a separate in-house usability department are seldom available. Few of the participants were familiar with methods like *user profile analysis* or *cognitive walkthroughs* which are regarded as fundamental from a usability engineer's point of view.

The UE methods that are considered to be reasonable to apply by the developers are often not used for the following interrelated reasons:

- There is no time allocated for UE activities: they are neither integrated in the development process nor in the project schedule.
- Knowledge needed for the performance of UE tasks is not available within the development team.
- The effort for the application of the UE tasks is estimated to be too high because they are regarded as time consuming.

From an analysis of the interviews, we derived high level requirements for a software tool to support the improvement of UE processes. These high level requirements are summarized in the claims below:

Claim 4 *Support flexible UE process models*

The tool should not force the development organization to adopt a fixed UE process model as the processes practiced are very diverse. Instead, the tool should facilitate a smooth integration of UE methods into the individual software development process practiced by the organization. Turning technology-centered processes into human-centered processes should be seen as a continuous process improvement task where organizations learn which of the methods available best match certain development contexts, and where these organizations may gradually adopt new UE methods.

Claim 5 *Support evolutionary development and reuse of UE experience*

It was observed that the staff entrusted with interface design and evaluation often lack a special background in UE methods. Yet, as the need for usability was recognized by the participating organizations, they tend to develop their own in-house usability guidelines and heuristics. Recent research (Weinschenk and Yeo, 1995, Billingsley, 1995, Spencer, 2000, Rosenbaum et al., 2000) supports the observation that such usability best practices and heuristics are, in fact, compiled and used by software development organizations. Spencer (Spencer, 2000), for example, presents a streamlined cognitive walkthrough method which has been developed to facilitate efficient performance of cognitive walkthroughs under the social constraints of a large software development organization. From experiences collected in the field of software engineering (Basili et al., 1994) it must be assumed that, in most cases, best practices like Spencer's ones are unfortunately not published in either development organizations or the scientific community. They are bound to the people of a certain project or, even worse, to one expert member of this group, making the available body of knowledge hard to access. Similar projects in other departments of the organization usually cannot profit from these experiences. In the worst case, the experiences may leave the organization with the expert when changing jobs. Therefore, the proposed tool should not only support existing human factors methods but also allow the organizations to compile, develop and evolve their own approaches.

Claim 6 *Provide means to trace the application context of UE knowledge*
UE methods still have to be regarded as knowledge-intensive. Tools are needed to support developers with the knowledge required to effectively perform UE activities. Furthermore, tools should enable software development organizations to explore which of the existing methods and process models of UE work best for them in a certain development context and how they can refine and evolve basic methods to make them fit into their particular development context. A dynamic model is needed that allows organisations to keep track of the application context of UE methods.

3. EXISTING APPROACHES FOR CAPTURING HCD KNOWLEDGE

HCI has a long tradition developing design guidelines. Their purpose is to capture design knowledge into small rules, which can then be used when constructing or evaluating new user interfaces. (Vanderdonckt, 1999) defines a guideline by a design and/or evaluation principle to be observed in order to get and/or guarantee the usability of a UI for a given interactive task to be carried out by a given user population in a given context.

A detailed analysis of the validation, completeness and consistency of existing guideline collections has shown that there are a number of problems (Vanderdonckt, 1999) (Welie and Traetteberg, 2000), e.g. guidelines are often too simplistic or too abstract, they can be difficult to interpret and select, they can be conflicting and often have authority issues concerning their validity. One of the reasons for these problems is that most guidelines suggest a general absolute validity but in fact, their applicability depends on a specific context.

Based on these problems with guidelines, a different approach for capturing design knowledge has been developed, called interaction patterns (Welie and Traetteberg, 2000). A pattern is described in terms of a problem, context and solution. The solution of a pattern is supposed to be a proven solution to the stated problem. Patterns represent pieces of good design that are discovered empirically through a collective formulation and validation process, whereas guidelines usually are defined normatively by a closed group. Guidelines are mostly presented without explanations or rationale. Another difference is that patterns make both the context and problem explicit and the solution is provided along with a rationale. Compared to guidelines, patterns contain more complex design knowledge and often several guidelines are integrated in one pattern. Patterns focus on "do this" only and therefore are constructive. Guidelines are usually expressed in a positive and negative form; do or don't do this. Therefore guidelines have their strength for evaluation purposes. They can easily be transformed in questions for evaluating a UI. A typical example of a guideline-based evaluation approach is the ISO-9241 evaluator (Oppermann and Reiterer, 1997).

Another interesting approach to capture HCI design knowledge are claims (Sutcliffe, 2001). Claims are psychologically motivated design rationales that express the advantages and disadvantages of a design as a usability issue, thereby encouraging designers to reason about trade-offs rather than accepting a single guideline or principle. Claims provide situated advice because they come bundled with scenarios of use and artifacts that illustrate applications of the claim. The validity of claims has a strong grounding in theory, or on the evolution of an artifact which demonstrated its usability via evaluation. This is also a weakness of a claim, because it is very situated to a specific context provided by the artifact and usage scenario. This limits the scope of any one claim to similar artifacts.

All existing approaches for capturing HCI knowledge have in common that their use is largely focused on a small part of development process for interactive systems, namely interface design and evaluation. They are still not integrated in important parts of the software development lifecycle such as requirements analysis.

4. THE EVIDENCE-BASED USABILITY ENGINEERING APPROACH

To address the shortcomings and to meet the requirements described in our claims, we advocate an evidence-based approach to the improvement of HCD processes.

We define evidence-based usability engineering as follows:

- *Evidence:* Something, such as a fact, sign, or object that gives proof or reasons to believe or agree with something.
- *Usability engineering:*

(1) The application of systematic, disciplined, quantifiable methods to the development of interactive software systems to achieve a high quality in use; and

(2) The study of approaches as in (1).

- *Evidence-based usability engineering:* An approach for establishing HCD methods in mainstream software development processes, that uses:

(1) qualitative and quantitative feedback on the efficiency of HCD methods collected in projects and integrates this data across project boundaries for controlling and improving the quality and productivity of HCD activities, and

(2) concepts of organizational learning for integrating HCD knowledge, gathered as in (1), into software development processes.

The essence of the evidence-based approach is that we do not cling to a fixed process model of the usability engineering process, but instead follow a paradigm of situated decision making. In this approach HCD methods are selected for a given engineering task, e.g. contextual task analysis, based on the available evidence that they will match to the development context at hand.

After performing a method, it should be evaluated if the method was useful for the development context or if it must be modified or discarded. The modification of the method should be recorded and stored for later reuse. Once a certain body of HCD knowledge is accumulated in that way, we have sound evidence for selecting an optimal set of HCD best practices for given development contexts. By continuously applying this procedure of conducting, evaluating and adapting HCD methods in a number of projects, an organization gradually adapts a set of HCD base practices to a wide variety of development contexts. This directly contributes to the general idea of software maturity models such as UMM (Earthy, 1999). According to these models, organizations are highly ranked on a maturity scale, if they are capable of tailoring a set of base practices according to a set of constraints such as available resources or project characteristics to solve a defined engineering problem.

So far we argue that the evidence-based approach requires four ingredients:

- A process meta-model, which guides the selection of HCD methods for a given development context and their integration in an overall software development process in a flexible, decision-oriented manner. The model must as well provide a strategy for evaluating, refining and capturing experiences for new development contexts thus promoting continuous process improvement and organizational learning in HCD.
- A semi-formal notation for structuring knowledge relating to HCD activities allowing it to be saved in an experience base. The experience base allows developers to keep track of documented best practices and their application context even if the underlying context factors such as processes, technologies, domains and quality standards are still evolving. A model is needed to formally relate the best practices of the experience base to a development context.
- A CAUSE (Computer-Aided Usability Engineering Environment) for managing the experience base and allowing developers to predict optimal sets of HCD methods based on the available evidence and the experience of the development organization.
- An organizational concept for deploying, maintaining and evolving the experience base.

4.1 The Evidence-Based Meta-Model

Our evidence-based model comprises a set of organizational tasks to support the introduction, establishment and continuous improvement of HCD methods throughout the whole software engineering lifecycle. It helps to manage and tailor the HCD base practices defined in usability maturity models such as UMM (Earthy, 1999) and the related methods practiced by the development organization according to specific constraints of the respective project and the experiences collected by the organization. The meta-model is based on our findings of experience-based improvement of user interface development processes (Metzker and Offergeld, 2001a). We refined the model to the extent that we now use a formal model to relate a defined development context to a set of best practices. So the selection of an optimal set of HCD methods is guided by a model of the development context and the evaluation results of the HCD methods in real projects within the organization. In more detail the model consists of the following four logical steps:

- Step 1: Define, revise and extend the reference model.

In the first step the reference model for the organization's HCD approach must be defined. If no reference model exists in the organization, one of the existing frameworks such as the process descriptions of UMM (Earthy, 1999) could be used as a starting point for a reference model. After performing one or more projects, the reference model, should be revised based on the experience collected in the projects.

- Step 2: Select suitable HCD base practices and related methods and integrate them into the software development process practiced.

In this step base practices are selected from the reference model to be integrated in the overall software development process. However, further important factors have to be considered, e.g. the type of system to be developed and project constraints like budget and schedules. This information must be mapped into a context model and guides the selection of appropriate HCD methods for the selected base practices. The HCD methods which have been selected for the improvement of the development process have to be integrated in the model of the practiced software development lifecycle and the project plan and complement the overall engineering process used in the project.

- Step 3: Support effective performance of the defined HCD methods.

Generally, at this step in the model, resources have already been allocated for HCD activities, e.g., a usability engineer was nominated, who is responsible for coordinating and supporting the execution of the various HCD activities of the new process. However, the efficiency and impact of the proposed HCD methods must be increased by providing the development team with best practices, tools and reusable deliverables of past projects, such as templates for usability test questionnaires, results of conceptual task analysis or user interface mockups. These facilitate effective performance of the selected HCD methods.

- Step 4: Collect and disseminate best practices and artifacts concerning HCD tasks.

The HCD methods applied in a project should be rated by the project team members. These ratings form the rationale for following projects to adopt or reject HCD methods. Methods poorly rated by project team members in a project have a low likelihood of being reused in later projects.

During the execution of HCD activities, artifacts with a high value for reuse are generated by the participants of HCD activities, for example, templates for usability tests, reusable code fragments, or an experience on how to most efficiently conduct a user profile analysis for assistance systems. Observations like these comprise HCD experience that have to be captured and organized in best practices along with the development context in which they apply to allow for easy reuse in the same or subsequent projects.

The evidence-based meta-model contains two cycles: The inner cycle between step 3 and 4 supports the introduction and establishment of HCD activities and methods within the practiced software development process on the project level. It supports the effective utilization and improvement of the HCD methods selected by fostering the application of best practices which are tailored to the needs of the development organization. This cycle is continuously iterated during the development process.

The outer cycle between step 4 and 1 guides the improvement process on the organizational level. The organization's HCD experience base, available methods and reusable artifact are tailored to the needs of the projects. Experiences collected on the project level are used to improve and evolve the organization's reference model. Ratings of methods provided by project team members guide and simplify the selection of methods in subsequent projects.

The steps of the evidence-based meta model are depicted in Figure 1.

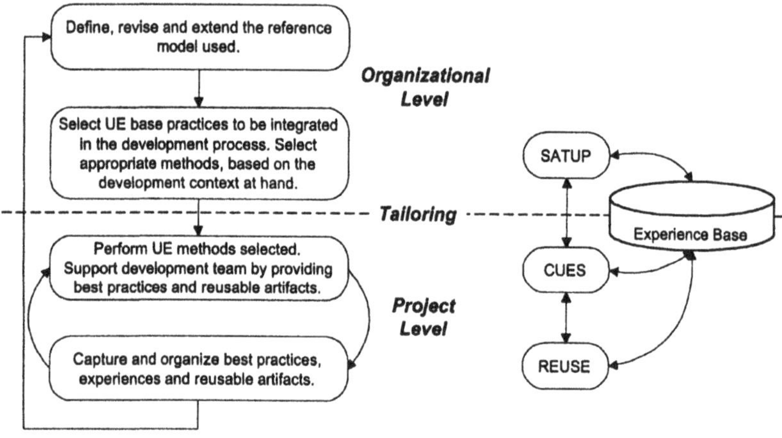

Figure 1 : Tool Support for Evidence-Based Usability Engineering

4.2 USEPACKs and the HCD Experience Base

The main focus of the evidence-based Usability Engineering methodology presented in this paper is to capture and evolve HCD knowledge for reuse and process improvement. Therefore we have developed a semi-formal notation for structuring *process* knowledge relating to HCD methods. For this purpose we use the concepts of USEPACKs (Usability Engineering Experience Package) and a context model. While USEPACKs are used to capture HCD methods, the context model is used to formally relate these methods to a development context. The main difference between USEPACKs, guidelines, interaction patterns and claims is that USEPACKs are primarily focused on process knowledge. The aim is to present context specific process knowledge, structuring the whole HCD process in different generic base practices. In these different base practices guidelines, interaction patterns or claims could be very helpful to represent specific HCI design knowledge. The design knowledge is embedded in HCD activities with the help of a set of reusable artifacts. Therefore a USEPACK encapsulates best practices on how to most effectively perform certain HCD activities and includes the related artifacts like documents, code fragments or templates that facilitate the compliance with the best practice described.

4.3 A Computer-Aided Usability Engineering Environment

To increase the impact of our approach we developed a CAUSE (Computer-aided Usability Engineering Environment) called ProUSE (Process Centred Usability Engineering Environment). ProUSE consists of an HCD experience base and three logical components for planning, selecting, applying, evolving and assessing HCD methods and reusable artifacts.

The experience base is seeded with an initial set of best practices in the form of USEPACKs. In our case we have adopted a variety of usability engineering methods from Nielsen (Nielsen, 1994) and Mayhew (Mayhew, 1999) but in general any HCD approach should be appropriate. The REUSE (Repository for Usability Engineering Experience) (Metzker and Offergeld, 2001b) component is used to capture, manage and evolve best practices related to HCD activities. It assists in documenting best practices using the USEPACK concept and relating them to a formal development context using a context model and storing them in the experience base. SATUP (Setup Assistant for Usability Engineering Processes) is used to plan HCD activities for a software development project. Given all available context information on the process (e.g. which HCD base practices should be performed), project (e.g. duration, budget, team size), domain and technology context factors, SATUP will propose optimal HCD methods and reusable artifacts based on the accumulated experience of the development organization stored in the experience base. If there are alternative USEPACKs available for a defined context situation, SATUP will compare the available ratings for all USEPACKs using a fuzzy multi-criteria decision making approach and propose the optimal USEPACK. Once an optimal HCD process was planned, CUES (Cooperative Usability Engineering Workspace) can be used by a distributed development team to access, perform and assess the HCD methods selected. The ProUSE prototype is based on Java technologies and integrated via a web portal concept which makes the modules available through intranet and web browser.

5. DEPLOYMENT OF PROUSE IN AN INDUSTRIAL SETTING

Before the ProUSE environment is deployed in a development organization for the first time, the systems experience base should be seeded as described in section 4.3. After this first step, the experience base contains a set of USEPACKs that describe methods for each base practice of the reference model used. These USEPACKs will usually have a poor context situation. Imagine now that a large software development organization is developing assistive, interactive home entertainment components and has recognized that usability aspects will play a major role in a new project. In that project, an intelligent avatar for assisting users in programming their video recorders should be created. The organization decides that the overall development process should be supplemented with usability engineering activities. One usability engineer is available for the project but the rest of the development team is inexperienced in usability engineering.

When the project is planned, the usability engineer uses SATUP to create a new project and maps the project's usability constraints to the context factors of the context model thereby creating a context situation for the project. After the usability engineer modelled the development context, the project is accessible to the development team.

Members of the development team can now access the new project via CUES. CUES creates a workspace where the USEPACKs relevant for the defined context situation can be accessed by the development team to support their usability engineering activities. CUES provides the development team with a tailored view on the experience base, shielding them from irrelevant information.

If a certain method was not useful to the development team, the team members can assign a poor rating to the respective USEPACK. This will reduce the likelihood for the USEPACK being selected in subsequent projects with the same context situation. On the other hand team members can assign high ratings to USEPACKs which had a positive impact on their work, thus increasing the likelihood that the respective USEPACK being reused in subsequent projects. By applying the best practices described in a USEPACK members of the development team will make valuable experiences. These experiences can be captured as extensions or comments of an existing USEPACK or can be captured in a new USEPACK.

Assume that the development team used the USEPACK "Contextual Task Analysis" to perform the contextual task activity. Though they found the general guideline useful, they soon discovered that the contextual task analysis for designing an intelligent avatar is fundamentally different from the general method they found in the USEPACK. To capture the modifications to the general method they create a new USEPACK 'Contextual Task Analysis for Intelligent Assistants' using REUSE. They enter their experiences in the USEPACK and attach documents and templates that can be reused when performing a contextual task analysis for an intelligent assistant.

The next time a project team has to design an intelligent assistant, it will have access to the improved contextual task analysis method and the reusable artifacts. These improvement activities will prevent subsequent development teams from encountering similar problems and will enable them to perform the task more efficiently.

How the tool support provided by ProUSE is related to our evidence-based usability engineering approach is depicted in Figure 1.

6. EVALUATION OF PROUSE

The goal of the evaluation was to get initial feedback on the validity of the underlying concepts and acceptance of the support tool ProUSE by development teams.

6.1 Test Subjects and Procedure

Twelve employees of five large to small size companies (Siemens (Munich), Sony (Stuttgart), Grundig (Nuernberg), Loewe (Kronach) in Germany) who are developing interactive software systems in domains such as home entertainment and telematics took part in this evaluation. The experiments were designed as semi-structured interviews. First, the general idea of the approach was presented and a short introduction to the ProUSE support tool was given to each participant. A questionnaire was handed out to collect personal data and data on the work experience of the interviewees. Each person was confronted with a scenario as described above and walked-through this scenario with the test supervisor. At defined points in the scenario, the interviewees had to solve tasks such as defining a projects usability attributes or creating a new USEPACK. At the end of the interviews, the subjects were asked if they would like to integrate the tool in their software development process and which modifications to the approach and the tool they would like.

6.2 Results

The evaluation of the pre-test questionnaire showed that the interviewees

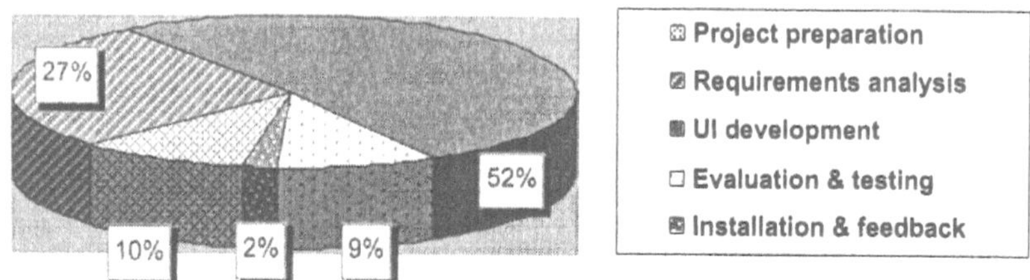

Figure 2 : Involvement of interviewees in phases of UI developmemt process

are largely involved in the development of the user interface, followed by requirements analysis and project preparation. Figure 2 shows the degree of involvement of the interviewees in the various phases of the development process. Eight of the twelve developers interviewed would like to integrate the approach into their development process. Four interviewees would not integrate ProUSE into their development process without major modifications. As indicated in Figure 3, three of the four developers who rejected the approach had no or little experience in the development of user interfaces.

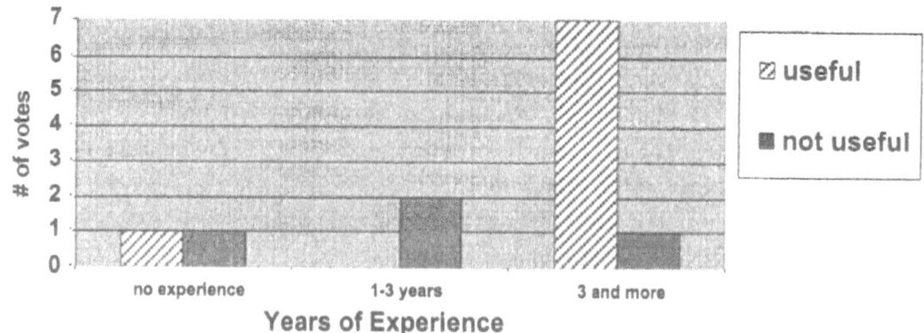

Figure 3 : Perceived usefulness of ProUSE during development depending on experience of subjects in UI design and development.

The votes for the evidence-based usability engineering approach might be linked to the long experience of the respective interviewees. They appreciate the idea of reusing existing HCD knowledge and methods for recurring design tasks. The rejection of the approach by less experienced developers suggests that we should emphasize the benefits that new employees get from accessing and reusing an existing body of HCD knowledge.

7. DISCUSSION

Recently the idea of process maturity was introduced to the field of usability engineering (ISO/TC 159 Ergonomics, 1999, DATech Frankfurt/Main, 2001). The rationale behind usability maturity models is that there are direct dependencies between an organization's capability to tailor its HCD processes according to various constraints, the quality of the development process performed and the quality in use of the interactive software system. Generally an organization has reached the maximum usability maturity level when it is able to perform, control, tailor and continuously improve its usability engineering activities. Our approach as discussed above is geared to support software engineering organizations in reaching high usability maturity levels. At a low usability maturity development organizations can use the experience base as a repository for base practices which are found in the initial set of USEPACKs (seed of the experience base) and which enable the engineering teams to perform those base practices. By applying the base practices in various projects, the development organization is able to derive USEPACKs for each base practice which capture project constraints such as 'size of development team' or 'available budget'. Thus the organization develops a set of more contextualized methods for each base practice, which will enable the organization to control its usability engineering activities. That means it can select the appropriate method for a given resource constraint from the set of USEPACKs available in the experience base.

By applying these controlled methods in future projects the organization collects experience on how to apply the available methods in different domains or for different technologies. By capturing these experiences in more contextualized USEPACKs and feeding them into the experience base the organization will increase its capability to tailor the set of available methods to a development context at hand. It will for example be able to have an optimized set of usability engineering methods for developing intelligent assistants with the avatar technology using a medium size budget with a small development team. By evaluating and eventually refining each method after applying it a continuous improvement process is triggered.

8. ACKNOWLEDGEMENTS

This research was sponsored in part by the BMBF award #01 IL 904 B7 of the EMBASSI project. We would like to thank all participants of our studies.

9. REFERENCES

Basili, V. R., Caldiera, G. and Rombach, H. D. (1994) *Experience Factory,*In *Encyclopedia of Software Engineering*, Vol. 1 (Ed, Marciniak, J. J.) John Wiley & Sons, New York, pp. 528-532.

Beyer, H. and Holtzblatt, K. (1998), *Contextual Design: Defining Customer-Centered Systems,* Morgan Kaufmann Publishers.

Billingsley, P. A. (1995), *Starting from Scratch: Building a Usability Programm at Union Pacific Railroad, Interactions,* **2,** 27-30.

Constantine, L. L. and Lockwood, L. A. D. (1999), *Software for Use: A Practical Guide to the Models and Methods of Usage-Centered Design,* Addison-Wesley.

DATech Frankfurt/Main (2001) In *DATech Prüfbaustein: Qualität des Usability Engineering Prozesses*, Vol. 2001 Deutsche Akkreditierungsstelle Technik e.V., .

Earthy, J. (1999), *Human Centred Processes, their Maturity and their Improvement International Conference on Human-Computer Interaction (INTERACT),* **2,** 117-118.

Henninger, S. (2000), *A Methodology and Tools for Applying Context-Specific Usability Guidelines to Interface Design, Interacting with Computers,* **12,** 225-243.

ISO/TC 159 Ergonomics (1999) In *Human-centered Design Processes for Interactive Systems*, Vol. ISO International Organization for Standardization, .

Mayhew, D. J. (1999), *The Usability Engineering Lifecycle: A Practioner's Handbook for User Interface Design,* Morgan Kaufman Publishers.

Metzker, E. and Offergeld, M. (2001), *An Interdisciplinary Approach for Successfully Integrating Human-Centered Design Methods Into Development Processes Practiced by Industrial Software Development Organizations.* in Eighth IFIP Conference on Engineering for Human Computer Interaction (EHCI'01). 2001. Toronto, Canada: Springer: pp. 21-36.

Metzker, E. and Offergeld, M. (2001), *Computer-Aided Improvement of Human-Centered Design Processes.* in Mensch und Computer, 1. Fachübergreifende Konferenz des German Chapter of the ACM, 2001. Bad Honnef, Germany: Teubner Verlag: pp. 375-384.

Nielsen, J. (1994), *Usability Engineering,* Morgan Kaufman Publishers.

Norman, D. A. (1998), *The Invisible Computer,* MIT Press.

Oppermann, R. and Reiterer, H. (1997), *Software evaluation using the 9241 evaluator, . Behaviour & Information Technology,* **16,** 232-245.

Rosenbaum, S., Rohn, J. A. and Humburg, J. (2000), *A Toolkit for Startegic Usability: Results from Workshops, Panels and Surveys.* in Conference on Human Factors in Computing Systems 2000. The Hague, Netherlands: ACM press: pp. 337-344.

Spencer, R. (2000), *The Streamlined Cognitive Walkthrough Method: Working Around Social Constraints Encountered in a Software Development Company.* in Conference on Human Factors in Computing Systems 2000. The Hague: ACM Press: pp. 353-359.

Sutcliffe, A. (2001), *On the Effective Use and Reuse of HCI Knowledge, ACM Transactions on Computer-Human Interaction,* **7,** 197-221.

Vanderdonckt, J. (1999), *Development Milestones Towards a Tool for Working with Guidelines, Interacting with Computers,* **12,** 81-118.

Weinschenk, S. and Yeo, S. C. (1995), *Guidelines for Enterprise-wide GUI design,* Wiley, New York.

Welie, M. v. (1999), *Breaking Down Usability.* in International Conference on Human-Computer Interaction (INTERACT). 1999. Endinburgh, UK: IOS Press: pp. 613-620.

Welie, M. v. and Traetteberg, H. (2000), *Interaction Patterns in User Interfaces.* in 7th. Pattern Languages of Programs Conference. 2000. Monticello, Illinois, USA: Washington University Technical Report number: wucs-00-29.

Usability: Gaining a Competitive Edge
IFIP World Computer Congress 2002
J. Hammond, T. Gross, J. Wesson (Eds)
Published by Kluwer Academic Publishers

Analyzing the Role of Organizational Culture in the Implementation of User-Centered Design:
Disentangling the Approaches for Cultural Analysis

Netta Iivari
University of Oulu, Department of Information Processing Science, Finland

Abstract: Usability is an important quality characteristic of a software product or system. User-centered design (UCD) is an approach focusing on making systems usable. Improving the position of UCD in organizations has proven to be a challenge. Organizational culture has been identified as an influential factor affecting the successes and failures of organizational improvement efforts. However, there does not exist studies of the effects and consequences of organizational culture in the implementation of UCD. In addition, there exists a lack of methods and theoretical models with which to reliably, systematically and meaningfully analyze organizational culture in relation to improvement efforts. This paper examines existing research within organizational studies, and proposes three approaches - comparative, interpretive and clinical - within which the role of organizational culture can be examined in relation to implementation of UCD. Implications for prospective research are outlined.

Key words: organizational culture, user-centered design, approaches for cultural analysis

1. INTRODUCTION

This paper examines existing research on organizational culture, and proposes approaches through which it could be utilized in relation to research on implementing "User-Centered Design" (UCD) or "Human-Centered Design" defined in (ISO 13407, 1999) and interpreted by Jokela (2001) into organizations. UCD as a systems design approach is characterized by its goal of producing usable systems and principles of user participation, an appropriate allocation of functions between users and technology, iterative design and multi-disciplinary design. UCD activities include: 1) understanding and specifying the context of use; 2) specifying the user and organizational requirements; 3) producing design solutions; and 4) evaluating designs against requirements. (ISO 13407, 1999). However, it might be more appropriate to speak about usability-centered design than user-centered design since many earlier systems design approaches, which do not share all the above goals and principles, are user-centered (e.g. the socio-technical design approach). UCD is defined method independently in the standard. Design approaches focusing on users and usability, e.g. contextual design (Beyer & Holtzblatt, 1998) and usability engineering (Mayhew, 1999), are interpreted as offering specific methods and techniques for UCD activities.

This research effort is part of a KESSU-research project, which aims to introduce and implement UCD in software development organizations, in which the position of UCD is often nonexistent or ineffective (Jokela, 2001). In addition, the improvement of the position of UCD has been widely recognized as a challenge (Axtell & Waterson, 1997; Jokela, 2001; Rosenbaum, 1999). There exists a need for more thorough understanding of the process of implementing UCD into organizations. We suggest that organizational culture is a factor that is intimately intertwined with the organizational change effort of introducing UCD into organizations.

Organizational culture has lately been a popular focus of analysis in studies on organizational change and development (Denison & Spreitzer, 1991). Studies have also examined the part culture plays in achieving total quality through total quality management (TQM). Culture is seen as a major cause of failure in the implementation of TQM (Detert et al, 2000: Kekäle, 1998). However, there still exist severe problems in understanding why so many change programs fail or do not diffuse into the organizations (Schein, 1996). In addition, there exists a need for methods and theoretical models with which to reliably, systematically and meaningfully analyze organizational culture in relation to improvement efforts (Denison & Spreitzer, 1991; Hatch, 1997; Smircich, 1983).

This research effort began with a literature search on several electronic on-line databases. Not a single study was found addressing the role of organizational culture in relation to implementing UCD into organizations. This paper takes a step toward that direction. First the concept of culture is specified. In cultural anthropology, culture denotes the socially transmitted patterns for behavior characteristic of a particular social group (Keesing & Strathern, 1998; Kroeber & Kluckhohn, 1952). It refers to a way of life among particular people. Culture is historical, learned, taken for granted, shared, and ideational. (Keesing & Strathern, 1998; Kroeber & Kluckhohn, 1952.) Culture is a symbolic system. A socio-cultural system is made up of routinized, adaptive, patterned forms of interaction. A symbolic system, on the other hand, consists of learned, shared, patterned sets of meanings. The distinction is between patterns *of* behavior and patterns *for* behavior - culture refers to the realm of ideas. (Keesing & Strathern, 1998; Lett, 1987.) Organizational culture, consequently, refers to the shared patterned sets of meanings for behavior in organizations.

The paper is organized as follows. The next section outlines the existing approaches in organizational culture studies, and highlights the epistemological, methodological and ethical differences in the approaches. Afterwards, three different approaches for cultural studies - comparative, interpretive and clinical - are presented in more detail, and their implications for studies on the implementation of UCD are outlined. The final section discloses the central themes and observations of the paper.

2. APPROACHES IN ORGANIZATIONAL CULTURE STUDIES

Organizational culture is a versatile concept (Smircich, 1983). In order to understand and meaningfully study organisational culture, it is paramount to comprehend its relationship with the evolution of thought in organization theory. Hatch (1997) identifies four perspectives in the development of organization theory. The first one is the classical period, which began in the beginning of last century. The modern perspective emerged in the 1950s. The symbolic interpretive perspective gained attention in the 1980s. The postmodern perspective emerged in the 1990s. Especially the modern and the symbolic interpretive perspective are widely used in organizational culture studies. (Hatch, 1997; Schultz, 1994.)

During the modern period the researchers focused on organizations through objective measures. The methods used were statistical. Results achieved were comparative studies and multivariate statistical analyses. Relying on notions of the positivist research tradition, scientific methods were preferred and scientific objectivity was emphasized. Surveys were commonly used for data gathering. (Burrell & Morgan, 1979; Hatch, 1997.) The symbolic interpretive perspective, on the other hand, aimed at counterbalancing the functionalist-positivist (Burrell & Morgan, 1979; Hatch, 1997) paradigm. This perspective relies on thoughts developed within cultural anthropology. The organizations were now approached through subjective perceptions and the analysis was contextualized; the phenomena were studied in situations in which they naturally occurred, from the 'natives point of view'. (Burrell & Morgan, 1979; Hatch, 1997.)

Schultz and Hatch (1996) outline two paradigms - functionalism and interpretivism - in organizational culture studies. Culture studies following the functionalist paradigm are based on an analytical framework that is defined prior to entering an organization. The framework used is generalized for all organizations studied. The analysis is conducted by filling in predefined variables and mapping causal relations between them. The aim is to condense and bring elements of cultural analysis together. Interpretivism, relying on the symbolic interpretive tradition on the other hand, offers the greatest contrast to functionalism's assumptions. It approaches culture from the 'native's point of view'. The constructs for describing the culture are suggested by the analysis. Focus is on the active creation of meanings and on the ways in which meanings are associated in organizations. Analysis is context-sensitive and concentrates on local, specific meanings.

Table 1. outlines three approaches in organizational culture studies - comparative, interpretive and clinical – and summarizes their underlying epistemological, methodological and ethical assumptions.

Approach	Epistemology	Methodology	Ethics
1. Comparative: Survey instruments: culture is approached as comparative traits and dimensions, measured as values or attitudes Influenced by modern perspective, quantitative organizational climate studies (Denison, 1996; Hatch, 1997; Schultz & Hatch, 1996)	Positivism: seeks to explain and predict what happens in social world by searching for regulaties and causal relationships between constituent elements. (Burrell & Morgan, 1979) Scientific knowledge consists of regulaties, causal laws and explanations (Burrell & Morgan, 1979)	Nomothetic methods (Burrell & Morgan, 1979): - Experiments - Field studies and surveys Formal mathematical analysis	Means-end oriented: culture is studied in order to derive cause and effect relationships (Chua, 1986) Serves the interests of the research
2. Interpretive: Ethnographic case studies: culture is approached as a pattern of meanings. Influenced by the symbolic interpretive perspective, tradition of cultural anthropology (Czarniawska-Joerges, 1992; Hatch, 1997; Schultz & Hatch, 1996; Smircich, 1983)	Antipositivism: social world can only be understood from the point of view of individuals who are directly involved in the activities which are to be studied. (Burrell & Morgan, 1979) Scientific knowledge consists of human interpretations and understandings (Burrell & Morgan, 1979)	Idiographic methods (Burrell & Morgan, 1979): - Case studies Context and organization specific, interpretive analysis	Interpretive: culture is studied in order to enrich people's understanding of their action (Chua, 1986) Serves the interests of the research Sympathetic to the cultural community studied

3. Clinical:	Epistemology:	Methodology:	Ethics:
Consultant oriented investigations: culture is approached as a tool for problem solving Influenced by systems approach & contingency view, organizational psychology, tradition of organizational development (Czarniawska-Joerges, 1992; Denison & Spreitzer, 1991; Schein, 1985; Smircich, 1983)	Either positivist or antipositivist	Either nomothetic or idiographic Universal analytical framework Clinical analysis	Means-end oriented (Chua, 1986); culture is studied in order to solve organizational problems Ideology of managerialism (Burrell & Morgan, 1979; Czarniawska-Joerges, 1992) – organization and management oriented, serves the needs of the client

Table 1, Three approaches in organizational culture studies

The approaches are identified following the division of paradigms in organization theory presented in (Burrell & Morgan, 1979; Hatch, 1997; Schultz & Hatch, 1996). The comparative approach reflects the modern perspective, following the functionalistic paradigm (Burrell & Morgan, 1979; Schultz & Hatch, 1996). The functionalist paradigm implies positivist epistemology and nomothetic research methodology. The interpretive approach follows the interpretive paradigm (Burrell & Morgan, 1979; Schultz & Hatch, 1996). The interpretive paradigm implies antipositivist epistemology and idiographic research methodology. The clinical, consult-oriented approach (Schein 1985; Deal & Kennedy, 1982; Peters & Waterman, 1982), also discussed by Czarniawska-Joerges (1992), is included in the functionalistic paradigm in (Schultz & Hatch, 1996). We interpret, however, that it has followed both the functionalist and interpretive paradigm. Even if it is often applied in a functionalist spirit when measuring organizational cultures; it has also been intermingled with the interpretive approach (methodologically in Schein, 1985). Therefore we suggest that the comparative and the clinical approach should be distinguished.

The ethics of research allows highlighting further differences between the three approaches. In his analysis of paradigmatic assumptions of information systems development approaches, Iivari (1991) interprets the ethics as the role and values of research. In relation to the role of the research, both the clinical and comparative approaches are means-end oriented approaches, in which "scientists aim at providing means knowledge for achieving certain ends without questioning the legitimacy of the ends" (Iivari, 1991), while the interpretive approach aims at "enriching people's understanding of their action and of how social order is produced and reproduced" (Iivari, 1991). Also the values of the research, whose interests the research serves (Iivari, 1991), differ between the approaches. The comparative and interpretive approaches aim at serving those of the academia, but in the clinical approach the needs of the client are the main motivators for the research, the clients often being the management of the organization studied. In an extreme, the managers are conceived as creators and manipulators of the organizational culture and the cultural analysis only assists the managers in the pursuit for excellence. (Czarniawska-Joerges, 1992; Schein, 1985). This clearly conflicts with the anthropological notion of understanding, not interfering with, applied in studies within an interpretive paradigm. Within the interpretive approach the researchers consider carefully the implications of the research for the lives of the researched. Self-reflection of the researchers and ethics of research are in a central position.

Next the approaches are presented in more detail and their implications for research on the role of organizational culture in the implementation of UCD are outlined.

3. THE COMPARATIVE APPROACH

3.1 Introduction to the comparative approach

Within the comparative approach, culture is studied as comparative traits or dimensions. Culture is measured as values, norms or attitudes. The measurement relies on certain typology based on general characteristics of organizational culture. The aim is not to highlight the unique qualities of cultures, but rather to group and profile them. The comparative approach relies on survey instruments to categorize and measure cultures. The instruments position cultures on a certain scale or typology. (Denison, 1996; Denison & Spreitzer, 1991; Kekäle, 1998.)

Competing values model has been popular in diagnosing organizational cultures from the comparative cultural perspective (e.g. Denison & Spreitzer, 1991; Quinn & Spreitzer, 1991; Tata & Prasad, 1998; Zammuto & Krakower, 1991; Iivari & Huisman, 2001). The model consists of two axes that reflect different value orientations. The vertical axis is flexibility - control dimension. Flexibility-oriented cultures support decentralization and differentiation, control-oriented support centralization and integration. The horizontal axis is internal - external dimension. Internal-focused cultures support maintenance of the existing system, while externally focused seek improvements and track changes in their environment. By positioning organizations within the axes they can be defined within four organizational culture types: group, developmental, rational and hierarchical culture. (Denison & Spreitzer, 1991.)

From the viewpoint of implementing UCD the competing values model has been applied in two relevant fields: to study the implementation of TQM and to analyze the deployment of systems development methodologies (SDMs). The former studies suggest that the developmental type of culture is most strongly linked to a TQM success (Dellana & Hauser, 1999; Tata & Prasad, 1998). This implies that the congruent organizational culture for TQM is that of a flexibility-oriented, emphasizing decentralization, differentiation and external orientation. (Dellana & Hauser, 1999; Tata & Prasad, 1998.) On the other hand, research on the relationship between organizational culture and the deployment of SDMs, Iivari and Huisman (2001) show that the SDM deployment, as perceived by systems developers, was primarily associated with the hierarchical culture type. The hierarchical culture is oriented towards security, order and routinization (Denison & Spreitzer, 1991). At the same time, the deployment, as perceived by the management, was negatively associated with the rational culture (Iivari & Huisman, 2001). The rational culture is focused on productivity, efficiency and goal achievement (Denison & Spreitzer, 1991).

Accordingly, the studies indicate that different types of organizational culture are more responsive to TQM, and to the SDMs on the other hand. Iivari and Huisman (2001) study the relationship between organizational culture and SDMs without making a distinction between different methodologies. They use the term "methodology" in a very broad sense to cover the totality of SD approaches, process models, specific methods and specific techniques. In order to evaluate whether their results concerning SDMs are valid in the case of UCD, one should explore the relationship between UCD and SDMs in more detail. Similarly, the connection between UCD and TQM need to be explored before deriving hypotheses of the suitable culture type for the UCD and its implementation.

Also another kind of instruments exists for the cultural studies. Kekäle (1998) has measured organizational culture in relation to TQM implementation. He assumes that the implementation of TQM should rely on different TQM tools in different culture types. He has used a categorization of TQM tools into hard, soft and mixed. Hard TQM tools emphasize written work procedures and accurate measurement of performance. Soft tools promote innovative solutions, teamwork and employee empowerment. Kekäle suggests that there is no one-size-fits-all approach in the implementation of TQM. The approach should be tailored – compatible tools selected for the implementation - so that the approach fits the target culture. Cultural change should be kept the smallest possible.

This is an interesting point of view that relates also to the implementation of UCD. It could be assumed that different tools and methods in relation to UCD are accepted differently. Probably there is no one-size-fits-all approach in relation to UCD either. This viewpoint is in accordance also with the theory of diffusion of innovations, in which it is suggested that the compatibility of the innovation with the existing practice, values and norms contribute positively to the rate of adoption.

3.2 Implications of the comparative approach

A considerable strength of the comparative approach is that the instruments developed to measure organizational culture can be used for collecting comparable data from organizations implementing UCD. Data gathering may be initiated relatively easily with these types of instruments. The instruments can also be used for follow up analyses. In addition, through use of the instruments the validity of the findings derived within other approaches can be enhanced.

The comparative approach to organizational culture has both theoretical and practical implications from the viewpoint of UCD. From a theoretical viewpoint it leads to the following research questions:

- Does the success of UCD differ in organizations with different cultures?
- Does organizational culture explain differences in the success of UCD?
- Do some types of organizational cultures facilitate or constrain the implementation (adoption) of UCD?
- What is the nature of the concept of "cultural fit" of UCD and its implementation?

The studies of the relationship between organizational culture and TQM implementation (Dellana & Hauser, 1999; Kekäle, 1998; Tata & Prasad, 1998) and between organizational culture and SDM deployment (Iivari & Huisman, 2001) suggests that the success UCD and its implementation may differ in organizations with different cultures. Research reviewed above also leads us to the question of whether "cultural fit or misfit" is a singular concept in the sense that there is an ideal organizational culture for UCD and its implementation and that UCD is totally incompatible with some types of organizational cultures. The proposals (Dellana & Hauser, 1999; Tata & Prasad, 1998) that the developmental type of culture is most strongly linked to TQM reflect this view. Alternatively, the findings in (Kekäle, 1998), when applied to UCD, would suggest that "cultural fit or misfit" could be a plural concept in the sense that it is specific to different UCD tools and methods.

From a more practical viewpoint one may raise a number of questions:

- What kind of values and norms constitute an 'ideal UCD culture'?
- What are the compatible culture types for UCD implementation?
- How can UCD be aligned with the type of the organizational culture?
- Should one introduce different UCD tools and methods for different types of organizations?

The first question rephrases the idea of cultural fit in more concrete terms. For the analysis of ideal assumptions, values and norms supporting UCD culture, similar kinds of research in the field ideal TQM culture is available (Detert et al, 2000; Kekäle, 1998). The second question points to a distinction between cultural fit of UCD and its implementation. Assuming UCD is sensitive to the organizational culture and that the client organization has a certain culture that is neither totally ideal nor totally incompatible with UCD, the question is how to align UCD with the organizational culture? Does UCD have cultural flexibility so that it can be adapted to different types of organizational cultures?

4. THE INTERPRETIVE APPROACH

4.1 Introduction the interpretive approach

An interpretive approach is the traditional approach within cultural studies. It relies on the use of ethnography as the main method for data gathering. Ethnography is derived from the tradition of cultural anthropology. Cultural anthropology studies local small-scale communities on a basis of intimate participation in the daily lives of the members of the community. Distinctive features are holism, comparison, participative observation, appreciation of both cultural differences and human commonalities, and emphasis on cultural context. Anthropology highlights the importance of interpretations of collective action, understandings from the 'native's point of view' and constant search for new meanings and interpretations through problematizing the familiar. Researchers' assumptions and predefined categories do not restrict the data gathering to certain traits or dimensions that are of interest to the researcher, but not necessarily to the cultural members studied. Qualitative data is to be gathered and subsequently mapped, but only after data gathering. (Czarniawska-Joerges, 1992; Keesing & Strathern, 1998.)

The researchers spend long periods of time in organizations, participating in the daily activities with the cultural members, and trying to understand the culture from the native's point of view. The data collection concentrates on qualitative data. Material from in-depth interviews, participant observation and field notes written by the researchers are typical. During the fieldwork period the aim is not to disturb the everyday life in the organization. The research effort may however lead to reflection done by cultural members. Due to this self-reflection of the researchers, the ethics of the research are in a central position. (Czarniawska-Joerges, 1992; Schultz, 1994.)

4.2 Implications of the interpretive approach

The interpretive approach is useful since it provides grounded, specific, context sensitive data and understandings from the native's point of view. It addresses issues important to the cultural members, not those predefined as important by the researchers. It has both theoretical and practical implications from the viewpoint of UCD and its implementation. For example, the following theoretical research questions are of interest:

- How is UCD encultured in organizations?
- What meanings are attached to UCD in practice?
- Is there "symbolic uses of UCD"?

One can claim that in order to become an effective part of the everyday systems design practice; UCD should become part of the organization's design culture. This leads to the question of how UCD is encultured in practice. We have examined (Iivari & Abrahamsson, 2002) the interpretations and understandings of UCD and its implementation in relation to different organizational subcultures interacting in the implementation of UCD in one software development company participating in the KESSU project. The subcultures identified were: 1) the usability specialists actively involved in the improvement; 2) the software engineers representing the viewpoint of the software development, who are a significant target of the improvement effort; and 3) the (senior) managers who sponsor the improvement.

The focus of our study was on the perceptions of the nature of UCD, the motives for implementing it, and the experiences while using it in relation to each subculture. The results reveal that there exist clear differences in the perceptions in relation to each subculture. Software engineers and managers especially had attached quite surprising meanings to UCD and its implementation (Iivari & Abrahamsson, 2002):

- The software engineers viewed UCD to be difficult to understand, too theoretical in nature, and containing too complicated terminology. They had a skeptical attitude towards the improvement effort and suspicions about the usefulness of UCD methods.
- The (senior) managers also deemed UCD to be too theoretical in nature and to contain complicated terminology. However, the managers had a very enthusiastic attitude towards the improvement. They conceived UCD as a tool for taming the customers, for keeping customers out of the

development, and for improving the image of the company. They also viewed the implementation effort as a tool for spreading knowledge and skills organization wide.

The results reveal that the subcultures have incongruent views, attitudes, expectations and assumptions concerning UCD and its implementation. Software engineers' very skeptical attitude and the managers' 'symbolic uses of UCD' are factors likely to influence the implementation of UCD (Iivari & Abrahamsson, 2002). However, the interpretations and understandings of UCD, the symbolic uses of UCD, and the process of enculturation of UCD into organizations need all to be empirically explored further.

5. THE CLINICAL APPROACH

5.1 Introduction to the clinical approach

The clinical approach has sometimes been dismissed as an unscientific endeavor, but it has been applied also in research efforts of a scientific nature. (Czarniawska-Joerges, 1992). Within the clinical approach, culture is conceived as a tool for problem solving. Schein defines organizational culture to be "a pattern of basic assumptions - invented, discovered, or developed by a given group as it learns to cope with its problems of external adaptation and integral integration - that has worked well enough to be considered valid and, therefore, to be taught to new members as the correct way to perceive, think, and feel in relation to those problems" (Schein, 1985). Schein presents a detailed description of different steps of his approach, within which the mode is clinical, therapeutic. (Schein, 1985).

In the clinical approach there exists a psychological contract between the client and the consultant. The organization needs to be motivated for the joint discovery. Due to this there needs to be a problem before the intervention. The aim of the approach is to address organizational problems and dysfunctions, and how they contribute to the survival of organization. (Schein, 1985; Schultz, 1994.) The research effort is guided by the needs of the client. The clients are usually the managers of the organization. Within this approach an extreme is that managers are seen as creators and manipulators of organizational culture, and the research effort only assists in the pursuit for excellence. (Deal & Kennedy, 1982; Peters & Waterman, 1982). This type of clinical approach, however, has been criticized as being an unscientific endeavor (Czarniawska-Joerges, 1992).

Czarniawska-Joerges (1992) warns that within the clinical approach the studies on organizational culture are often connected to cultural anthropology, but in many cases the reference to anthropology is used just as a label, not as an approach. Consultant-oriented researchers have used anthropological concepts, but only as attractive metaphors. This has nothing to do with analytic purposes, but instead with the purposes of control. However, the clinical approach, when relying on the approach defined by Schein (1985), conceives organizational culture in more depth than just as an attractive metaphor, and applies many anthropological viewpoints.

5.2 Implications of the clinical approach

The clinical approach provides guidance on how to help an organization. In all, the clinical approach does not result in very interesting theoretical research questions. Its main contribution is the consultant-oriented, client-focused research mode, which might offer visible, practical benefits for target organizations during the implementation effort. Furthermore, the approach in (Schein, 1985) is useful since with it:

- The basic assumptions can be analyzed with detailed guidelines
- The organizational problems and dysfunctions can be addressed
- The effects of the basic assumptions on the implementation of UCD, and the effects of the implementation of UCD on the problems of external adaptation or internal integration can be considered

6. CONCLUDING REMARKS

Organizational culture has been recognized as an important topic of study since the early 1980's. It has been acknowledged as an influential factor affecting the successes and failures of organizational improvement programs. However, there do not exist organizational culture studies in relation to the implementation of UCD. Undoubtedly studies of this kind are needed, since the implementation of UCD has proven to be challenging. However, culture is a versatile concept, and thus there exists controversies in both defining and applying it. Therefore this paper has analyzed the existing paradigms in organizational culture studies and outlined three approaches - comparative, interpretive and clinical – for the purposes of the culture studies. Finally, the implications of the three research approaches for the research on the implementation of UCD have been presented.

All the approaches should be acknowledged as useful in the pursuit of understanding the role of organizational culture in the implementation of UCD. This kind of multi-paradigmatic research into organizational culture benefits from triangulation and the use of a variety of methods. Through this the researchers can develop grounded, but general theories. Therefore, the approaches should be seen as complementary, not incompatible ones.

(Czarniawska-Joerges, 1992; Denison, 1996; Denison & Spreitzer, 1991; Schultz & Hatch, 1996; Zammuto & Krakower, 1991.)

The comparative approach contributes to the research effort by offering:

- Comparable data from different organizations – generalizations
- First hand information about the value orientation of the organization – possible guidelines for selection of an implementation strategy
- Easy and quick follow up analyses
- Triangulation: enhancement of the validity of the findings derived within interpretive or clinical approach, and
- Predefined frameworks for the analysis.

The interpretive approach provides:

- Thorough understandings from the native's point of view.
- A research approach concentrating on the issues important to the cultural members - grounded, specific, context sensitive data – provides
- A sound research approach for qualitative research.

Finally, the clinical approach is useful since:

- It focuses on the needs of the client and primarily assists the organization
- A therapeutic, client-centered mode may motivate an organization to undergo this self reflection process needed in cultural analysis.

Consequently, all the approaches - comparative, interpretive and clinical - study the same phenomena, but within different methodological, epistemological and ethical premises. It is our contention that a researcher should, while attempting to apply the approaches, be aware of their assumptions and underlying philosophies. The purpose of this paper has been to provide a condensed introduction to different approaches in organizational culture studies, and to their underlying assumptions. All the approaches suggested for trial should be viewed useful in the pursuit of understanding cultural context in the implementation of UCD. We will empirically experiment with the approaches presented in this paper within the KESSU project during future empirical research on the subject.

7. ACKNOWLEDGEMENTS

We would like to thank Prof. Juhani Iivari for his contribution to the paper. This research effort has been supported by INFWEST.IT Postgraduate Training Program.

8. REFERENCES

Axtell, C. M., Waterson, P. E. & Clegg, C. W. (1997): Problems integrating user participation into software development. *International Journal of Human-Computer Studies* **47**.

Beyer, H. & Holtzblatt, K. (1998): *Contextual Design: Defining Customer-Centered Systems*. San Francisco: Morgan Kaufmann Publishers, Inc.

Burrell, G. & Morgan, G. (1979): *Sociological Paradigms and Organizational Analysis. Elements of the Sociology of Corporate Life*. London: Heinemann Educational Books Ltd.

Chua, W.F. (1986): Radical developments in accounting thought. *Accounting Review*. **LXI**(5).

Czarniawska-Joerges, B. (1992): *Exploring Complex Organizations. A Cultural Perspective*. Newbury Park: Sage Publications.

Deal, T. E. & Kennedy, A. A. (1982): *Corporate Cultures: The rites and rituals of corporate life*. Reading MA: Addison-Wesley.

Dellana, S.A. & Hauser, R.D. (1999): Toward Defining the Quality Culture. *Engineering Management Journal*. **11**(2).

Denison, D.R. (1996): What *is* the difference between organizational culture and organizational climate? A native's point of view on a decade of paradigm wars. *Academy of Management Review*. **21**(3).

Denison, D.R. & Spreitzer, G.M. (1991): Organizational Culture and Organizational Development: A Competitive Values Approach. In Richard W. Woodman and William A. Pasmore (ed.). *Research in Organizational Change and Development. An Annual Series Featuring Advances in Theory, Methodology, and Research*. **5**. Greenwich: JAI Press Inc.

Detert, J.R., Schroeder, R.G. & Mauriel, J.J. (2000): A Framework for Linking Culture and Improvement Initiatives in Organizations. *Academy of Management Review* **25**(4).

Hatch, M.J. (1997): *Organization Theory. Modern, Symbolic, and Postmodern Perspectives*. New York: Oxford University Press.

Iivari, J. (1991): A Paradigmatic analysis of contemporary schools of IS development. *European Journal of Information Systems*. Vol. 1. No. 4.

Iivari, J. & Huisman, M. (2001): The Relationship Between Organizational Culture and the Systems Development Methodologies. *Advanced Information Systems Engineering, 13th International Conference CAiSE 2001 Proceedings*. Berlin: Springer-Verlag.

Iivari, N. & Abrahamsson, P. (2002): The Interaction Between Organizational Subcultures and User-Centered Design - A Case Study of an Implementation Effort. *Proceedings of the 35th Annual Hawaii International Conference on System Sciences*.

ISO 13407 (1999): Human-centered design processes for interactive systems. *International Standard*.

Jokela, T. (2001): *Assessment of user-centred design processes as a basis for improvement action. An experimental study in industrial settings*. Oulu: Acta Universitatis Ouluensis Scientiae Rerum Naturalium. A 374.

Keesing, R.M. & Strathern, A.J. (1998): *Cultural Anthropology. A Contemporary Perspective*. Third edition. Fort Worth: Harcourt Brave College Publishers.

Kekäle, T. (1998): *The Effects of Organizational Culture on Successes and Failures in Implementation of Some Total Quality Management Approaches. Towards a Theory of Selecting a Culturally Matching Quality Approach.* Vaasa: Acta Wasaensia No 65.

Kroeber, A. L. & Kluckhohn, C. (1952): *Culture: a critical review of the concepts and definitions.* Cambridge: Harvard University Press.

Lett, J. (1987): *The Human Enterprise. A Critical Introduction to Anthropological Theory.* Boulder: Westview Press Inc.

Mayhew, D..J. (1999): *The usability engineering lifecycle: a practitioner's handbook for user interface design.* San Francisco: Morgan Kaufmann Publishers, Inc.

Peters, T. J. & Waterman, R.H. (1982): *In search of excellence: lessons from America's best-run companies.* New York : Harper & Row.

Quinn, R.E. & Spreitzer, G.M. (1991): The Psychometrics of the Competing Values Culture Instrument and an Analysis of the Impact of Organizational Culture on Quality of Life. In Richard W. Woodman and William A. Pasmore (ed.). *Research in Organizational Change and Development. An Annual Series Featuring Advances in Theory, Methodology, and Research.* **5**. Greenwich: JAI Press Inc.

Rosenbaum, S. (1999): What Makes Strategic Usability Fail? Lessons Learned from the Field. *Proceedings of CHI '99.* Pittsburgh, USA.

Schein, E. (1985): *Organizational culture and leadership.* 2nd edition. San Francisco: Jossey-Bass.

Schein, E. (1996): Culture: The Missing Concept in Organization Studies. *Administrative Science Quarterly.* **41**.

Schultz, M. (1994): *On Studying Organizational Cultures. Diagnosis and Understanding.* Walter de Gruyter: Berlin.

Schultz, M. & Hatch, M.J. (1996): Living with Multiple Paradigms: the Case of Paradigm Interplay in Organizational Culture Studies. *Academy of Management Review.* **21**(2).

Smircich, L. (1983): Concepts of Culture and Organizational Analysis. *Administrative Science Quarterly.* **28**.

Tata, J. & Prasad, S. (1998): Cultural and structural constraints on total quality management implementation. *Total Quality Management.* **9**(8).

Zammuto, R.F. & Krakower, J.Y. (1991): Quantitative and Qualitative Studies of Organizational Culture. In Richard W. Woodman and William A. Pasmore (ed.). *Research in Organizational Change and Development. An Annual Series Featuring Advances in Theory, Methodology, and Research.* **5**. Greenwich: JAI Press Inc.

Usability: Gaining a Competitive Edge
IFIP World Computer Congress 2002
J. Hammond, T. Gross, J. Wesson (Eds)
Published by Kluwer Academic Publishers

The Importance of User Roles in Feature Bundling Decisions in Wireless Handheld Devices

Strategic User Needs Analysis (SUNA)

Sheila Narasimhan and Gitte Lindgaard
Human Oriented Technology Lab (HotLab)
Dept of Psychology, Carleton University, Ottawa, Ontario, Canada, K1S 5B6
snarasim@chat.carleton.ca and gitte_lindgaard@carleton.ca

Abstract: The bundling of features in wireless technologies is considered to be a significant issue by market analysts and service providers. Currently, there is a proliferation of handheld devices such as Personal Digital Assistants (PDAs) making it very difficult for users to select the devices that match their needs. A literature review suggests that although feature bundling in handheld sets and services is a critical decision in product and service development, it is often left to chance. This paper indicates that for a smooth deployment of wireless technologies, it is important to study the needs of users from the perspective of the roles for which they use the handheld device. Specifically, this paper describes the development and testing of a methodology for supporting the selection and bundling of features in wireless technologies such as Personal Digital Assistants (PDAs). The methodology, termed Strategic User Needs Analysis (SUNA), combines several investigative methods from HCI and market research with an emphasis on User Role Modelling (Constantine & Lockwood, 1999). Initial testing of SUNA on a small sample of users, representing two focal user roles, indicates that the methodology is effective in identifying features most needed for the two focal roles. It identified the relevant characteristics, usage patterns, similarities and differences between these, and their consequent implications for feature bundling by product designers and developers.

Key words: Personal digital assistants, wireless technologies, user needs assessment, role modelling, job analysis, features bundling.

1. INTRODUCTION

User needs and task analyses occupy an important position in Human Computer Interaction (HCI) literature. A review of several methods (Beyer & Holtzblatt, 1998; Hackos & Redish, 1998; Maguire, 1997; Mayhew, 1999) indicates that there is a strong focus on user task analysis techniques. These techniques describe user tasks, as they are performed (e.g. Shepherd, 2001; Kirwan & Ainsworth, 1992), in great detail, and are, therefore, not ideally suited to identifying the features and services critical to each group or segment of users. Secondly, these methodologies assume implicitly or explicitly that the purpose and functions of the system in question are already known and that the tasks it is intended to support have been determined. This assumption in turn renders them less appropriate for Greenfield applications. Even methodologies that take users' work context into account (e.g. Beyer & Holtzblatt, 1998) assume that users are readily accessible and that they can be interrupted while performing tasks. However, this tenet does not hold for mobile workers and travelling executives whose jobs do not lend themselves to intrusive inquiry methods proposed in task analysis methodologies. The selection and bundling of features is an important planning task in the product design and development stage, which requires strategic information on usage patterns, behaviour and needs of users within distinctive, identifiable groups. Since task analysis fails to provide this higher-level information, it is important to look at other methods.

A review of marketing literature was undertaken to identify appropriate investigative techniques for feature bundling. The review revealed that industry analysts mainly focus on market predictions (Yankee Group, 1999). Their methodologies are grounded in market research techniques, which are "about studying people as "customers" and "consumers" especially their own views of their needs and desires, their preferences and their reactions to new ideas" (Hackos & Redish, 1998, p.17).

Given that the HCI and market methods did not offer an immediate solution to the issue of feature bundling, it became necessary to develop and test a methodology, which would identify user needs at a strategic level based on product usage patterns, rather than on user performance in predetermined tasks. Specifically, it was important to identify those factors, which distinguish one group of users from another in terms of the desired bundle of features in Personal Digital Assistants (PDAs). Several investigative techniques were combined, adapted, and applied here to meet this challenge. We call the resulting approach Strategic User Needs Analysis (SUNA) to highlight the fact that it is a strategic planning tool. The paper outlines SUNA and its possible application to support PDA feature bundling.

2. METHODOLOGY

Constantine and Lockwood's (1999) notion of user role modelling offered a sound investigative technique to link usage patterns, user behaviour and user needs to their respective roles. The user role model is defined as an abstract collection of user needs, interests, expectations, behaviours, and responsibilities. This abstract collection of information about the user is used to describe the relationship of the user to the system (PDAs) and subsequently his or her needs stemming from the roles.

A brainstorming session was initiated to accomplish a variety of tasks in a group setting. The tasks are shown in Figure 1.

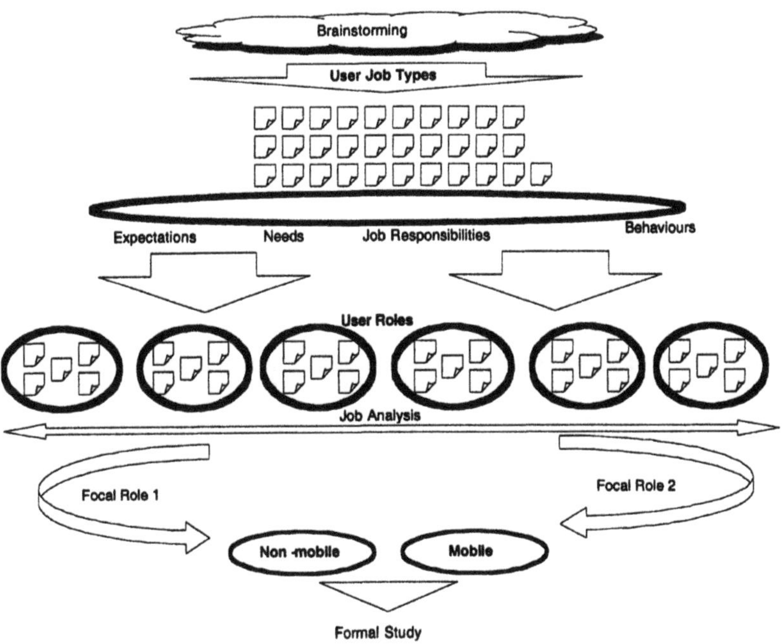

Figure 1: Brainstorming session tasks

The first step involved the listing of user job types. The user job types listed were then clustered into user roles on the basis of the needs, expectations, behaviours and job responsibilities of each job type. Six user roles were identified from 31 job types. A job analysis using job descriptions and specifications from two companies was undertaken to confirm that the clustering was in fact valid. Two focal roles were then selected for the formal field study.

In the field study, a sample of participants representing the user roles identified in the brainstorming session was observed to identify usage patterns and behavioural characteristics. An automatic software log on the participants' PDAs recorded their usage of the various functions over two days. Some users had to fill in their usage manually in a diary because their PDAs were not compatible with the software for automatic logging of usage. An open-ended interview was conducted with each participant using an instrument developed specifically for this purpose.

3. IDENTIFYING USER/JOB TYPES

Seven PDA users representing a variety of disciplines such as, human resources, administration, IT, marketing and software development in a large telecommunications company participated in the brainstorming session. The session commenced with a brief description of the research purpose as well as its significance in the bundling of PDA features using the role model approach. The concepts of user types and user roles were then described. Each participant was asked to read and sign an informed consent form. To generate as many user types as possible, participants were asked to write the names of as many user/job types as they could think of on post-it notes, with one type per note. Participants took turns pasting their roles on a board. Duplicates were eliminated, leaving a list of unique user/job type names. A total of 31 user types were generated in this fashion as shown in Table 1 below.

User Types		
Administrative Assistants	IT support	Security
Babysitters/Caregivers	Marketing Researchers	Servers
Delivery People	Military Personnel (RCAF)	Small Business Owners
Designers (R&D)	Paramedics	Stock Brokers
Dispatchers	Professors	Students
Doctor	Real Estate Agents	Team leaders and executives
Emergency Personnel	Reporters/Journalists	Transportation Personnel
Field technicians	Researcher	Travel Agents
Globe trotters	Restaurant/Hotel Clients	Travel/Tour Guides
HR Professionals	Sales representative	Travelling executives
		Ultra light Pilots

Table 1. User types generated by brainstorming

3.1 Deriving User Roles

Abstract user roles have to be derived from specific user/job types using a bottom-up approach (Constantine & Lockwood, 1999). The participants were asked to group the 31-user/job types on the basis of the perceived needs, expectations, behaviours, and job responsibilities associated with each job type. Needs were defined as requirements for the device, such as the need to receive e-mail or text messages. Behaviour reveals the expected frequency and volume of usage. Expectations reflect the user's expectations of device reliability and transmission speed, access to the network, and his/her mobility. Relevant job responsibilities are identified by listing typical activities that a person would perform in the particular role, such as contacting customers or the work base, checking inventory or accessing a given dynamic database. Grouping of user/job types continues until all similar roles are grouped together and the resulting roles are distinct.

The participants after much discussion grouped user/job types into generic or abstract categories of user roles. The resulting user roles were further validated through an analysis of the needs, expectations, behaviours, and relevant job responsibilities found in formal job classification documents obtained from the Human Resources departments of two organisations. The 31user/job types identified in this study were finally reduced to a set of six categories of user roles: field service, travel routing, database access, non-mobile professionals, mobile professionals, and multiple roles.

3.2 Designating Focal User Roles

From the six user roles, two focal user roles were to be selected for further study. Focal roles are those viewed to be critical for the PDA market, specifically with respect to the feature bundling of PDAs. Because PDAs are in the early stages of the product life cycle, the discussion focused on user roles representing early adopters. The corporate business market, as opposed to individual consumers, was identified in broad terms as a leading segment with a larger number of innovators and early adopters of PDAs.

Within the corporate business market sector, senior managers/executives were seen as early adopters given their high level of mobility and/or their constant need for time critical information for fulfilling their role. The two critical roles selected were thus mobile and non-mobile professionals. Examples of the perceived needs, expectations, behaviours and relevant job responsibilities pertaining to some representatives of these categories are shown in Table 2 below. Complete details may be found in Narasimhan (2001).

User role	User type	Needs	Expectatio ns	Behaviour s	Job re- sponsibility
Non-mobile	Administrative assistants	Scheduler Communicate with manager Manage meetings and events Travel info Contact lists	Scheduling capability Access to internal/ external databases Reliable device	Frequent usage Moderate volume	Carry out admin duties to free up time for the group
	Dispatchers	Routing information Contextual information Relay info to field personnel	Must be fast, reliable and have database access (wireless necessary?)	Frequent usage High volume	Communicat e and relay info to field personnel
Mobile	Stock brokers	Stock quotes Contact lists E-trade Client portfolio Stock analysis	Accurate, real-time, fast access, secure, portable, reliable	Frequent usage Moderate volume	Stay in touch with markets and clients Conduct transactions
	Reporters/ Journalists	Address book Contact list Schedule Travel logs Routing info Research info	Accurate, fast, real-time, global access, file transfer, secure intranet/ internet	Frequent usage Low-moderate volume	Gather news Report to news room in real time

Table 2. Needs, expectations, behaviours, and job responsibilities for a subset of mobile and non-mobile professionals

3.3 Analysing Usage Patterns

The usage patterns common to the six user roles were derived from the results of the brainstorming session and the job analysis. Three dimensions of usage emerged from the information: extent of mobility, volume of action/transactions in the field, and amount of information transferred. Each dimension was measured in a qualitative manner using a low, medium and high scale. A summary of this analysis for non-mobile and mobile professionals is shown in Table 3 below. Details of all others are available in Narasimhan (2001).

	Mobility			Action/ transaction			Amount of information		
	L	M	H	L	M	H	L	M	H
Non-mobile professionals	✓				✓				✓
Mobile professionals			✓			✓		✓	

Table 3. User role usage patterns

As the Table shows, the two focal user role categories differed on all three dimensions. While non-mobile professionals' usage patterns were indicative of transferring large amounts of information, hence a bandwidth issue, mobile professionals required the convenience of a portable, easy to carry PDA, with high speed of access, capable of completing transactions.

The results of the brainstorming session culminated in successful selection of two focal roles representing the early adopters of new wireless technological innovations such as PDAs. The methodological focus on user roles and their relationship to PDAs rather than on individual users enabled a higher level of abstraction necessary for the purpose of strategic bundling.

3.4 Initial Field Testing

The field study involved observing usage patterns of mobile and non-mobile professionals representing the two focal user roles selected at the end of the brainstorming session. Twelve users of mobile technologies, six from each focal user role group participated in the study. The participant's usage of the various functions of the PDAs was recorded automatically through the use of a software program that was beamed on to their device. Exceptions were made in the case of a cellular phone user and a RIM Blackberry user, since their PDAs were incompatible with the automatic usage logging software. These individuals recorded usage on a log sheet. The device usage of all participants was captured over a two-day period. At the end of the two days, participants were interviewed individually in their own office. The logged data was used as a reference to jog the user's memory with respect to the purpose of the use, the type of communications established, and the features necessary to assist the role. The data log thus provided a realistic setting for assessing the user role and the relationship of the PDA in assisting the user role. This is similar to Beyer and Holtzblatt's (1998) notion of an 'artifact model' in which an artifact is used to jog the user's memory for the analyst to understand the work the user is trying to accomplish with the system in question.

A set of 30 open-ended questions addressing six research questions was developed and administered in each interview:

1. What are users in this role trying to accomplish?
2. Which PDA functions are used most frequently?
3. What is the relationship of the PDA functions to the user role?
4. What other devices are used to accomplish what the user wants?
5. Gaps preventing the user from completing the work in the user role
6. Existing features and users' wish list

4. RESULTS

4.1 User Roles and Sub-Roles

Participants were asked to identify the four main functions, or sub-roles, they fulfil in their current job. Analysis of responses indicated that the following functions involved the use of PDAs: Communicator, Leader & Manager, Administrator, Analyst & Researcher, Creator & Developer, and Field operator. The description of sub-roles indicated that the non-mobile professionals' main functions tended to be internally oriented towards the organisation, whereas the mobile professionals' functions tended to be outwardly oriented towards clients. Since mobile professionals are away from the office, there seems to be a greater emphasis on communication capabilities of PDAs, whereas the non-mobile professionals focussed more on the PDA's administrative functions. It will also be recalled that the mobile and non-mobile professional roles varied in usage dimensions (volume and frequency of transactions). These differences in roles and usage patterns are indicative of two user roles that could form the basis for features bundling in PDAs and other wireless technological innovations. High-level functions that could be supported by PDAs were then identified from the participants' descriptions. These are presented in Table 4 below.

Main job function	PDA-supportable functions
Communicator	Time management, People management, Communication, People interaction (partner, secretary, staff), Customer contact, Client work (consulting), Client relationships, Presentations
Leader& Manager	Project management, Office management (finance, recruiting), Leadership role (manage marketing/sales group)
Administrator	Operational strategy, Hiring staff, Document management, Time management, Admin/Evaluation
Analyst& Researcher	N/A
Field operator	Design

Table 4. Possible PDA features supporting non-mobile and mobile professionals (n=12)

4.2 PDA Functions Used Frequently by Focal Roles

Based on the data logs and memory, the most frequently used features for non-mobile professionals included the date book, Quicksheet (spreadsheet), address book, memo pad, and calculator. On the other hand the frequently used features for mobile professionals included the date book, address book, e-mail, memo pad, to do list, and cell phone.

Given the high mobility of their roles, mobile professionals tended to use their PDAs as a mobile office to network with their own head office and their clients (e-mail, cell phone). It is interesting to note that the non-mobile professionals with their well-equipped offices with telephones and PCs did not use the networking functions in their PDAs. Even when these commonly used functions are available in mobile devices, these early adopters in the non-mobile category still primarily use traditional devices perhaps due to cost considerations.

4.3 Linkage of PDA Functions to the User Role

Table 5 provides the reasons for which the PDA functions are used by the two user roles. The information in the Table indicates that certain commonalities prevail across the two groups, although some functions are used differently. For example, whereas non-mobile professionals use the date book for administrative purposes, mobile professionals use it for time management. Similarly, the non-mobile user role uses the address book as much for addresses as for phone numbers, whereas the mobile user role uses it mainly as a quick reference to phone numbers. To the mobile user operating in an environment that allows integration of voice and data, access to remote and local databases, and linkage of the date book and address book with e-mail and telephone functions would add considerable value. Non-mobile professionals may not need these converging meta-functions unless they also changed their usage patterns to rely more on mobile than on desktop technologies. The observation that the non-mobile professionals do not use e-mail or the to do list in their PDA reinforces the notion that, at this point in time, they do not quite see the PDA as a substitute for traditional devices.

Function	Non-mobile	Mobile
Date book	Make appointments, schedule, reminder, coordinate meetings	Time management (alerts, beeps)
Address book	Internal/external addresses, phone	Quick reference to phone numbers
Memo pad	Business/personal use	Business notes in field
Calculator	Calculations	---
Quicksheet	Class attendance, marking	---
E-mail	---	Communicate with office, clients
To Do list	---	Organize business and personal affairs
Cell phone	---	sole phone contact

Table 5. PDA function usage in the two user roles

4.4 Other Devices Used In Concert With PDAs

Non-mobile professionals use computers (PC, laptop), telephones (terrestrial, cell), and paper in conjunction with the PDA. The address book is used in conjunction with telephones, linking the administrator and communicator roles. The memo pad is used in concert with the PC primarily to back up the memo pad entries, which may consist of items such as meeting and presentation notes.

Mobile professionals use the date book and the address book in conjunction with voice communication devices, again linking the administrator and communicator roles. The address book is also used with the laptop to update/backup administrative information. The laptop is used for e-mail, and the memo pad is backed up in a "Hotsync" operation.

4.5 Gaps In PDA Functions In Fulfilment Of User Roles

In the non-mobile role, the key gaps identified with the Palm and Handspring related to visual factors, battery life, and software-related functions. The following gaps in PDAs were noted:

- Handwriting difficulties, e.g. lack of an on-line reference for the graffiti language and poor character recognition
- Screen deficiencies, e.g. small size, poor back lighting, reflection, low resolution
- Poor battery life
- Difficulties finding, downloading, and integrating additional software

In the mobile role, the distinctive issues related to ergonomics, convenience, and absence of cross-functional and communication capabilities. Issues raised by mobile users (PDAs, Blackberry, cell phone) were:

- Handwriting/typing difficulties, e.g. poor character recognition, small keyboard, no graffiti (Blackberry), numeric keypad on the cell phone
- Screen deficiencies, e.g. small size, poor back lighting, reflection, low resolution
- Poor battery life
- Devices hard to grip
- Lack of inter-linking capabilities between functions, e.g. no link from date book to contact list
- Inconvenient e-mail function on the Blackberry and the cell phone, e.g. e-mails must be trimmed, cell phone and office e-mail addresses are different, and responding to e-mails is difficult because of scrolling
- Poor hotsync/synchronisation operation to the PC, e.g. fields are not matched

4.6 Perceived Value of PDA Features

A wish list of what participants would like to see in the later models of PDAs was obtained. Some differences between the non-mobile and mobile professional roles were noticed. Non-mobile professionals wanted to include phone, e-mail, voice memo, instant messaging, and banking features to facilitate the office role at home. The mobile professionals wanted to integrate the PDA with wireless connectivity and the Blackberry with Graffiti handwriting. They also mentioned GPS, unified messaging, information services for maps and stock quotes, e-wallet allowing credit or debit card information, and a high-speed broadband wireless connection. One can see from the wish list that both user roles tend to get more sophisticated with a key emphasis on convergence from mobile professionals.

In addition to a wish list, participants were also asked to rate existing and suggested new features for importance on a 5-point rating scale ranging from 'very unimportant' (1) to 'very important' (5). Results of this exercise are shown in Table 6 below. Features were grouped into 'ergonomics', functions', and 'access'. 'Ergonomics' refers to physical design issues, 'functions' refers to features that do not require network connectivity, and 'access' represents those features that require such connectivity.

Category	Element	Mobile (n=6)	Non-mobile (n=6)
Ergonomics	PDA size	6	5
	Screen size	6	4
Feature	Address book	6	5
	Scheduler	6	6
	Alarm	1	4
	To Do list	3	4
Access	Phone	6	3
	Voice mail	6	3
	Wireless connectivity	4	1
	Information services	4	0
	E-mail	4	2
	E-wallet	3	4
	GPS	2	1
	Internet	2	1
	Intranet	2	0
	E-commerce	1	1
	Banking	0	2
	Voice memo	0	3
	Fax	0	0
	Unified messaging	0	2

* Note: Features rated 4 or 5 by more than half of the participants are shaded

Table 6. * Number of participants rating features 'Important' (4) or 'Very important' (5)

As the Table shows, ergonomic issues were considered important to both groups of participants. All the features, such the address book, scheduler, alarm were considered important to the non-mobile user role. Only three users in the mobile user role considered the to do list as important eventhough the to do list was among the most frequently used functions. It seems surprising also that the alarm was considered important by most of the non-mobile professionals but only by one of the mobile professionals, as this had not been noted among the most frequently used functions. Clearly, those 'access' functions that enable direct person-to-person contact were important to the mobile, but not to the non-mobile professionals. It appears that relative to the access functions the administrative functions were less important to the mobile professional role. The observation that neither group found the information-rich access features, such as internet/intranet access, important probably reflects one of the limitations of small monochrome screens and the fact that both groups have access to PCs and/or laptops from their own or other offices and hotels. Thus, the PDA appears to play a role of convenience rather than being seen as a replacement of services that are also available via other means.

The above data should be interpreted with caution. The sample is small, the data collection period was only two days, and, although some data were collected from electronic logs, the lack of accuracy between people's wishes and their estimates of their own 'typical' usage is well documented (Lindgaard, 1993; Lindgaard & Ferguson, 1992).

5. DISCUSSION

While segmentation and feature bundling to differentiate a product or service on the basis of segment needs is the goal of every product manufacturer and service provider, the robustness of the research methods employed to identify the distinctive user groups and their needs often appear questionable. The objective of this research was to identify and test a methodology that would be helpful in relating features of wireless technological innovations such as the PDA to different groups of users with distinctive roles and usage patterns. The challenge was to identify target user groups who represent early adopters of new technology, to understand and document their needs such that information thus gleaned could be applied to selecting features for future technologies.

The notion of 'user roles' as described by Constantine and Lockwood (1999) was central to the methodology outlined above. The focus on roles allowed for a strategic abstraction of user needs from an individual level to a group level. Inherently, successful feature bundling very much depends on identifying segments that are not only early adopters but also are distinguishable so that they can be targeted. The proposed methodology rests on the role(s) users occupy rather than on their individual habits and preferences. It facilitates the subsequent selection of users for further study during the UNA, and it enables product & service designers to focus on the common elements of target user groups.

Within Constantine and Lockwood's (1999) framework, user roles are combined into user role maps revealing the interrelationships between the various roles. The present study revealed that the non-mobile professional was an abstraction of three sub-roles: internal communicator, in-office administrator/manager, and in-house operator. Since the non-mobile professional roles are mainly internally oriented, the PDA's date book assisting the administrator/operator sub-role is the most frequently used function. The mobile professional was an abstraction of four sub-roles: external communicator, business/sales developer, out of office administrator/manager, and field operator. The sub-roles of the mobile professional role are primarily oriented to the world outside the organization, for example, in contacting customers, developing business or building strategic partnerships. To support the various sub-roles of mobile professionals, communication functions supporting person-to-person contact are thus important, as shown in Figure 2.

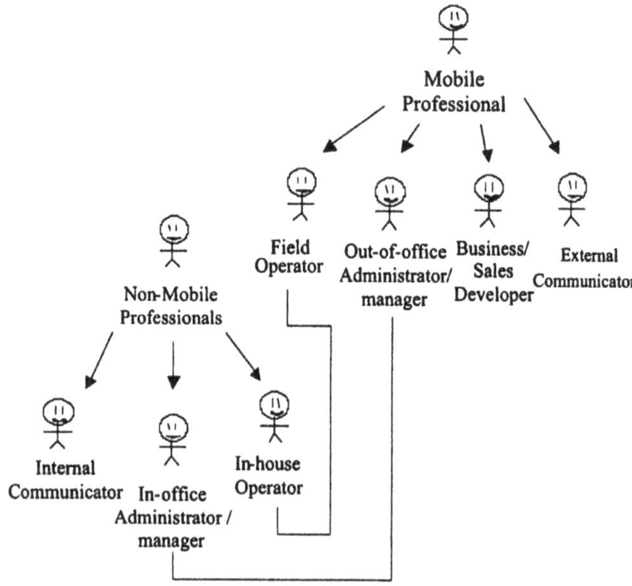

Figure 2. User Role Map For Mobile and Non-Mobile Roles (adapted from Constantine & Lockwood, 1999)

Some affinity or resemblance was noted between the in-office and out-of-office administrator/manager sub-roles as well as the in-house operator and field operator sub-roles.

It thus appears that the external communicator and business developer sub-roles differentiate the mobile professional role from the non-mobile professional role in relation to PDA usage. The external communicator sub-role within the mobile professional role manifests itself in the more common use of PDAs with communication capabilities such as the Blackberry and cellular phone with e-mail and Internet access.

If users in the mobile role have PDAs with wireless connectivity, then they complete the rest of their role functions with a laptop computer. Those in the mobile role with a Palm handheld use the cellular phone and regular phone to complete their role functions. In this context, the wireless connectivity of PDAs emerges as an important function for the mobile role. Another key point of difference in the use of PDAs in the mobile role is the interaction between the date book, the address book, the e-mail, and the phone in a dynamic field setting. The interaction among the PDA functions makes it extremely important to interlink the functions, rendering easy changeover from one function to another possible.

6. SUMMARY AND CONCLUSION

The SUNA methodology outlined here proceeded from a broad of user/job types enunciated at the beginning of a brainstorming session to an abstraction of job/user types into user roles distinct in terms of needs, behaviour, expectations and job responsibilities. The method also allowed analysis based on formal job classification data. The characteristics of the user roles were clear enough to select two focal roles based on the objective of identifying early adopters of a technology that was still in its early stage of development. The methodology included testing on a small sample of users with an automatic logging system where possible. In the context of the log, it was feasible to understand the PDA usage in relation to the user roles and sub-roles through an extensive face-to-face interview. Analysis of the collected information indicated that the difference and commonalties in PDA usage was related to the difference and commonalties in the sub-roles. The focus on user roles rather than on individual users supported a 'big picture' perspective on the one hand, while it also brought out important similarities and differences between the focal user roles investigated.

From a product development perspective, SUNA precedes a fully-fledged UNA in the sense that SUNA focuses on strategic identification and selection of functions and meta-functions for targeted user groups whereas

UNA's focus is on analysing well-defined tasks and specific user profiles underlying detailed interface design.

The next steps are clearly to test and refine the SUNA methodology on larger samples for different user roles requiring wireless technologies, and to integrate it together with Usability Engineering into software and product development methodologies. It would be very interesting also to explore its conceptual usefulness in a complete Greenfield context in which the technology in question is at a concept stage.

7. REFERENCES

Beyer, H. & Holtzblatt, K. (1998), *Contextual Design: Defining Customer-Centered Systems*, Morgan Kaufmann Publishers, Inc., San Francisco.

Constantine, L., & Lockwood, L. (1999), *Software for Use: A Practical Guide to the Models and Methods of Usage-Centered Design*, ACM Press, New York.

Hackos, J.T. & Redish, J.C. (1998), *User And Task Analysis for Interface Design*, John Wiley & Sons, Inc. New York.

Kirwan, B. & Ainsworth, L.K. (eds.) (1992), *A Guide to Task Analysis*, Taylor & Francis, London.

Lindgaard, G. (1993), Wow - 568 smart features on your PABX: What really determines the uptake of technology? *International Symposium Human Factors in Telecommunications Proceedings*, Darmstadt, Germany, May 11-14.

Lindgaard, G. & Ferguson, J. (1992), Value for money?: The wonderful world of versatile PABX systems, *Telecom Research Laboratories Report NO. 8209.*

Maguire, M. (1997), *User-Requirements Framework Handbook*, HUSAT Research Institute, Loughborough, UK.

Mayhew, D.J. (1999), *The Usability Engineering Lifecycle: A Practitioner's Handbook For User Interface Design*, Morgan Kaufman Publishers, San Francisco, CA.

Narasimhan, S. (2001), *A User Needs Assessment for Personal Digital Assistants*, Unpublished Honours Thesis, Department of Psychology, Carleton University, Ottawa, Canada.

Shepherd, A. (2001), *Hierarchical Task Analysis*, Taylor & Francis, London.

Yankee Group, The. (August 1999), *Wireless/Mobile Data Applied Vertically: A Business Segmentation Model*, (Nortel Intranet).

Usability: Gaining a Competitive Edge
IFIP World Computer Congress 2002
J. Hammond, T. Gross, J. Wesson (Eds)
Published by Kluwer Academic Publishers

Exploring the Use of the Mobile Phone

Nadine Ozkan
CSIRO / CMIS
Currently: Lanterna Magica Inc,.433 St-Joseph west, # 20, Montreal, QUE, Canada H2V 2P3
email: nadine.ozkan@lanternamagica.com

Abstract: The work reported here provides insight into the practice of mobile communication. Interviews with experienced mobile phone users were conducted on specific instances of communications they placed, and the corpus gathered was analysed from the following three perspectives: why was a mobile phone used rather than another communication device; what was the intent or the goal of the communication, and, when appropriate, why was text messaging chosen over voice communication.

Results reveal the various punctual reasons that motivate the use of the mobile phone (such as its functionality, its cost, its ease of access), as well as the type of communications placed from a mobile phone. These reasons and communication types all concur to make this device the support of fluid and flexible social interactions and coordination. As to text messaging, it is considered as a medium in its own right, whose use is largely governed by emerging social conventions.

Key words: mobile communication, user practices, technology appropriation

1. INTRODUCTION: RESEARCH QUESTION

Mobile phones have gained extraordinary popularity since their introduction a few years ago. For example, at the time of writing this paper, an Ericsson advertisement claims that some 200 million SMS messages are sent around the world every day. Mobile communication can truly be described as a social phenomenon. Surprisingly however, mobile communication has not been much studied in the literature. The work presented here addresses this gap. The objective is to gather an understanding of the current usage patterns of the mobile phone: What constitutes mobile communication? What factors account for the choice of mobile communication as opposed to stationary communication? What habits and conventions emerge in the community of mobile users, and are re-enacted by this community? In addition, given that mobile phones today allow communication either by voice or text, we also must address the question of the factors motivating mobile phone users' choice between these two channels.

In our investigations, we have chosen to focus specifically on mobile phone usage for communication of a personal nature, i.e., exclusive of work-related communication. This is motivated by two reasons. The first is that, while much work has been devoted to distance communication and collaboration in work settings, mobile communication for personal reasons is still a largely unexplored area. (Some of the studies that have provided insight include (Carroll et al., 2001; Ling and Yttri, 1999; Palen et al., 2000).) The second reason is that the mobile phone has become an ubiquitous device, whose initial use at acquisition time might be instrumental, i.e., motivated by specific tasks (either work-related or for use in the coordination of family life), but whose usage pattern quickly becomes in practice an integrated part of life (Ling and Yttri, 1999; Palen et al., 2000), supporting a diverse range of personal communication.

This is especially true of the population that is currently a great consumer of mobile communication, namely teenagers and young adults. This population does not perceive the use mobile phone as instrumental, but rather as a support for social integration, negotiation and networking (Carroll et al, 2001; Ling and Yttri, 1999). Our investigations must therefore also have a special focus on this important population segment.

2. METHOD DESCRIPTION

We chose to address our research question using a qualitative method. This is motivated by the fact that, as previously mentioned, very little has been published on the use of mobile phones which would have enabled us to approach the problem with an initial set of hypothesis. Given this lack of substantial and current information, we needed to uncover large trends of usage patterns. A qualitative approach, well suited to the detailed observation of a small number of cases and yielding contextually rich information that can be analysed from a number of perspectives, was therefore in order.

We interviewed 13 mobile phone owners, each day for a period of a week, asking them to tell us about each of the personal calls or text messages they placed in the last 24 hours. Note that because our study is focused on factors that motivate the choice of the mobile phone, we were only interested in out-going communications, not in in-coming ones. Indeed, users only make the choice to use the mobile phone when they place a call, not when they answer one. We had provided the informants with small, custom-made diaries in which they could record their outgoing communications and which they could carry around with their mobile phone. The role of these mini-diaries was to act as a memory jotter: the idea was for the informants to record enough of the conversation or message to remember it at the time of the interview.

The age range of the informants was between 19 and 33, with an average of 25. There were 6 females and 7 males. Three were full-time workers and parents and the other 10 were full-time students, living with their parents. Most of the latter were also part-time workers. All the participants, like most people today had busy lifestyles: students all had one or two part-time jobs, workers had families to attend to, and all had extensive social networks.

All the participants were experienced mobile phone users. Indeed, results from (Palen et al, 2000) show that early patterns of use and early perception of the mobile phone differs substantially from stabilized ones. We were interested in stabilized usage patterns.

Each interview gathered the following information:

- the reasons for the communication and its general content,
- the circumstances of the communication: when and from where it was placed, with a special focus on public or private spaces, its degree of urgency, of sensitivity, etc.,
- the background to the communication or its general circumstances – e.g., is it part of a regular pattern, was it pre-agreed or expected in some sense, what were the caller's set of motivations, etc.,
- the relationship between the sender and the recipient(s) (in decreasing order of familiarity: family, close friends, distant friends or acquaintances, service or goods provider),
- whether the communication was the only activity performed at the time (the main task), or whether it was performed in conjunction with or in support of another (a secondary task),
- the reasons for choosing the text channel when this was the case. We focused on the reasons for choosing text (as opposed to the reasons for either voice or text), because we quickly realised that voice is perceived by mobile phone users are the default, natural choice, while text messaging is a decision.

We also asked each informant the following general questions:

- their age,
- their family situation and their occupation (student, working part-time or full time, etc.),
- their experience as regular mobile phone users,
- their initial reason for buying a mobile phone,
- the cost structure for their mobile communications (i.e., their costing plans).

3. RESULTS AND ANALYSIS

We collected a total of 138 "stories" about specific mobile communications: 89 about outgoing calls, and 49 about outgoing text messages. As expected given our focus on personal communication, all but 2 instances were of communications with close friends or family.

We analysed the stories we gathered from three perspectives, each of which is discussed in detail in the next sections. First, we examined the reasons invoked by the informants for choosing mobile communication. Secondly we examined the nature of the communication itself – its contents and its intent (or goal). Thirdly, we examine the reasons for using text messaging (as opposed to a phone call).

3.1 Reasons for choosing a mobile communication device

Here, we report the reasons participants invoked for choosing to place a communication from their mobile phone, rather communicating in another way (including face-to-face and the use of a landline). The main reasons for using a mobile phone are discussed below (also see Table 1).

Reason	% of communications logged
phone functionality	28.3
cost structure	28.3
perceived only option	18.9
travelling	16.7
spontaneity of communication	15.2
appropriate for circumstances	7.2
spontaneity of event	6.5
urgency / time-criticality	5.8
fill dead time	5.1

Table 1. Reasons for choosing a mobile device

Note that any one communication could be motivated by a combination of several reasons.

Phone functionality. A good proportion of calls are made from mobile phones simply because they offer functionality that most land phones do not. Among these, the most cited are the call history, which automatically stores the phone numbers of incoming and outgoing calls, the personalized phone book and the fact that a stored number does not need to be dialled by the phone user. Even in situations where a landline is available and would be cheaper, the mobile phone can be preferred because users can look up a number easily and avoid dialling. Many participants also prefer to call back someone who called their mobile phone from their mobile phone, again because dialling can be done automatically.

Cost structure. The user's costing plan is an important reason for using the mobile phone. For example, under some circumstances (time of day, carrier company of recipient mobile, etc.) calls are free for some period of time (typically 20 minutes). Under other types of costing plans, users pay a fixed amount per month for a fixed allocated use time, and want to utilize this as much as possible (without going over, of course). Maximizing utility for cost is an important factor motivating calls from the mobile phone, including in non-mobile situations (e.g., from home, instead of the landline). Cost is also an important parameter in the choice of sending a text message, especially when the goal of the communication is not specific, but linked to "relationship maintenance" (see below, section 3.2).

Perceived only option. Even when other options are available, such as landlines or public phones, the mobile phone is often perceived as the "only option" because of its ease of access. For example, participants used the mobile phone from their bed, in order to avoid getting up, even if a landline was available in another room. Similarly, participants use the mobile phone while walking on the street, disregarding the option of public phones.

Travelling. Travelling (including walking, being in a car or public transport) here describes a reason for placing a communication, rather than as a description of the activity that occurred while communicating. To illustrate the difference, a call to finalize the details of a meeting place in order to plan one's route would fall in this category, while a call placed to chat while stuck in traffic would not. It is interesting to note that travelling is not a major reason for using the mobile phone. Even communications placed while travelling (i.e., travelling as a description of the circumstances of the call rather than as its reason) only make-up a minority of the communications we gathered.

Spontaneity of communicating. This category includes communications that had to be placed and were placed as soon as the participant thought of it. (It differs from the "spontaneity of event" category, described next, which includes communication to spontaneously arrange a meeting or event. Here, we refer to communications that had to be placed anyway.) The mobile phone allows users to avoid remembering to call and planning their communications in "batches".

Appropriateness for circumstances. We gathered several instances of a group sitting in a restaurant or café and deciding to contact a common friend who is not present, either to invite him or her or to just keep in touch. Here, the mobile phone enables seizing the opportunity as it presented itself.

Spontaneity of event. The mobile phone allows users to have unplanned encounters with friends (e.g., "I'm at the university coffee shop, come and meet me here"). This is valid for both text messaging and phone calls.

Urgency, time criticality. A small number of instances involved urgent or time-critical communications. The mobile phone enables communication in a reactive and timely manner. While issues of safety and urgency may initially motivate the acquisition of a mobile phone (Palen et al, 2000), they only accounted for a small proportion of actual use in stabilized practice in our study.

To fill dead time. Many calls are placed because "I was bored and decided to call a friend". This is typically the case on public transport, during a boring lecture or seminar, or while stuck in traffic. Sometime calling or sending a text message at a "dead time" is planned by the user, e.g., "I thought I would "text" him from the airport because I knew I would have time to kill there." The calls or messages which were placed in such "dead times" were mostly of the "relationship maintenance" type (see below).

These results show that the reasons why people use mobile phones are far from being only linked to mobility. As shown above, there are numerous reasons that motivate people to use their mobile phones, even when a landline is available.

It is also worth noting that teenagers and young adults often use the mobile phone as a personal line (instead of having a second home phone with a different number). Pragmatically, this type of arrangement keeps individual communication bills separate from household bills, and the mobile phone is viewed as a landline with additional capabilities and convenience. But there is also a social factor at play here. For people in this age range, social networking is vital and contributes in an important way to self-identity. Thus social communication is viewed as a highly personal activity. Having a personal, exclusive communication device re-enforces this feeling. (See (Carroll et al., 2001) for the role of the mobile phone on the formation of identity and a sense of belonging.)

Cost is an important consideration in the use of the mobile phone, and it plays a dual role: it can act as a motivator, for example when calls to a mobile phone are cheaper if placed from a mobile than if place from landline, but can also act as a barrier: several of the participants complained that they had problems controlling the costs of their mobile communications – use of the mobile phone is described as "addictive".

Finally, it seems many of the reasons invoked for using a mobile phone (as opposed to another communication device, or to face-to-face communication when it is possible) revolve around its enhanced capabilities as compared to a landline (e.g., the "functionality" category above), its ease of access (e.g. "perceived only option", "urgency", "fill dead time") and its flexibility and timeliness (e.g. "spontaneity of communication", "spontaneity of event", "appropriate for circumstances"). These attributes are especially well suited to the requirements of our participants for a "fluid" lifestyle. By "fluid", we mean flexible, reactive to changing circumstances with minimum effort.

3.2 Intents of mobile communication

We now turn to the intents or goals of the communications we gathered. We found two broad types of communications from a mobile phone: relationship maintenance and coordination of events. They are discussed here, and summarised in Table 2. (Note that the same communication could have several distinct intents.)

Intent	% of communications logged
Planning and coordination	71.1
organise a meeting or event	26.1
"plastic" plan	19.6
changes to firm plans	18.1
initiation of a regular plan	5.1
co-ordinate resource / task sharing	2.2
Relationship maintenance	27.5
Others - Miscellaneous	15.9

Table 2. Intents of mobile communication

A substantial proportion of the communications we logged concerned expressions of feelings, keeping in touch with friends, informing a partner of one's whereabouts, or simply chitchats. We refer to this type of communication as relationship maintenance. The use of the mobile phone for relationship maintenance is very diverse. It ranges from short text messages (e.g., one word to a girlfriend), to regular 20 minutes chats at times when the use of the mobile phone is free.

One type of relationship maintenance communications concerned what we term "loose keeping in touch". "Loose keeping in touch" concerns the general expression of friendship or love with no sense of urgency or timeliness – for example, daily long chitchats with a boyfriend or girlfriend. Some of these communications may also be short "drops" that do not require interactivity and hence are especially well suited to text messaging (e.g., "boring lecture, thinking of you"). For example, one participant told us she often "texts" people she sees every day just to say hello. Other examples include keeping friends and relatives informed of significant events in one's life (e.g. "just bought a new bike" or "got a good mark on my exam").

In this regard, we found that there seems to be an emerging "etiquette" for choosing the appropriate channel for "loose keeping in touch" communications: the channel chosen seems to depend on the closeness of the relationship between the conversing parties. For example, to express good wishes (for a birthday, travel, etc.) to close friends, our participants would call, while they would favour sending a message to distant friends.

Another type of relationship maintenance communication we gathered concerned more pressing or compelling motivations. In these cases, calling is chosen over "texting", probably because voice communication is "richer" than text (it has more cues, it conveys presence better) and because interactivity is important. Let us report two revealing examples of this. In the first instance, a student phoned her boyfriend before entering an exam room because "I was nervous and talking to him calms me down". In the second instance, a young child was disturbed by that fact that her mother was away at work one afternoon, and asked her father to ring up Mom from the day-care "just to hear her voice". In these cases, emotional support and reassurance were sought, and vocal mobile communication was appropriate in addressing these needs in a flexible, time-sensitive way, regardless of location.

The other large category of intent concerned the coordination of actions and events, especially of meetings and rendezvous. This has been referred to elsewhere as the micro-coordination of life events (Ling and Yttri, 1999). There are several types of coordination which have emerged from our study, and which seemed typical of mobile communication. They are described below.

Organising an event. An important proportion of the communications we logged were placed to organize meetings or event (of other types than "plastic planning" – see below). Text messaging is frequently used for organizing group events since users can take advantage of the "group-send" functionality. In these cases, the communication is terse, resting on a good deal of common knowledge among the parties.

The "plastic plan". We borrow the term "plastic plan" from one of our participants to refer to a plan that is only sketched when first established, and gradually refined over several communications. Access to mobile communication allows people to have initially vague plans (e.g., "Meet me for lunch in the city"), which are refined gradually or on the spot (e.g., "I'm on my way to the city now, meet you in half an hour at Town Hall."). "Plastic planning" definitely constitutes a strongly emerging way of coordinating social rendezvousing. This finding echoes the "softening of time" referred to in (Ling and Yttri, 1999). One participant told us that the reason he acquired a mobile phone was that he missed several rendezvous' with his friends, all mobile phone users, because he could not be reached at the time of "firming up the plan". Plastic planning allows flexibility and reactivity, and thus is well suited to the lifestyle of the young population.

Changes to firm plans. This especially concerns notifications of delays when a firm plan was made, but unexpected events prevent it from happening as planned (e.g., traffic delays). Other instances are change of plans (e.g., "I've changed my mind about the lift, have you left the parking lot yet?"), and people losing each other in a crowd (e.g., "I've lost you, where are you?").

Initiation of a regular plan. Text messaging is used to trigger or confirm regular meetings with minimum communication content. Again, this type of message relies heavily on implicit, shared knowledge among the participants, hence its brevity. For example, the message "meet me before the lecture" is understood to mean "meet me at the university café, 15 minutes before the lecture and bring your lecture notes so I can photocopy them". The place, precise time and purpose of the rendezvous are known to the participants through previous shared experiences, and therefore don't need to be specified. The communication serves as either a trigger or a confirmation of a regular plan.

Coordinate resource or task sharing. This concerns for example coordinating the sharing of the household car in a flexible and time-sensitive way. Tasks also are distributed in this way (e.g., "I'll pick up food on the way home")

In synthesis, most communications with mobile phones pertain to relationship maintenance or to coordination. "Plastic planning", which. allows for fluid social coordination and can only be possible with a mobile phone, seems to be a growing phenomenon, as it is especially well suited to the life style of the young population. These observations indicate that the mobile phone is an essential element supporting the elaboration and maintenance of social life for our participants.

3.3 Reasons for text messaging

Note that while land phones (private or public) are competing devices to mobile phones, there is no competitor to text messaging. (Email and instant messaging are far from being the stationary equivalent to text messaging, as they are very different in terms of overheads, accessibility, length and complexity of messages, functionality, etc. They are perceived as other mediums altogether.) Still, sending a text message is generally perceived as the secondary use of the mobile phone, while phoning is its primary use, the "default" option. Consequently, sending a text message require an actual choice from our participants (contrary to phoning).

Below are the characteristics of text messaging which were specifically invoked as motivations for its use (see also Table 3).

Reason	% of textual communications logged
recipient friendly	36.7
avoid conversation	28.6
channel consistency	20.4
non-instrumental info. drop	20.4
socially acceptable to text	12.2
cost vs. calling	8.2
fall back option	8.2
"send to group" functionality	6.1

Table 3. Reasons for text messaging

Recipient-friendly. Because it is not interactive, text messaging is perceived as more "recipient-friendly" than calling: it leaves the recipient in charge of when to take the communication, and whether to answer it or not. It has been described by our participants as more "discreet" and more "appropriate" than calling, especially when the recipient is thought to be unavailable (e.g., busy or sleeping). Hence, non urgent communications are often transmitted through text rather than voice.

Avoid conversation. Our participants often send a message when they do not want to engage in conversation but still want to communicate. In many cases, this may be for the sake of time or efficiency. Here, text messaging seems to have the equivalent function to calling someone's vocal mailbox. In addition, probably because it is not interactive, messaging is also perceived as providing a "social distance" relatively to a phone call. As mentioned above, this is considered appropriate when the communicating parties are not in a close relationship.

Channel consistency. An important number of text messages were sent because "I was answering a previous text message so I didn't want to call". Text messaging is often used in response to an in-coming text message. This refers to a phenomenon that may be termed "channel consistency", whereby someone prefers to return a communication in the same channel as it was received. Reasons behind this may involve a sense of social appropriateness: if the initiator of a communication has chosen one channel, then it is considered appropriate that follow-up communications should be made using that same channel.

Non-instrumental information drops. Text messaging is also used for one-way "non-instrumental" information drops, i.e., for communications that are merely informative, not urgent, and do not specifically contribute to a task (e.g., "got a good mark on my exam"). There is often a pre-existing arrangement, implicit or explicit, that information will be sent, but this is not necessarily the case. Again, text messaging is preferred here because no interaction with the interlocutor is required.

Socially acceptable to text. For the sender, text messaging is also more discreet and, not being interactive, less demanding in terms of attention. It is used in "public" situations, or in situations where talking on the phone would not be socially appropriate: during a lecture, on busy public transport or in small group settings without isolating oneself from the conversation. For example, we encountered instances of participants sending text messages while with a group of friends – sending a message allowed them to continue interacting with the group, while isolating one self to place a phone call would have been perceived as rude to the group.

Cost compared to calling. Text messaging is also used as the cheaper alternative to calling. We see again that cost is a consideration for mobile phone users, but, surprisingly given that "texting" is considerably cheaper than calling, it did not emerge as a major factor for our participants.

Fall back option. In a minority of cases, a text message is sent when calling fails. Here, reasons might be that the recipient's mobile phone has poor reception or is switched off.

Group communication. Text messaging is used to communicate to a group in a succinct way, taking full advantage of abbreviations and pre-established codes. Here, users take advantage of the "send to group" functionality of the phone.

In conclusion, it is interesting to note that text messaging is mostly used as a communication channel in its own right, not merely as a fall back option. In addition, the use of text messaging seems to be guided by emerging social conventions: in some circumstances, it is judged more appropriate either for the sender or the recipient, than calling. Finally, and contrary to the general findings regarding the use of the mobile phone (section 3.1), text messaging is only marginally motivated by phone functionality (e.g. the "group send") and costs.

4. CONCLUSION: WHAT HAVE WE LEARNED AND HOW IS IT USEFUL?

The various factors which were uncovered by this study as motivating the use of the mobile phone, such as its functionality, its cost, its ease of access and its flexibility, as well as the types of communications that are placed from a mobile phone (coordination and relationship maintenance) all contribute to support what we have termed "fluid" social interaction and coordination. The mobile phone is not exclusively used in mobile situations.

Indeed, its use is much larger than strictly linked to one set of circumstances: it has a major role in supporting today's lifestyles.

Another interesting results of this survey is the fact that the use of the mobile phone is governed by an emerging "mobility etiquette", which, albeit probably still in formation, has nonetheless a definite influence in how and when to communicate. This is especially true for text messaging.

Thirdly, findings pertaining to the use of text messaging show that it is considered as a medium in its own right, not only as a fall back option.

Understanding the practices around the use of a particular technology is useful in many ways. Firstly, this understanding helps to design new enhancements to that technology. For example, mobile phone companies have announced that they will shortly release a miniature camera to be hooked on the mobile phone, thereby adding video communication, synchronous and asynchronous, to the two channels (text and voice) currently available to the mobile phone user. Undoubtedly, the uptake of the "mobile videophone" will be rooted in the current practices of mobile phone users. Understanding the latter can therefore give clues to forecast the former, and thus help in the definition and positioning of mobile video communication.

Another benefit of understanding user practices is to add to current knowledge regarding technology adoption. The investigation presented here is an exploration into the factors that lead to voluntary technology adoption (notwithstanding the social factors in play) for "recreational" or personal purposes, (i.e., not work-related). We have not referred, in this study, to theoretical frameworks of technology adoption or acceptance, for example as those defined in (Davis, 1993; Rogers, 1995), because these frameworks pertain to the work place and to technologies that support work functions. We submit that "recreational" technologies are perceived, assessed and used in ways that are very different to work-related ones. Hence, a theory of technology adoption for personal use still needs to be built, based on case studies such as this one.

5. ACKNOWLEDGEMENTS

Many thanks to Robert Tot, from CSIRO/CMIS, for his participation to this study.

6. REFERENCES

Carroll, J., Howard, S., Vetere, F., Peck, J. & Murphy, J. (2001), Identity, Power and Fragmentation in Cyberspace: Technology Appropriation by the Young People. Working Paper 01/IDG/2001, Dept. of Information Systems, University of Melbourne, Australia. Available at http://www.dis.unimelb.edu.au/staff/idgroup/workingpapers.htm

Davis, F.D. (1993), User acceptance of information technology: system characteristics, user perceptions and behavioral impacts, *International Journal of Man-Machine Studies*, Vol. 38, No. 3, pp. 475-487.

Lenhart, A., Rainie, L., Lewis, O. (2001), Teenage Life Online: The rise of the instant-message generation and the Internet's impact on friendships and family relationships. Pew Internet Project report, June. http://www.pewinternet.org/reports/toc.asp?Report=36

Ling, R. & Yttri, B. (1999), Nobody sits at home and waits for the telephone to ring: Micro and hyper-coordination through the use of the mobile telephone. Telenor R&D report 30/99. ISBN 82-423-0505-6.

Palen, L. Salzman, M. & Young, E. (2000), Going Wireless: Behavior and Practice of New Mobile Phone Users. *Proceedings of the Computer Supported Collaborative Work (CSCW)'00 Conference* (Philadelphia, Pennsylvania Dec.), ACM Press, pp. 201-210.

Rogers, Everett, M. (1995), *Diffusion of Innovations*. Free Press, New York, (fourth edition).

Usability: Gaining a Competitive Edge
IFIP World Computer Congress 2002
J. Hammond, T. Gross, J. Wesson (Eds)
Published by Kluwer Academic Publishers

Usability Engineering Milestones In Complex Product Development - Experiences At Nokia Mobile Phones

Industrial Experience

Pekka Ketola
Nokia Mobile Phones, Finland

Abstract: How can usability engineering be managed in highly complex innovative product development? When usability engineering is performed in Concurrent Engineering (CE) product development, there are stages where usability engineering needs to be refocused in order to perform successfully in the changing project environment. The focusing points follow the product development milestones but are not identical with those. From usability engineering perspective those points are critical for achieving effectiveness and efficiency in the product development.

Key words: Usability engineering, concurrent engineering, industry experience

1. INTRODUCTION

Product development of information appliances is often based on fast Concurrent Engineering (CE) (Valjus, 1994) due to need for cost, time and quality efficiency. The pace is given by strong competition and business situation in the industry and markets.

The phases of sequential product design, for example the Waterfall method (Royce, 1970), are requirement analysis, specification (definition), design, implementation, integration and testing. In Concurrent Engineering there are several parallel sequential design areas, for example mechanics, hardware and software, synchronized via common milestones in order to ensure an optimal timetable and to minimize implementation risks. Milestones are places where the organization decides whether it is time to continue to next phase, and sometimes design compromises need to be done (acceptable design is preferred instead of best design).

Efficient usability engineering works in an effective and competent manner in the current development phase with little wasted effort. Efficiency can be measured by comparing realization (output) against usability engineering goals, plans and amount of work (input).

Effective usability engineering aims to produce an adequate or desired result. It can be measured by studying how usable the final product is, or by analysing field feedback. During product development the effectiveness can be estimated, for example, by comparing the performed usability work against the number of usability engineering originated design changes. Planning benefits, in general, are difficult to assess using objective measures. Perceptual measures, such as fulfilment of planning objectives as a measure of planning effectiveness, have better success (Premkumar and King, 1994).

It is important to understand the particular product development environment and to know the opportunities and limitations that different product development phases and concurrency set for usability engineering, in order to perform effective and efficient usability engineering. The objective of this study is to examine what kinds of usability improvements are possible in smart phone (Figure 1) development phases and how product development stages actuate usability engineering. This research problem has been addressed in Keinonen et al. (1996). Our approach to usability engineering is holistic, i.e. it views the product usability as an entity that is built from the user interface (hardware and software), the external interface and the service interface (Ketola and Röykkee, 2001).

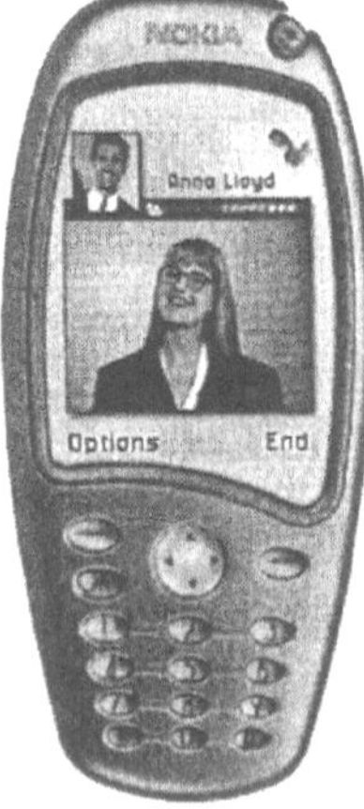

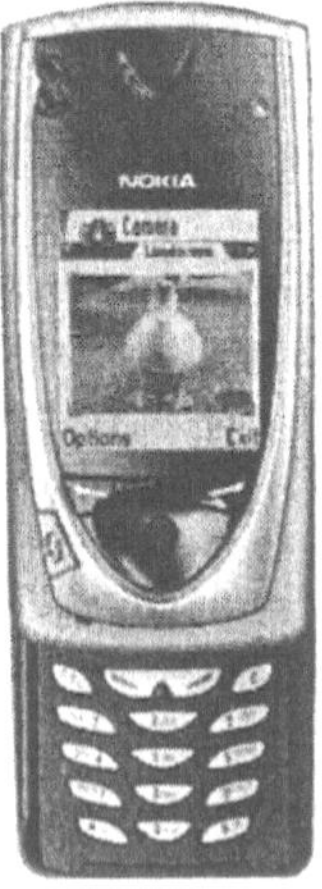

Figure 1. An example of a smart phone concept (left) and a smart phone (right) (Nokia 7650).

Research reports and literature (Keinonen et al., 1996; Trenner and Bawa, 1998; Mayhew, 1999; Raddle and Young, 2001), describe the practical usability engineering problems in product development and solutions for those problems. The two basic problems are:

- usability engineering is done too late and
- lack of management support for usability engineering.

If the development organization is not well adapted to human-centred design these problems are likely to appear. In addition to these problems, in fast paced CE it is simply difficult to usability engineer all needed parallel design and engineering areas. Concurrent product development is a complex engineering environment. The complexity results from (Tianfield, 2001):

- complexity of the product's (technical) structure,
- complexity of development organization and
- complexity of user requirements (late and difficult-to-identify user requirements).

Current understanding and description of sequential product development phases does not give much support for serious usability engineering in a Concurrent Engineering project. It does not match with human-centred design. Hakiel (1997b) emphasizes the need for product engineering across disciplines rather than software engineering. This raises a practical problem in concurrent product development: If the product is complex and resources limited, what usability activities should be performed and when?

Though the usability engineering lifecycle is well defined and known, it is often difficult to apply human-centred design in concurrent product development lifecycle due to the fast development pace, complexities and because the product development is not fundamentally based on human-centred approach. However, the more complex the product is technically or conceptually, the more important it is to involve elements from human-centred design and to usability-engineer the product (Keinonen et al., 1996).

1.1 Previous work

Standards and guidelines (ISO 13407; Mayhew, 1999; Daly-Jones et al., 1999) define how human-centred design should be performed to provide usable systems. The assumption is that the product development process is based on human-centred design or the desired development mode is human-centred. Hakiel (1997) claims that though we have the knowledge how to do it, the problem is that we do not routinely do what we know.

Hakiel discusses how usability engineering can be integrated with software engineering. He notes that though key development principles and processes are the same in software and usability engineering, they apply to different domains. In software processes, the emphasis is on the quality of code, i.e. defect free code, while the emphasis in usability engineering is on user requirements. Hakiel presents two contrasting approaches to product engineering: (1) usability design deliverables are aligned with software design deliverables (upper part in Figure 2) and (2) usability design deliverables are contributing to software requirements (lower part in Figure 2). He emphasizes the distinction between design for use, which leads to the specification of an information technology artefact, and software development, which leads to the implementation of the artefact in software.

Usability design deliverables aligned with SW design deliverables

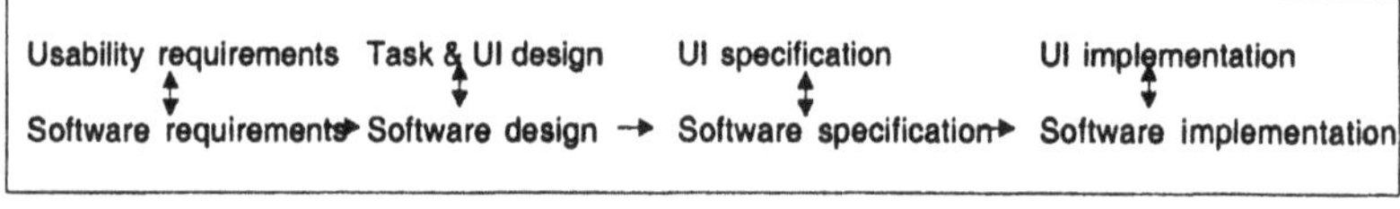

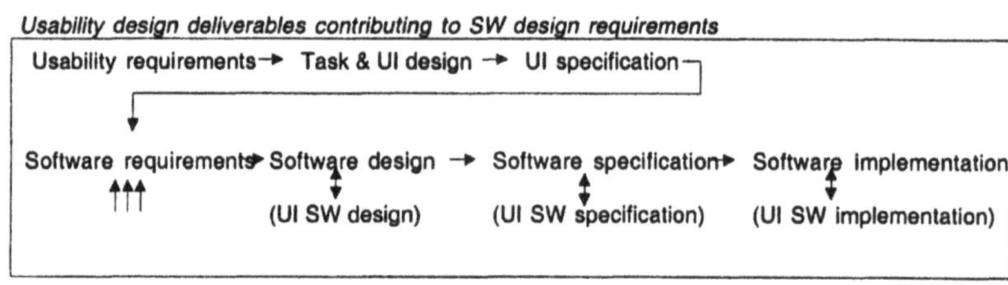

Figure 2. Contrasting usability and software engineering approaches.

It would be ideal to perform all design for use before software development. However, my observations from mobile phone development indicate that Concurrent Engineering forces UI and SW design to be aligned to concurrent development phases, especially when innovative features are designed.

Keinonen et al. (1996) studied the problem of designing increasingly complex devices. They concluded that usability can be embedded in the product development, but there must be a market-driven or intra-organizational need for change. The need for intra-organizational demand pull is also noted by Kaderbhai (1998). An industry review during 1996 showed that usability is basically a familiar concept but the essential part of usability engineering, user involvement, is still a non-utilized resource (Nieminen and Parkkinen, 1998).

While my study describes experiences at Nokia Mobile Phones, Korhonen (2000) gives an overview of usability research at Nokia Research Center. This overview gives a basic understanding of the various usability engineering activities in the research areas that precede the actual product development.

1.2 Project Approach

The findings of this study are based on several mobile phone development projects (Table 1) that were based on Concurrent Engineering and where usability was a design goal. One project served as a case project for usability engineering. In the case project, the usability work was based on a particular Usability Plan (Ketola, 2001). The results were further assessed in three other projects by doing a hands-on trial. This approach provides reliability of the results, at least, in the mobile phone development.

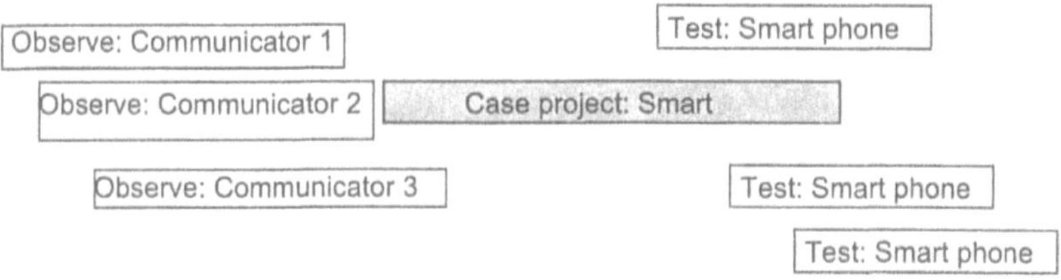

Table 1. Projects followed in the study

The research problem was to answer the following questions:

- What are the critical points for usability engineering in a concurrent product development?
- How should usability engineering be refocused in those points in order to perform effective and efficient design and usability actions?
- What is the exact difference (turning point) when moving from early to late design in Concurrent Engineering product development?

Concurrent product development sets both limitations and opportunities for usability engineering. During the projects it became clear that there are predictable turning points in product development where the usability engineering needs to be refocused. I call those usability engineering milestones. In addition, concurrency gives the perspective that there is no single early and late design phase, but one product development lifecycle contains at least two early and late phases in different engineering areas.

1.3 Description of the case project

This case study is based on one project (a smart phone product development cycle at Nokia Mobile Phones) where CE product development process is improved by integrating usability engineering activities with the process. The aim of the product development project is to create a new "leading edge" smart phone product with several novel technologies, new form factors and new interaction styles. Key functions of the phone are quality with excellent messaging and imaging capabilities, exciting and easy-to-use interfaces, compact concepts, attractive designs and entertaining. The product enables the users to create and manage personal visual content (digital pictures) in a way that enables easy picture messaging from phone to phone and from phone to any network service.

2. CONCURRENT ENGINEERING

In a CE project, several product development teams work in parallel. The aim is to provide agreed deliverables in agreed timeframes, and finally integrate the components. It must be noted that parallel design defined by Nielsen (1994) is a different concept. Nielsen handles parallel design as a method for developing and evaluating competing designs.

Figure 3 describes the basic concurrent development process model from Fujitsu (Ayoama, 1993). Concurrent Engineering is highly applicable in product development where the final product consists of multiple integrated technologies or engineering outcomes, for example integrated software, hardware and mechanics.

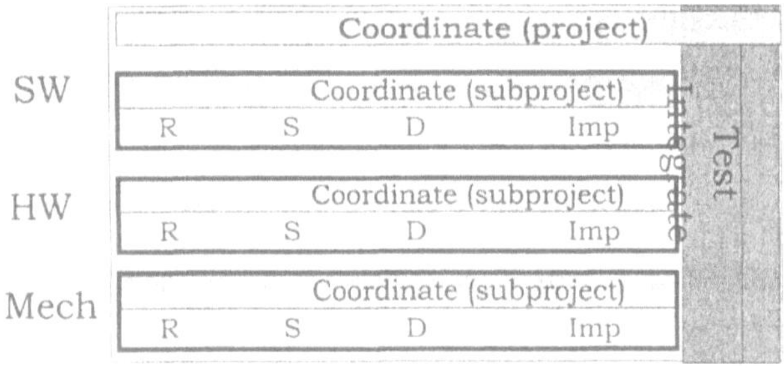

Figure 3. Concurrent development model with coordination between Requirements (R), Specification (S), Design (D) and Implementation (I).

The engineering practice inside a development team need not be sequential, but it can follow other more efficient processes. For example, incremental development may be appropriate for SW engineering, while waterfall design works better with hardware engineering. Thus, CE is more product development coordination than product implementation method.

Coordination and execution activities are performed both in the main process (project level) and sub-processes (engineering teams). The execution processes can be independent, i.e. they are not directly dependent on other sub-processes. The coordination processes are often tightly interconnected, especially in the late development phases.

2.1 Concurrent Engineering Dependencies

In mobile phone product development there are several practical dependencies between engineering areas.

- product requirements, product concept, technical product platform and industrial design define the initial development frames for all engineering areas.
- industrial design defines the overall dimensions of the product and the main factors for mechanical design.
- mechanical design defines the position and size of all product components and the available dimensions for hardware.
- hardware defines main performance issues, such as display capabilities, memory size and processor efficiency. Hardware enables certain software performance.
- software defines the software-based user interface capabilities.

The above-mentioned engineering areas have a final effect on user interface and so are potential subjects for usability engineering. From a user perspective, the product should provide quality of use. This implies that usability engineering should be done in areas that have an effect on quality of use and usability. In a mobile phone, the areas extend from software to, for example, hardware, mechanics, ergonomics, out-of-box readiness, even network services.

3. USABILITY ACTIVITIES IN PRODUCT DEVELOPMENT PHASES

Following the product development phases, the already known project milestones (M) with usability activities are:

- M0: Start of usability engineering. The milestone is typically followed (or preceded) by requirements analysis and product specification.
- M1: Start of product design. This milestone starts (or continues) early design and formative usability evaluation. Usability engineering is done with low fidelity prototypes. The units for measuring effectiveness and efficiency are the number of identified design improvements and the capability to propagate the improvements to product design.
- M2: Start of detailed design and implementation. Usability engineering is performed with high fidelity prototypes.

- M3: Start of summative usability evaluation. This milestone starts usability evaluation in order to produce summative data about the product. The measuring units for effectiveness and efficiency are the number of found usability problems and the usability of the final product.
- M4: Start of field feedback.
- M5: End of usability engineering. In most cases in the scope of this study, product usability engineering was ended before M4.

A notable observation is that the dimensions for measuring efficiency and effectiveness are different in M1 (capability to propagate the improvements to product design) and M3 (usability of the final product). The milestones (M0 to M5) and their position in product development phases are presented in Table 2.

M0		M1		M2		M3		M4		M5
	Specify product		Design		Implement and integrate		Test		Launch	

Table 2. Milestones and development phases.

Usability engineering milestones are product development stages where usability engineering needs to be refocused in order to provide efficiency and effectiveness in the changing development environment. A milestone is identified, for example, from the following characteristics:

- the project priorities or goals are defined or changed.
- a usability activity starts or ends (new usability activity starts, old activity is changed or ended).
- formal design support changes to summative design evaluation.
- target setting changes to planning, planning changes to follow-up.
- project practices for coordinating design changes is changed.
- usability engineering tool changes (for example from simulation to product prototype).

4. NEW USABILITY MILESTONES VIA HORIZONTAL AND VERTICAL REVIEW

Concurrent product development increases the number and changes the content of previously introduced usability engineering milestones. In the following the CE process is studied horizontally and vertically.

4.1 Horizontal review

By horizontal project review (lifecycle perspective) it is possible to identify the actual product development phases and their characteristics, and to estimate the potential effectiveness of usability engineering.

Figure 4 shows how many design *changes* were made in different design phases and design areas in the case project. The data was created by interviewing designers and engineering managers of the specific design areas, and by analysing the proposed and implemented design changes. The bottom line in the figure presents the situation where no changes are done.

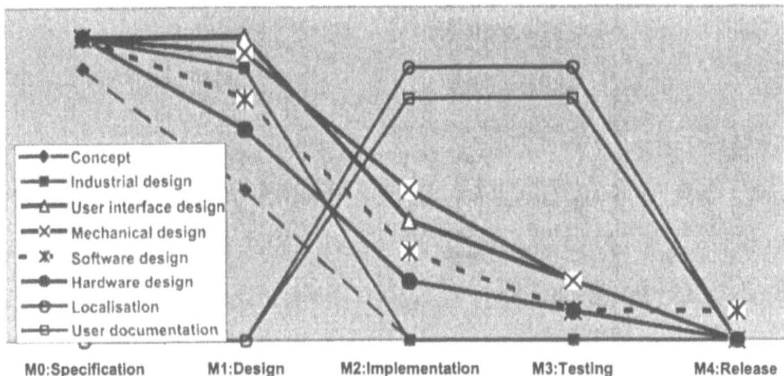

Figure 4. Doable product design changes in CE milestones

The findings based on a horizontal project view are:

1. Most product design (industrial, user interface, mechanical, software and hardware design) changes are made between M0 and M2.
2. Some changes are made even in very late design phases (software, localization, user documentation).
3. Near M2 the product concept freezes. In this milestone the development team knows exactly for the first time what the product should be like. Before concept freezing, the organization is defining the product, i.e. there are design options. After concept freezing the organization focuses on implementing the concept and there are minimal design options. The product requirements are defined much earlier (M0), but in order to design and implement new features or technologies for the first time it is necessary to leave the possibility for design changes to late design (Hakiel, 1997b). This increases design uncertainty and design teams must be alert for implementing even surprising design needs.

4. The turning point from early design (creating the design) to late design (design changes and improvements) can be estimated. The turning point can be seen at M2. In the observed projects, this was the point when the development organization started to use a design change management control mechanism.
5. Supporting engineering areas (localization, user documentation) have early and late design phases.
6. Two freezing patterns can be detected. First, the main engineering areas (software, mechanics, hardware) freeze gradually from M0 to M2. Secondly, supporting engineering areas have a main design phase between M2 and M3 with fast freezing speed. Hence, product development has two separate design phases: product design and support material design.

From this horizontal review, the following new milestones (M) can be proposed:

- M (EarlyToLate): Early design changes to late design.
- M (ConceptFreeze): Concept freezes. This gives us two important conceptual phases: pre-concept-freeze and post-concept-freeze design
- M (EarlyToLateSupportMaterial): Early design of user support material and localization changes to late design.

4.2 Vertical review

By studying a project from a vertical perspective (concurrency perspective) it is possible to identify the concurrency in product development phases, the effects of concurrency, and the potential usability engineering efficiency. The vertical findings based on Figure 4 are:

1. Development concurrency is real. For example, user interface design is concurrent with software design. User interface design is aligned with the software design instead of being a preceding action (compare Figure 2).
2. Designs freeze in a predictable order (1. concept, 2. hard design, 3. soft design, 4. Supporting designs).
3. Design changes are accepted in all design areas until M2.

4.3 Definition of early and late design phases

Product development can be divided into early and late design. The early design phase is characterized by interaction design and formative usability evaluations. Late design is characterized by detailed design and summative usability evaluations. Kiljander (1999), Nielsen (1994) and Mayhew (1999) emphasize the importance of focusing on early design phases instead of late phases due to high costs of changes in late phases. The estimate of increasing design change costs is based on findings in software engineering.

Earlier studies identify early design and late design as separate design phases. However, there is no definition of how a practitioner can identify the turning point from early to late design. Based on the observations above, I define early and late design phases for Concurrent Engineering project, and the milestone between these phases, as follows:

- **early design phase** is identified by high capability and interest of an organization to create new design, and accept and implement design changes to existing design. In the early design phase, the target of product development is to maximize the number of design improvements in the given timeframe.
- **early design phase changes to late design** when the organization decides to apply a (systematic) method for handling design change proposals.
- **late design phase** is identified by low capability and interest of an organization to create new design, and accept and implement design changes to existing design. In the late phase, the product development target is to minimize the number of design changes in order to manage project timetables and risks.

The ultimate goal of usability engineering is to support the project in achieving the project goals of cost, quality and time-to-market. The distinction and implication of early and late design phases are important: maximise design efficiency, effectiveness and quality before M1 and minimize design changes after M1.

5. MILESTONES AND SIMULATIONS

The primary usability engineering tool is a product simulation or prototype. Depending on the product development phase, different simulations and prototypes are available, low-fidelity, high-fidelity or product prototypes.

The product entity is composed from the engineering results in the late development phase (Figure 3). When a new product is developed, there is not a working product prototype before integration phase. The implication is that usability engineering on the product entity is not possible in the early phase without the aid of advanced hardware or software simulation. Meanwhile, usability engineering is possible in the non-integrated engineering areas.

In typical mobile phone development phases, the following prototypes can be produced:

- Early design: low-fidelity (and high-fidelity) prototype, design mock-up, mechanics simulation
- Late design: (low-fidelity and) high-fidelity prototype, hardware prototypes, mechanics prototypes, partially working software
- Integration phase: partially working product prototype
- Testing phase: fully working product prototype.

The availability of prototypes and prototype functionality/maturity are major factors for usability engineering. Based on the prototype availability we can set prototype-based milestones (Mp) accordingly:

- Mp1: Low-fidelity prototypes and mock-ups available.
- Mp2: High-fidelity and mechanical prototypes available.
- Mp3: Partially working product prototype available.
- Mp4: Fully working product prototype available.

Kiljander (1999) discusses the importance of prototypes for mobile phone development. In order to perform efficient usability engineering in the early development phase, a product simulation is required. Thus, the development of simulation is an essential part of early product development and should be an integral part of product development process.

6. NEW MILESTONES AND JOB DESIGN

Milestones are important for job coordination. We have now seen that there are several possible milestones where the changes in design environment have an effect on usability engineering (Figure 5). Those places are related to:

- general product development stages
- capability to accept and implement design changes
- capability to perform iterative design
- current design environment, availability of prototypes.

New usability milestones do not mean that we need more bureaucracy in the project. Knowledge and awareness about milestones and turning points can be used in planning the usability work and job design, in the same way as landmarks, map and compass are needed for navigation. In the planning phase, by identifying the opportunities such as available prototyping tools, and limitations such as project state, the usability practitioner can prepare to work in an optimal way, effectively and efficiently.

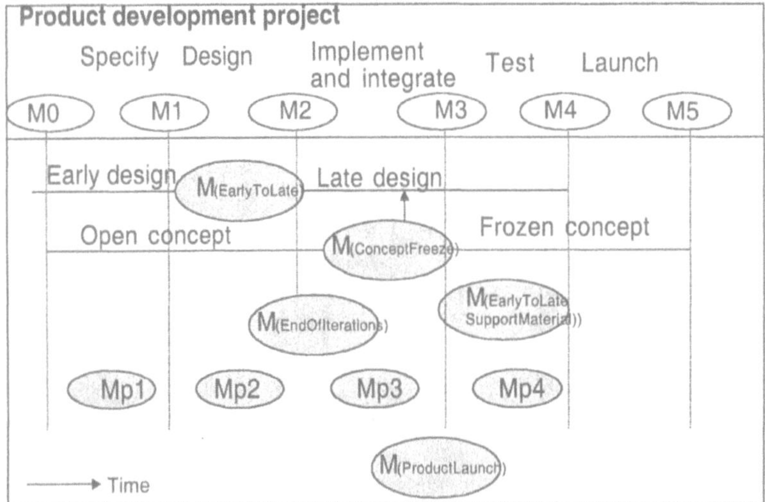

Figure 5. The effect of milestones during product development on usability engineering.

By taking milestones into consideration it is also possible to improve cost efficiency of usability engineering by focusing on areas where changes are possible and where usability engineering is mostly needed. New milestones have two practical consequences related to work organization:

- new usability engineering control points and follow-up mechanisms are needed.
- to some extent, job design or redesign is needed in each milestone. Earlier tasks can disappear and new ones arise (Järvinen, 1980).

The identification and definition of milestone M(EarlyToLate) is especially useful. The spontaneous tendency of designers is to improve the designs as long as possible, while the will of project management is to minimize all changes after M(EarlyToLate). An explicit definition of this milestone provides improved understanding of the common goals and helps to organize the design work in a better way.

The positive effect of new milestones is the improved ability to coordinate usability engineering. The negative effect of new milestones and job design is the unproductive nature of tasks. Control and job organization do not contribute to actual product development (Järvinen, 1999).

Usability engineering could also be coordinated with less milestones. Removing milestones would potentially lead to improved capability in following the principles of human-centred design, especially iterative design. The drawbacks would be weaker capability to organize the work in fast product development, and weaker visibility and linkage to the product development entity.

7. DISCUSSION AND CONCLUSIONS

The challenge of usability engineering in complex product development is to verify that the final product is usable and that sufficient usability engineering is done in all design areas that have an effect on user experience. We need efficient but simple ways to integrate usability engineering activities into the concurrent development process following the principles of human-centred design.

In this study, I have introduced a new concept (usability milestone) that can be useful in concurrent usability engineering. Based on this new concept, I have identified and analysed several new usability milestones and discussed their effect on usability engineering.

The main result of this study is that usability engineering can be successfully performed in fast concurrent product development but it may require better control mechanisms than described by current research. The control mechanisms can be based on identified new milestones.

Concurrent Engineering projects are time-critical. The attitude towards usability activities is often that they delay product development and cause extra work (Kaderbhai, 1998). An important objective for usability engineering is to support the project in achieving the milestones in the planned timetable. This can be achieved when usability engineering is an integral part of the design process and adapted to the project limitations and opportunities.

A common problem in complex product development is timetable delays. By decreasing the design phase time and increasing the design quality and efficiency with usability engineering, it is possible to provide either more optimal or more reliable timetables and time-to-market. On the other hand, usability engineering typically requires time-consuming iterative design.

This study has taken a look to concurrent usability engineering from the perspective of only one industry and with a limited number of case projects. The introduced usability engineering milestones may be only partially applicable to other product development practices. The timing of milestones is dependent on the particular project.

By analysing potential usability milestones in the beginning of a project it is possible to make a usability plan enabling efficient and effective usability engineering within the given project targets and timetables.

New usability milestones are useful if they improve or verify the quality of the product. The efficiency and usefulness of usability engineering milestones can be measured, for example, with effort metrics (Höglund, 1999): time, cost and results. This kind of measurement is possible when there is reference data from other projects.

Based on the findings in this study, I propose questions that lead to further study. Can usability engineering decrease the uncertainty or delays in product development? How applicable and useful is the M(EarlyToLate) milestone? Are the findings of this study applicable in other industries and in other models of product development, for example Waterfall-based software engineering? And finally, can we develop better usability engineering practices for Concurrent Engineering using defined usability milestones and knowledge about the turning points?

8. REFERENCES

Ayoama M. (1993), *Concurrent Development Process Model*, IEEE Software 1993 Vol. 10, No 4, pp. 46-55.

Daly-Jones O., Bevan N. and Thomas C. (1999), *Handbook of User-Centred Design*. D6.2.1. Version 1.2.

Hakiel S. (1997), Usability Engineering and software engineering: How do they relate? in Smith M.J., Salvendy G. and Koubek R.J (eds.), *Advances in Human Factors/Ergonomics, 21B Design of Computing Systems: Social and Ergonomic Considerations*, in Proc. Seventh Int. Conf. on Human-Computer Interaction, San Francisco, California, USA. Vol. 2, pp. 521-524. Elsevier.

Hakiel S. (1997b), Delivering ease of use, *Computing & Control Engineering Journal* April 1997, pp. 81-87.

Höglund M. (1999), Efficient and Effective Use of Effort Metrics, *The European Conference on Software Process Improvement (SPI 99)*, Barcelona, Spain.

ISO 13407. (1999), *Human-centred design processes for interactive systems*, International standard.

Järvinen P. (1980), On Structuring Problems of Job Design Met, *in The Development and Maintenance of Information Systems*, BIT 20, pp. 15-24.

Järvinen P. (1999), *Oman työn analyysi ja kehittäminen*, Opinpaja Oy, Tampere.

Kaderbhai T. (1998), Overcoming Inertia within a Large Organization, in Trenner L. & Bawa J. (eds.), *The Politics of Usability*, Springer Verlag London, pp. 35-48.

Keinonen T., Nieminen M., Riihiaho S. & Säde S. (1996), *Designing Usable Smart Products*, Helsinki University of Technology, Dept. Computer Science. Report TKO-C81, Otaniemi.

Ketola P. (2001), The Usability Plan as Part of the Concurrent Engineering (CE) Process: An Empirical Study, in Callaos N., Audestad J.A. & Sanchez M. (eds.), *Proc. World Multiconference on Systemics, Cybernetics and Informatics, SCI 2001, Volume IV Mobile/Wireless Computing*. IIIS, pp. 225-230.

Ketola P. & Röykkee M (2001), Ergonomics and Usability Factors In a Mobile Handset. Proc. Annual Congress of the Nordic Ergonomics Society NES 2001, Publications 7, University of Tampere, School of Public Health, Finland, pp. 240-243.

Kiljander H. (1999), User Interface Prototyping Methods in Designing Mobile Handsets, *Human-Computer Interaction INTERACT '99*, pp.118-125.

Korhonen P. (2000), Usability Research in Nokia: Evolution, Motivation and Trust, *CHI 2000 Extended Abstracts*. ACM, pp. 219-220.

Mayhew D.J. (1999), *The Usability Engineering Lifecycle*, Morgan Kaufmann.

Nielsen J. (1994), *Usability Engineering*, Academic Press.

Nieminen M & Parkkinen J. (1998), Usability activities in product development, in Vink P., Koningsveld E.A.P. & Dhondt S (eds.), *Human Factors in Organizational Design and Management – VI*. Elsevier Science B.V, pp. 433-438.

Premkumar G. & King W.R. (1994), Organizational characteristics and information systems planning: An empirical study, *Information Systems Research* 5, No 2, pp. 75-109.

Raddle K. & Young S. (2001), Partnering usability with development: How three organizations succeeded, *IEEE Software January/February 2001*, IEEE, pp. 38-45.

Royce W. (1970), Managing the development of large software systems, IEEE WESCON, reprinted in *Proc. 9th Int. Conf. On Software Engineering (ICSE)*, Monterey, CA 1987, IEEE Computer Society Press, Washington D.C, pp. 328-338.

Tianfield H. (2001), Advanced life-cycle model for complex product development via stage aligned information-substitutive concurrency and detour, *Int. J. Computer Integrated Manufacturing*, 2001, Vol. 14, No. 3, pp. 281-303.

Trenner L. & Bawa J. (1998), *The politics of usability. A practical guide to designing usable systems in industry*, Springer, London.

Valjus P. (1994), Limittäinen tuotekehitys valtaa alaa, *Tekniikan näköalat 1*, pp. 26-27.

Usability: Gaining a Competitive Edge
IFIP World Computer Congress 2002
J. Hammond, T. Gross, J. Wesson (Eds)
Published by Kluwer Academic Publishers

Use Case Maps: A Roadmap for Usability and Software Integrated Specification

A. Alsumait, A. Seffah, and T. Radhakrishnan
Computer Science Department, Concordia University,
Maisonneuve Blvd. W. Quebec, Canada.
seffah Email: @cs.concordia.ca

Abstract: The purpose of this paper is to explore use case maps as a medium for integrating task analysis and usability requirement into the traditional software requirement engineering process. The paper responds to major gaps in user interface specification in HCI, in software development methods for interactive software, and in the communication between usability specialists and software developers. We illustrate, via a concrete example, the usage of use case maps as an approach for specifying user interface and usability requirements. The Use Case Maps (UCMs) is a scenario-based notation for describing, in an abstract way, how the organizational structure of a complex system and the emergent behavior of the system are intertwined. It provides a first-class design model for the "how it works" aspect of both object-oriented and real time systems. Use case maps give a road-map-like view of the cause-effect paths traced through a system by scenarios or use cases (Buhr, 1998).

Key words: Use cases, use case maps, task analysis, user requirement, usability requirement, user interface requirement, functional requirement.

1. INTRODUCTION

It has been reported that a large number of change requests to modify an application are made after its deployment. Several studies have shown that 80% of total maintenance costs are related to problems of users with the system and not technical bugs (Randolph and Mayhew, 1994; Landauer,

1995). Among them, 64% are usability problems (Landauer, 1995). In a survey of 8,000 projects, the Standish Group found that the lack of user involvement and incomplete user requirements represent the major reason of project success or failure (Standish Group, 1995). One of the major reasons for this situation is that software engineering methodologies, when used for developing highly interactive software with a significant user interface, have a major limitation. Most of them do not propose, at least explicitly, any mechanisms for: empirically identifying and specifying user needs and usability requirements, or testing and validating requirements with end-users (Forbrig, 1999; Nunes and Falcãoe Cunha, 1999; Seffah and Hayne, 1999).

Among the software engineering techniques, use cases have been investigated as a potential approach for user requirement (Constantine and Lockwood, 1999; Forbrig, 1999; Krutchen, 1999; Nunes and Falcãoe Cunha, 1999). A use case is a collection of possible scenarios between the system and actors, characterized by the goals the primary actor has, while a scenario is a sequence of interactions happening under certain conditions (Cockburn, 1997). Although, in theory, use cases have the potential to gather the non-functional requirements that are a simplified description of the context of use, in practice, use cases have been used for gathering the system functionalities and features including technical capabilities and constraints. They attempt to describe representative ways in which the user will interact with the software but not in comprehensive format (Constantine, 1995). Another limitation of use case-driven requirement approach is that the main people involved in this process are stakeholders and technical persons including use case specifiers and user interface developers. End-users are not directly involved (Seffah and Hayne, 1999) and the notation used is not easily understandable.

User-centered requirement techniques and in particular task analysis suggested by the human-computer interaction (HCI) community has the power to complement traditional software engineering approaches and in particular use cases (Nunes and Falcãoe Cunha, 1999; Seffah and Hayne, 1999). User-driven requirement approaches are used for gathering a complete description of the context of use and usability goals including user characteristics, task analysis, as well as the physical, technical and organizational environments in which the system will be used (Setten et al, 1997; Arnowitz et al, 2000). However, most of the currently available HCI techniques are not intended for dialog modeling: system reactions are not represented, and error-free, non-interrupted action sequences are assumed (Jambon, 1996; Setten et al, 1997).

Therefore, both HCI and software engineering approaches each have their own strengths and weaknesses; in addition their objectives overlap in some areas but differ in others. For example, in model-based task analysis in HCI, the objective is normally to achieve a generic and thus abstract model of the task, typically in a hierarchical form of goals and sub-goals (Dayton et al, 1998). In object-oriented development, use cases are often employed in gathering functional requirements (Constantine, 1995; Krutchen, 1999). HCI techniques enhance functional requirement descriptions by adding information that improves the users' understanding of the future system. Basically, this additional information concerns the context of use and takes into account usability problems that may be encountered by end-users when performing certain tasks.

Here, we discuss our investigations on the use of use case maps as an approach for specifying user interface and usability requirements as well as for bridging the current gap between software and usability engineering methods. The Use Case Map (UCM) is a scenario-based notation for describing graphically how the organizational structure of a complex system and the emergent behavior of the system are intertwined. It provides a first-class design model for the "how it works" aspect of both object-oriented and real time systems (Buhr, 1998). Use case maps give a road-map-like view of the cause-effect paths traced through a system by scenarios or use cases. Already, UCMs have been used in a number of areas (Buhr, 1998):

- Requirements engineering and design such as real-time systems, object-oriented systems, telecommunication systems, distributed systems, multimedia systems, agent systems.
- Detection and avoidance of undesirable feature interactions.
- Performance analysis and prediction.
- Evaluation of architectural alternatives.
- Functional testing.

UCMs are intended to be a useful tool for functional requirement, scenario-based software development, as well as for stakeholders-to-developers communication (Buhr, 1998; Seffah and Hayne, 1999; Amyot and Mussbacher, 2001). However, their support for designing user interfaces is still acknowledged to be insufficient. There is a common misconception that the same models developed to support the design of the application internals are not adequate to support interaction design, supporting the usability aspects of the applications. In this paper, we propose an extension of UCMs for user interface systems. This extension provides the necessary integration between user interfaces and underlying functionalities. In fact, by having a single modeling notation, common structures and behaviors of user interfaces and the underlying functionalities can be shared at design time among usability engineers and developers. Furthermore, user interface developers can have the benefits of designing user interfaces in a declarative, systematic, and also standard way. Our starting position is that a good proportion of user interface (usability) design problems may be served by scenarios and use cases, as perhaps the primary design representation. We should keep in mind that our proposed extension should not be tied to a specific view of the design process. It should try to serve the needs of user interface designers within the framework of the UCM model.

2. BACKGROUND AND RELATED WORK

The following are only some of the many investigations that, over the last few years, have tried to study use cases and task analysis for requirement engineering and in general build a bridge between object-oriented development and task analysis techniques.

Forbrig (1999) introduced a framework for combining task models, user models, and object models. These multiple dimensions require tools enabling the manipulation of all these models along the different phases of software development. Related to this work, Seffah and Hayne (1999) and Antunes et al. (2001) also investigated the similarities of task analysis and use case techniques via an attempt to recast the results of a task analysis into the format of use cases as well as software-to-usability communication, which is not explicitly described in use cases-driven development. Paternò (2001) discussed an approach to integrating the Unified Modeling Language (UML) for designing interactive systems based on the use of use cases, class diagram, ConcurTaskTrees (CTT) task models and scenarios. The logical framework that has been presented gives an indication of the types of representations to use in the various phases and their relationships.

Constantine and Lockwood (1999) suggest that use case specifiers should first prepare lightweight use case model descriptions (essential use cases) that do not contain any implicit user interface decisions. Later on, user interface designers can use these essential use cases as input to create the user interface without being bound by any implicit decisions. Related to this work, Krutchen (1999) introduces the concept of use case storyboard as a logical and conceptual description of how a use case is provided by the user interface, including the interaction required between the actor(s) and the system.

Theoretically, having a unique and consistent model that provides simple views for any actor and automatically includes user's concerns should be enough to enable the software engineers to keep track of user needs during their design process. However, as Artim and Van Harmelen (1998) pointed out in their case study, the culture of the software engineer does not include collaborating with the user in the process of building a better system. These sociological forces within development teams limit and even discard any impacts of the user in the development of the system, thus providing a system that fits to static user specifications, rather than fitting the best to user needs. We can deduce from this case study that even though the process of development determines directly the product being created, it is not the only factor. Jarke (1999) tries to clarify the purpose and manner to use scenarios in the modeling process, since this concept can be used in very different ways. He defines the scenarios as constructs that describe possible sets of events that might reasonably take place; they offer "middle-ground abstraction between models and reality".

3. USE CASE MAPS – A BRIEF INTRODUCTION

Use Case Maps (UCMs) is a visual notation developed at Carleton University (Buhr, 1998). The key idea of UCMs is to describe scenario paths in terms of causal relationships between responsibilities. A causal relationship between components can be interpreted in many ways, depending on the component structure. As shown in Figure 1, UCMs are composed of:

- **Start points** (filled circles representing pre-conditions or triggering causes)
- Causal chains of **responsibilities** (crosses, representing actions, tasks, or functions to be performed)
- **End points** (bars representing post-conditions or resulting effects).

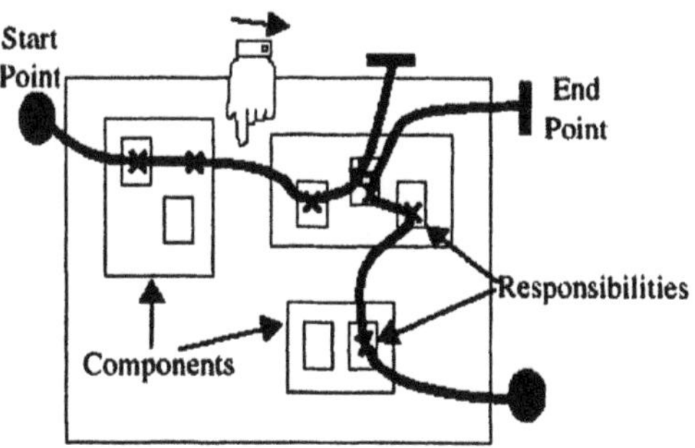

Figure 1. An example of a Use Case Map (Buhr, 1998).

Start point, responsibilities, end points, and components are the basic elements of the UCM. The responsibilities can be bound to **components**, which are the entities or objects composing the system. The wiggly lines are **paths** that connect start points, responsibilities, and end points.

UCMs are used to describe and integrate use cases representing the requirements (Amyot and Mussbacher, 2001). The construction of UCMs can reveal problems with the use cases, which may be incomplete, incorrect, ambiguous, inconsistent, or at different levels of abstraction (Amyot and and Mussbacher, 2001; Buhr, 1998). In fact, the usefulness of UCMs is broader than their name suggests. They aim to support human understanding of the entire picture of requirements during all phases of the lifecycle, and not just to specify scenario sequences by combining a set of scenarios in a single diagram that enables designers to express scenarios and scenario interactions in a graphical manner (Amyot and Mussbacher, 2001). UCMs provide a mechanism that can be used by designers to analyze the overall system behavior that emerges from scenario combinations (Buhr, 1998). Moreover, UCMs provides a bird's-eye, path-centric view of system functionality. It allows for dynamic behavior and structures to be represented and evaluated, and these in turn improve the level of reusability of scenarios (Buhr, 1998). For more information, readers may visit the UCMs web site at www.UseCaseMaps.org.

3.1 UCMs Extension for Usability Requirements

One important goal of user interface and usability requirements engineering is to ensure that a consistent and feasible requirements specification can be developed, while ensuring that the specification is a valid reflection of user requirements. To achieve this goal, we investigated the possibility of making use of the prospective standard Use Case Maps (UCMs) for the support of user interface and usability requirements.

Our strong belief that UCMs are powerful for user interface and usability requirements is based on the simplicity of UCMs notation. Based on previous studies (Buhr, 1998; Amyot and Mussbacher, 2001), we believe that the UCMs notation is easily understandable by both the user (customer) and the software developer. In fact, this helps user interface designers to handle different users' understanding and expectation of the interface, and bridge the gaps by refining the requirements earlier. If the software developer is using UCMs, this will support the idea of concurrent engineering where a whole overview of the system (functionality and user interface) can be presented using one abstract model. Consequently, this improves the probability that software and the interface will be correct when it is finally put together, since contradictions in the requirement can be captured in early stages, which shortens the overall time required and makes it correct. It will also help to reduce the chances of introducing errors when changes are made. Furthermore, many studies are focusing on how to integrate UCMs to UML and how to formalize UCMs in XML (Amyot and Mussbacher, 2001).

Finally, a major strength in the extended UCMs is its ability to capture most of the user interface requirements. We found that UCMs can be used in the following three dimensions:

- **Task Dimension** seeks to represent tasks that are relevant for interactions. Thus, UCMs are used as a simple and expressive visual notation that allows describing task scenarios at an abstract level in terms of sequences of responsibilities and tasks over a set of components. Tasks can be split up into subtasks (actions, operations) or inherited from 'super'-tasks.
- **Dialog Dimension** is intended to explain the style of human-computer interaction and also describes the sequence of dialogs that can take place between the user and the system.
- **User Interface Dimension** identifies the objects comprising the user interface, their grouping and specifies their layout, e.g. by indicating approximate placement or by indicating topological relations between groups. This dimension represents the space within the user interface of a system where the user interacts with all the functions, containers, and information needed for carrying out some particular task or set of interrelated tasks. Moreover, successive displays of different screens and interactive objects are presented.

The 'look and feel' of an interactive system concerns the detailed reactive behavior of interactive objects that make up the interface. Using UCMs, these objects can be described in a range of forms. Use cases can provide a description that abstracts away from the software structure, while the dialog dimension can provide a more detailed account of this interaction. Figure 2 introduces the extended notation to provide UCMs with more expressive power for interaction design. These notations are described below:

a. System initiates a dialog.
b. The initiator of the dialog could be the system or the user.
c. Dialog between the system and the user is repeated until one of them ends the dialog.
a. _Same as 3 except that the dialog is repeated *n* times.
e. The dialog is optional.
f. Proactive message; message passed from the system to the user.
g. A question-and-answer dialog
h. A form-filling dialog
i. A menu dialog.

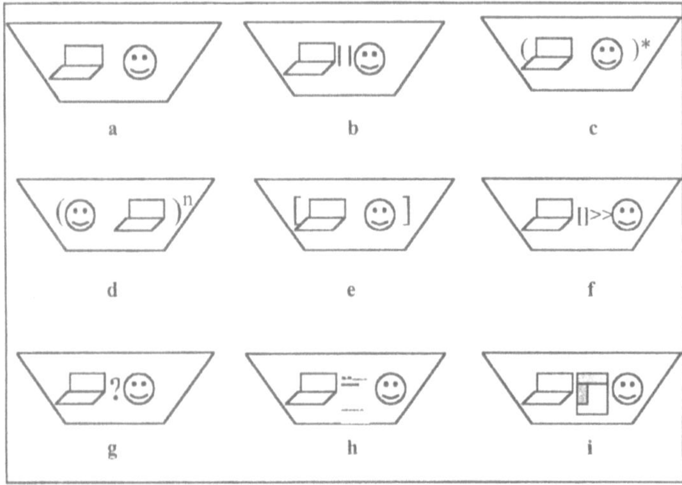

Figure 2. Extended notation for UCMs

In short, our proposal for the extended UCM framework for user interface systems should include a new UCM interaction model to accommodate the three dimensions. Therefore, the user interface model encompasses the task, dialog and layout structure dimensions, clearly mapping the conceptual architectural models for interactive systems, while maintaining the desired separation of concerns.

1.2 AN ILLUSTRATIVE EXAMPLE

Filter Agent (FA) aims to assist the user with email management using a memory based learning technique. The interface agent (FA) learns by continuously "looking over the shoulder" of the user as the user is performing actions. The interface agent monitors the actions of the user over long periods of time, finds recurrent patterns and offers to automate them. If the user drags and drops a particular electronic mail message to a specific folder, the mail agent adds a description of this situation and the action taken by the user to its memory of examples. The agent keeps track of the sender and receiver of a message, the Cc: list, the keywords in the Subject: line, whether the message has been read or not, whether it is a reply to a previous message, and so on. If a new mail arrives, the agent predicts which action is appropriate for the current situation and also measures its confidence in each prediction by determining how many examples the agent has memorized. If the agent is confident, then it will autonomously take the action on behalf of the user. Otherwise, the agent either offers suggestion to the user and wait for the user's confirmation to automate the action, or wait and observe the user action.

1.2.1 Task and Dialog Dimension

The behavior of the filter agent and consequently the relationship among the functions mentioned earlier are better understood by following UCMs flows shown in Figure 3. Based on the root map in Figure 3, users and designers can consider early decisions regarding the sequence in which functions are performed. This map describes the system behavior that starts when a pre-condition is satisfied, for example, new email arrives (filled circle labeled **MA**).

A dialog illustrates that a conversation between the user and the agent is taking place where details are delayed to a sub-UCMs. The dialog notation is applied to our work not only to hide details, but also to decompose the system into small manageable units. This scenario ends when one or two of the following triggering events occur: user exits the email application (bar labeled **E1**) or an email is filed (bar labeled **E2**). These events are represented by post-conditions in the UCMs. A route is a path that links an initial cause to a final effect. For example, **<S, [a2], [a4], D, E2>** represents a route that starts when new email arrives, user reads the mail and sends it to a specific folder, followed by a dialog between the user and the agent.

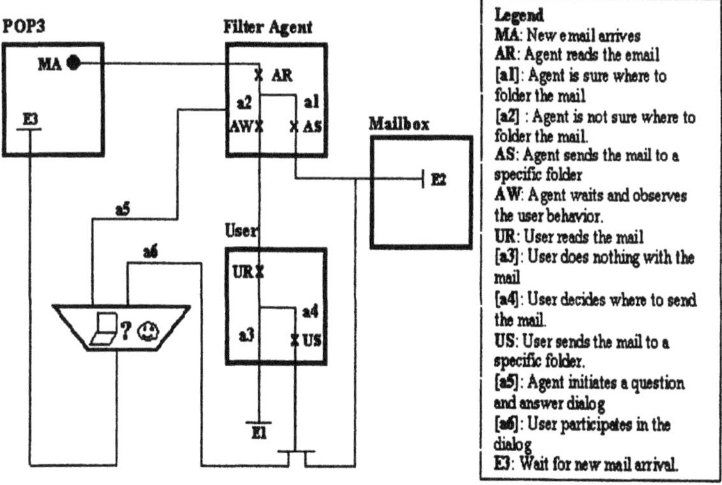

Figure 3. The Root Use Case Map

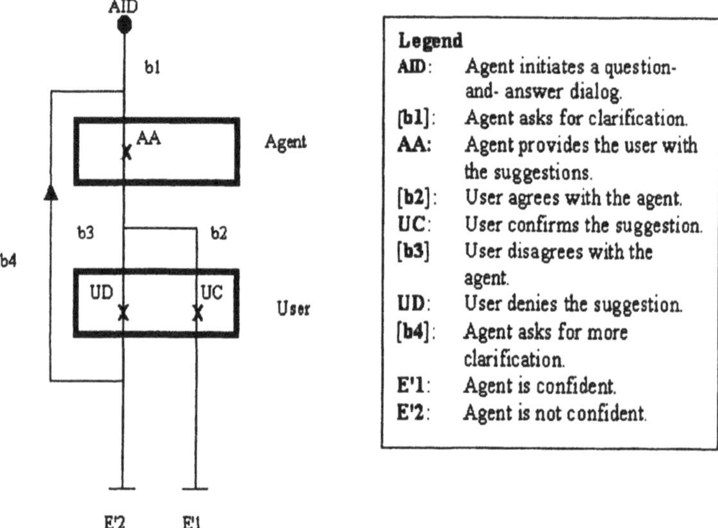

Figure 4. UCM explaining the dialog between the agent and the user

Figure 4 depicts the second level of the requirement model when a conversation or a dialog goes on between the agent and the user. The agent offers it suggestion to the user waiting for a confirmation. The user either confirms the suggestion or denies it. Alternative paths (called OR-forks) represent composite UCMs that can be split into two different paths (no level of concurrency is associated with them). For instance, a responsibility point (cross-labeled **AA** in the figure) is activated along the **[b1]** path to decide whether the user confirms the suggestion or deny it. The alternative sub-paths (labeled **[b2]** and **[b3]**) are generated after this suggestion.

1.3 Task and Structural Dimension

The enriched UCMs not only describe the sequence of tasks and dialogs that can take place between the user and the system, but also help to understand and reason about the requirements of the user interface, including usability aspects.

Figure 5 shows the user interface structure of the email application that consists of a tool bar, folder menu, mailbox, and an agent window.

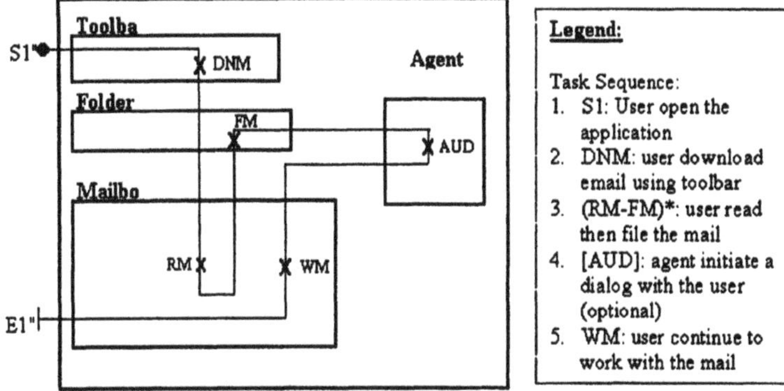

Figure 5. Structured UCMs for the user interface of the email application

Figure 5 describes the approximate position of the components of the user interface and the user/system behavior that starts when a user opens the email application. The user downloads new arrived mails using the tool bar menu. Then the user continuously reads a mail then folders it until either the agent initiates a dialog or the user quits the application.

2. CONCLUSION AND FURTHER INVESTIGATION

The most valuable contribution of this ongoing research effort is the development and analysis of a complete UCMs notation for high-level requirements of user interfaces. Our enriched UCMs put together three dimensions of user interface requirements including the task, the dialog, and the structure of the user interface. In this manner, functions and tasks are distributed over the use case map defining how the users will be permitted to move among various tasks and how and when the user will move from one object to another in the interface. Moreover, the enriched UCMs capture the initiator and style of interactions between the user and the system.

The improved UCMs have also the potential to capture a complete picture of user interface requirements by describing how a system will be used and to what ends. However, the amount of work it generates shows the vital need of a CASE tool to manage the use-case descriptions along with additional information pertinent to user interface analysis and design. This tool should also manage many views of the same model, and is able to generate five types of reports on a model corresponding to the needs of different actors and steps of the development process:

- A "user's view" of the use cases,
- A "developer's view" of the use cases,
- A glossary of terms,
- A more focused user interface analyst's report,
- An actor-system interaction report.

5. REFERENCES

Amyot, D. & Mussbacher, G. (2001), Bridging the requirements/design gap in dynamic systems with Use Case Maps (UCMs). In: *23rd International Conference on Software Engineering -ICSE'01*, May 12-19. Toronto, Canada. 743-744.

Antunes, A., Seffah, A., Radhakrishnan, S. & Pestina, S. (2001) Improving and mediating software-to-usability communication. In: *Workshop on Multiple User Interfaces over the Internet: Engineering and applications Trends In conjunction with HCI-IHM'2001*, http://www.cs.concordia.ca/~faculty/seffah/ihm2001/index.shtml, May 10-14, Lille, France.

Arnowitz, J., Fijma, D. & Verlinden, J. (2000), *Communicating a task analysis with task layer maps*. ACM Press New York, NY, USA, 346-353.

Artim, J.M. & Van Harmelen M. (1998), Incorporating work, process and task analysis into commercial and industrial object-oriented system development. In: *Proceedings of the conference on CHI 98 summary: human factors in computing systems*, ACM Press, 198.

Buhr, R.J.A. (1998), Use case maps as architectural entities for complex systems, *IEEE Transactions on Software Engineering*, 24(12), 1131-1155.

Cockburn A. (1997), Structuring Use Cases with Goals. *Journal of Object-Oriented Programming*, Sep/Oct, 1997, 35-40, and Nov/Dec, 1997, 56-62.

Constantine, L. & Lockwood, A.D. (1999), Software for use: a practical guide to the models and methods of usage-centered design. Reading, Massachusetts: Addison-Wesley.

Constantine, L. (1995), Essential modeling: use cases for user interfaces. *Interactions*, ACM Press, 2(2), 34-46.

Dayton, T., McFarland, A. & Kramer, J. (1998), Bridging user needs to object-oriented GUI prototypes via task object design. In: L. Wood (ed.), Design: User Interface Design: Bridging the Gap from User Requirements to Design, Boca Raton, FL: CRC Press, 15-56.

Forbrig, P. (1999), Task and object-oriented development of interactive systems - how many models are necessary?. In: *Proceedings of Design Specification and Verification of Interactive Systems Workshop-DSVIS'99*, Braga, Portugal, 225-237.

Jambon, F. (1996), Formal modeling of task interruption. In: *Proceedings of the CHI '96 conference companion on Human factors in computing systems: common ground*. ACM Press, 45-46.

Jarke, M. (1999), Scenarios for modelling. *Communications of the ACM*, 42(1), 47-48.

Krutchen, P. (1999), Use case storyboards in the rational unified process. In: *Workshop on Integrating Human Factors in Use Case and OO Methods-13th ECOOP*. June 14-19, Lisbon, Portugal.

Landauer, T.K. (1995), The trouble with computers: usefulness, usability and productivity. MIT Press.

Nunes, N.J. & Falcãoe Cunha, J. (1999), Detailing use-cases with activity diagrams and object views. In: *Workshop on Integrating Human Factors in Use Case and OO Methods-13th ECOOP*. June 14-19, Lisbon, Portugal.

Paternò, F. (2001), Towards a UML for interactive systems. In: M.R. Little, L. Nigay (eds.), *8th International Conference of EHCI 2001*, Toronto, Canada, May 2001, 7-18.

Randolph, G.B. & Mayhew, D.J. (1994), *Cost-justifying usability*. Academic Press.

Seffah, A. & Hayne C. (1999), Integrating Human Factors in Use Case and OO Methods. . In: *Workshop on Integrating Human Factors in Use Case and OO Methods-13th ECOOP*. June 14-19, Lisbon, Portugal.

Setten, M., van der Veer, G. & Brinkkemper, S. (1997), Comparing interaction design techniques: a method for objective comparison to find the conceptual basis for interaction design. In: *Proceedings of the Conference on Designing Interactive Systems: Processes, Practices, Methods, and Techniques*. August 18-20, Amsterdam, The Netherlands, 349-357.

Standish Group. (1995), *CHAOS: A Recipe For Success*, The Standish Group International, INC.

Usability: Gaining a Competitive Edge
IFIP World Computer Congress 2002
J. Hammond, T. Gross, J. Wesson (Eds)
Published by Kluwer Academic Publishers

User Requirements Analysis

A Review of Supporting Methods

Martin Maguire
Research School in Ergonomics and Human Factors
Loughborough University, UK
m.c.maguire@lboro.ac.uk

Nigel Bevan
Serco Usability Services, UK
nbevan@usability.serco.com

Abstract: Understanding user requirements is an integral part of information systems design and is critical to the success of interactive systems. However specifying these requirements is not so simple to achieve. This paper describes general methods to support user requirements analysis that can be adapted to a range of situations. Some brief case studies are described to illustrate how these methods have been applied in practice.

Key words: user requirements, user-centred design, usability methods

1. INTRODUCTION

Understanding user requirements is an integral part of information systems design and is critical to the success of interactive systems. It is now widely understood that successful systems and products begin with an understanding of the needs and requirements of the users. As specified in the ISO 13407 standard (ISO, 1999), user-centred design begins with a thorough understanding of the needs and requirements of the users. The benefits can include increased productivity, enhanced quality of work, reductions in support and training costs, and improved user satisfaction. Requirements analysis is not a simple process. Particular problems faced by the analyst are:

- addressing complex organisational situations with many stakeholders
- users and designers thinking along traditional lines, reflecting the current system and processes, rather than being innovative
- users not knowing in advance what they want from the future system (Olphert & Damodaran, 2002)

- rapid development cycles, reducing the time available for user needs analysis
- representing user requirements in an appropriate form.

This paper considers how these problems can be addressed by selecting appropriate methods to support the process of user requirements generation and validation. It describes each method briefly and shows how it contributes to the requirements process.

The basis for the application of different user requirements methods is a simple process as shown in Figure 1 below encompassing 4 elements:

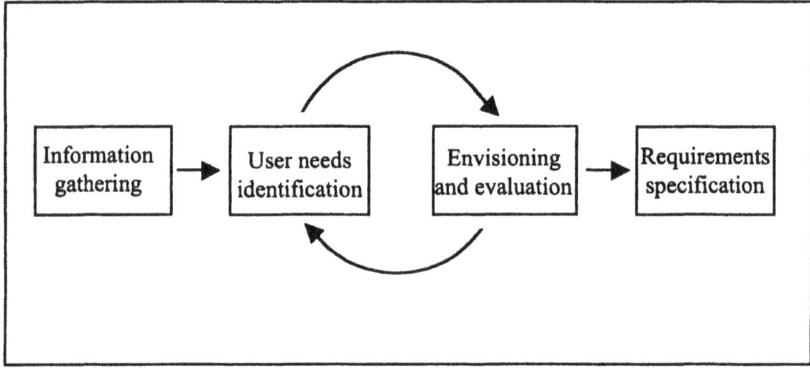

Figure 1: General process for user requirements analysis

The four stages, and methods used to support the stages, are described in the next sections, followed by a summary table highlighting the advantages and disadvantages of each technique.

2. INFORMATION GATHERING

The first step in user requirements analysis is to gather background information about the users and stakeholders and the processes that currently take place. The following methods may be adopted:

Stakeholder analysis identifies all the users and stakeholders who may influence or be impacted by the system. This helps ensure that the needs of all those involved are taken into account. If required, the system is tested by them. User groups may include end users, supervisors, installers, and maintainers. Other stakeholders include recipients of output from the system, marketing staff, purchasers and support staff (Taylor, 1990). Stakeholder analysis identifies, for each user and stakeholder group, their *main roles, responsibilities and task goals* in relation to the system. One of the main issues is how to trade-off the competing needs of different stakeholder groups in the new system (see 4.5 Allocation of function and user cost-benefit analysis).

Secondary market research involves researching published sources such as research reports, census data, demographic information, that throw light upon the range of possible user markets. Websites representing special groups of users such as that for the Royal National Institute for the Blind (www.rnib.org.uk/digital) give information about the nature of the user population they represent (Mander & Smith, 2002).

Context of use analysis is used when a system or product is developed. The quality of a system, including usability, accessibility and social acceptability factors, depends on having a very good understanding of the context of use of the system. For example, a bank machine (ATM) will be much more usable if it is designed for use at night as well as during the day, in bright sunlight as well as normal light, and by people in wheelchairs as well as those able to stand. Similarly in an office environment, there are many characteristics that can impinge on the usability of a new software product e.g. user workload, support available, or interruptions. Capturing contextual information is therefore important in helping to specify user requirements. In order to gather contextual information, stakeholders attend a facilitated meeting, called a Context Meeting. Here a questionnaire is completed to capture the characteristics of the users, their tasks and operating environment (see main headings in Table 1 below).

User group	Tasks	Technical environment
• System skills and experience. • Task knowledge. • Training. • Qualifications. • Language skills. • Age & gender. • Physical and cognitive capabilities. • Attitudes and motivations.	• Task list. • Goal. • Output. • Steps. • Frequency. • Importance. • Duration. • Dependencies.	• Hardware. • Software. • Network. • Reference materials. • Other equipment.
Physical environment	**Organisational environment**	
• Auditory environment. • Thermal environment. • Visual environment. • Vibration. • Space and furniture. • User posture. • Health hazards. • Protective clothing & equipment.	• Work practices. • Assistance. • Interruptions. • Management & communications structure. • Computer use policy. • Organisational aims. • Industrial relations. • Job characteristics.	

Table 1. Context of use factors

Context of use analysis was one of the outcomes of the ESPRIT HUFIT project and developed further in the ESPRIT MUSiC project (Bevan and Macleod, 1994). Context of use analysis within usability activities are also reviewed in Maguire (2001c).

Task analysis involves the study of what a user is required to do in terms of actions and/or cognitive processes to achieve a task. A detailed task analysis can be conducted to understand the current system, the information flows within it, the problems for people, and opportunities that indicate user needs. There are many variations of task analysis and notations for recording task activities. One of the most widely used is hierarchical task analysis, where high level tasks are de-composed into more detailed components and sequences. Another method creates a flow chart showing the sequence of human activities and the associated inputs and outputs (Ericsson 2001). Kirwan & Ainsworth (1992) provide a guide to the different task analysis methods, while Hackos & Redish (1998) explain some of the simpler methods for user interface design.

Rich pictures can help stakeholders map, explore and understand a complex problem space and thereby help to identify hidden requirements (Checkland, 1981). The technique involves creating a series of sketches to show how people and systems relate to each other in an organisation. They may show peoples' roles, power structures, communications and reporting mechanisms. Drawing simple figures of people with thought and speech bubbles linked to them can show particular problem areas in the current environment that may lead to new user requirements.

Field study and observational methods involve an investigator viewing users as they work and taking notes of the activity that takes place. Observation may be either direct, where the investigator is actually present during the task, or indirect, where the task is recorded on videotape by the analysis team and viewed at a later time. The observer tries to be unobtrusive during the session and only poses questions if clarification is needed. Obtaining the co-operation of users is vital so the interpersonal skills of the observer are important. For further information see Preece et al. (1994).

Diary keeping provides a record of user behaviour over a period of time. They require the participant to record activities they are engaged in throughout a normal day that may lead to the identification of user requirements for a new system or product. Diaries require careful design and prompting if they are to be employed properly be participants.

Video recording can be used to capture human processes in a stakeholder's workplace or other location. The results can then be revised for the purpose of understanding more about the work and generating relevant questions relevant to user needs. Video can also be a useful supplement to other method e.g. to demonstrate new system concepts to users during user/stakeholder discussion groups.

3. USER NEEDS IDENTIFICATION

Once user data has been collected, user needs can start to be identified. A number of methods exist for identifying such needs.

User surveys involve administering a set of written questions to a sample population of users. Surveys can help determine the needs of users, current work practices and attitudes to new system ideas. Surveys are normally composed of a mix of 'closed' questions with fixed responses and 'open' questions, where the respondents are free to answer as they wish. This method is useful for obtaining quantitative as well as some qualitative data from a large number of users about the problems of existing tasks or the current system. For further information see Preece et al. (1994).

Focus groups bring together a cross-section of stakeholders in a discussion group format. This method is useful for requirements elicitation and can help to identify issues that need to be tackled. The general idea is that each participant can act to stimulate ideas in the other people present, and that by a process of discussion, the collective view becomes established which is greater than the individual parts. For further information see Bruseberg & McDonagh-Philp (2001).

Interviewing is a commonly used technique where users, stakeholders and domain experts are questioned to gain information about their needs or requirements in relation to the new system. Interviews are usually semi-structured based on a series of fixed questions with scope for the user to expand on their responses. They can also be used as part of task analysis. For further information see Preece *et al.* (1994) and Macaulay (1996). Interviews on a customer site by representatives from the system development team can be very informative. Seeing the environment also gives a vivid mental picture of how users are working with the existing system and how the new system can support them (Mander and Smith, 2002).

Scenarios and use cases give detailed realistic examples of how users may carry out their tasks in a specified context with the future system. The primary aim of scenario building is to provide examples of future use as an aid to understanding and clarifying user requirements and to provide a basis for later usability testing. Scenarios can help identify usability targets and likely task completion times. The method also promotes developer buy-in and encourages a human-centred design approach. Scenarios of use are sometimes called 'use cases', although the term is also used by software engineers to refer to the use of functions.

In a related method called **personas,** a caricature is created with a name, personality and picture, to represent each of the most important user groups. Potential design solutions can then be evaluated against the needs of a particular persona and the tasks they are expected to perform. Personas are used by innovative design groups to stimulate creativity rather than refine a design solution (Cooper 1999).

Future workshops are a way to help users and designers 'break out' from a current situations and thinking. Essentially they involve gathering participants and posing questions such as: 'Where do you want to be 10 years from now'. Once participants have agreed a suitable goal, they then seek to establish a process by which it can be achieved. Another variation is to define new technological developments, discuss when they might be attainable and what implications this might have for the user organisation.

Evaluating an existing or competitor system can provide valuable information about the extent to which current systems meet user needs and can identify potential usability problems to avoid in the new system. Useful features identified in a competitor system can also be fed into the design process as potential user requirements. Measures of effectiveness, efficiency and satisfaction can be used as a baseline for the new system. To obtain accurate measures a controlled user test should be used, but valuable information can still be obtained from less formal methods of testing.

4. ENVISIONING AND EVALUATION

Once an initial set of user requirements has been developed, it is important to develop a prototype to illustrate them. User feedback can then be obtained on the prototype to validate and refine the user requirements. Potential techniques are described in this section

Brainstorm sessions bring together a set of design and task experts to inspire each other in the creative, idea generation phase of the problem solving process. They are used to generate new ideas by freeing the mind to accept any idea that is suggested, thus allowing freedom for creativity. The method has been widely used the early phases of design. The results of a brainstorming session are, it is hoped, a set of good ideas and a general feel for the solution area to meet user needs.

Card sorting is a technique for uncovering the hierarchical structure in a set of concepts by asking users to group items written on a set of cards. This is often used, for instance, to work out the organisation of a website. Users would be given cards with the names of the intended web pages on the site and asked to group the cards into related categories. After gathering the groupings from several users, designers can typically spot clear structures across many users. Statistical analysis can uncover the best groupings from the data where it is not clear by inspection. IBM (2002) is an example of an analysis programme.

Affinity diagramming is a related technique that can be used for organising the structure of a new system, and allows participants to work as a group. Designers or users write down items such as potential screens or functions on sticky notes and then organise the notes by grouping them, to uncover the structure and relationships in a domain. Affinity diagrams are often a good next step after a brainstorming session. See Beyer & Holtzblatt (1998) for more information.

Storyboards, also termed "Presentation Scenarios", are sequences of images that show the relationship between user actions or inputs and system outputs. A typical storyboard will contain a number of images depicting features such as menus, dialogue boxes and windows. Storyboard sequences provide a platform for exploring and refining user requirements options via a static representation of the future system by showing them to potential users and members of a design team (Andriole, 1989).

Prototyping is where designers create paper or software-based simulations of user interface elements (menus, buttons, icons, windows, dialogue sequences, etc.) in a static or dynamic way. When a ***paper prototype*** has been prepared, a member of the design team sits before a user and 'plays the computer' by moving the paper and card interface elements around in response to the user's actions. The difficulties encountered by the user and user comments, are recorded by an observer. ***Software prototypes*** provide a greater level of realism than is normally possible with simple paper mock-ups. Here, the aim is to create a rapid prototype that is used to establish an acceptable design for the user but is then thrown away prior to full implementation. Some design processes are based on a rapid application development (RAD) approach. Here a small group of designers and users work intensively on a prototype, making frequent changes in response to user comment. The prototype evolves into the full system. Hall (2001) discusses the merits and cost-benefits of varying fidelity levels of prototypes.

Allocation of function is an important element for many systems. As ISO 13407 (1999) states in clause 7.3.2, allocation of function is "the division of system tasks into those performed by humans and those performed by technology" to specify a clear system boundary. A range of options is established to identify the optimal division of labour, to provide job satisfaction and efficient operation of the whole work process. **User cost-benefit analysis** can then be carried out to determine how acceptable each user group will find the new arrangement. The use of task allocation charts and cost-benefit analysis is most useful for systems that affect whole work processes rather than single user, single task products. They also provide the opportunity to rethink the system design or user roles to provide a more acceptable solution for all groups. A process for performing a user cost-benefit analysis is described by Eason (1988).

Design guidelines and standards are referred to by designers and HCI specialists for guidance on ergonomic issues associated with the system being developed. The ISO 9241 standard (ISO, 1997) covers many aspects of hardware and software user-interface design, and contains a widely agreed body of software ergonomics advice. See Bevan (2001) for more information on ISO standards. Style guides embody good practice in interface design. Following a style guide will increase the consistency between screens and can reduce the development time. For a GUI (graphic user interface) an operating system style guide should be followed to implement good practice and to provide consistency. For websites, design guidelines are evolving but good web design principles are gradually being established (Nielsen, 2000). Nicolle and Abascal (2001) discuss issues and present guidelines to make systems accessible by people with disabilities.

Parallel design sessions involve a few small groups of designers working independently, to generate a range of diverse solutions. The aim is to develop and evaluate different system designs before choosing a solution (possibly drawing from several solutions) as a basis for the implemented system

5. REQUIREMENTS SPECIFICATION

General guidance on specifying user and organisational requirements and objectives is provided in ISO 13407. The following should be documented within the specification: identification of the range of relevant users and other stakeholders, a clear statement of design goals, the requirements with an indication their priority levels, measurable benchmarks against which the emerging design can be tested, evidence of acceptance of the requirements by the stakeholders, acknowledgement of statutory or legislative requirements, e.g. for health and safety. It is also important to manage changing requirements as the system develops.

The following sections describe techniques and methods to support user and organisational requirements specification.

Task/function mapping specifies the system functions that each user will require for the different tasks that they perform. By showing the relationship between the tasks and the corresponding functional requirements linked in matrix form, trade-offs can be made between different functions, or to add and remove functions depending on their value for supporting specific tasks. It is also useful for multi-user systems to ensure that the tasks of each user type are supported.

Requirements categorisation

User requirements: It is important to establish and document the user requirements so that they lead into the process of designing the system itself. User requirements will include summary descriptions of the tasks that the system will support and the functions that will be provided to support them.

Usability requirements: It is also necessary to describe the detailed usability requirements in order to set objectives for the design team, and help prioritise usability work. Generally agreed usability goals to define are: effectiveness: the degree of success with which users achieve their task goals: efficiency: the time it takes to complete tasks; and satisfaction: user comfort and acceptability; see ISO 9241, part 11 'Guidance on Usability' (ISO, 1997).

These are most easily derived from the evaluation of an existing system. Other more detailed usability issues provide more specific design objectives e.g. understandability, learnability, supportiveness, flexibility and attractiveness. Having established usability requirements, it is then necessary to translate the requirements into a specification (specification = requirement + measure). ISO 9126-4 (ISO, 2002) provides a framework for specifying measurable requirements (see also section 6.3).

Organisational requirements: A third element is to specify the organisational requirements for the user-system complex, i.e. those that come out of a system being placed into a social context. An understanding of organisational requirements will help to create systems that can support the management structure of the organisation and communications within it, as well as group and collaborative working. Defining and grouping the tasks in an appropriate way will help to create motivating and satisfying jobs, ideally allowing users autonomy, flexibility, provision of good feedback on their performance and the opportunity to develop their skills and careers. Statutory or legislative requirements may also be classed as organisational requirements.

The information needed to specify user, usability and organisational requirements will be drawn from the context of use and user needs activities described in previous sections. Maguire (1998) and Roberston & Roberston (1999) provide frameworks for user requirements specification.

Prioritisation of user requirements is important so that development resources can be directed appropriately. The DSDM development method uses 'time boxes' where the functions and features in each phase of a system's release are defined by the resources available. This helps control the risks in system development, and allows the customer to redirect future effort to meet the user's needs more closely.

Criteria setting relates to the need for criteria to help decide whether the user requirements have been achieved. This can be done by an inspection team or by user testing, where a representative user sample performs typical tasks with the system and the performance scores and attitude ratings help decide if the system can be accepted. Defining acceptance criteria in advance can be achieved by performing pre-tests on the existing system or on a competitor system, to specify criteria that the new system must be at least as good as these current systems.

6. COMPARISON SUMMARY

Table 2 below presents the advantages and disadvantages of each method presented in this paper to assist in method selection.

Method	Benefits	Drawbacks
2. INFORMATION GATHERING		
Stakeholder analysis	Ensures that all relevant stakeholders are considered.	-
Secondary market research	Low cost and provides good overview of potential market.	Information may be too general or out of date.
Context of use analysis	Provides framework for documenting all factors that may affect the usability of the product.	May be lengthy process. Not all headings applicable to project. Could be short-circuited for smaller systems.
Task Analysis	Defines and models tasks that can highlight user needs directly.	May be over-formal for simple tasks or open-ended tasks.
Rich pictures	Allows complex user environments to be mapped out and potential requirements to be identified	Pictures may highlight indicative factors but may lack sufficient detail.
Field study and observational methods	Allows viewing of what users actually do in context and may discover unnoticed processes.	Time consuming to perform. User commentary and analyst observation may disturb tasks.
Diary keeping	Allows user to record activities throughout the day.	Users may forget to complete diaries or summarise activities at the end. Analyst reminders may be annoying.
Video recording	Captures real current activities without the intrusiveness of direct observation.	Time consuming to perform. Requires users to explain activities post-observation.
3. USER NEEDS IDENTIFICATION		
User surveys	Relatively quick method of determining preferences of large user groups and allows for statistical analysis.	Does not capture in depth comments and may not permit follow-up.
Focus groups	Allows analyst to rapidly obtain a wide variety of user views and possibly a consensus.	Recruitment effort to assemble groups. Dominant participants may influence group disproportionately.

Table 2. Comparison of user requirements methods

3. USER NEEDS IDENTIFICATION continued		
Interviewing	Interviews allow for quick elicitation of ideas and concepts. Customer visits brings user context to life.	Need to negotiate access and to combine range of possibly differing opinions from different users.
Scenarios, use cases and personas	Effective way of thinking about future system use in context. Personas can bring user needs to life.	Scenarios may raise expectations too much. Personas may over simplify user population.
Future workshops	Way of thinking creatively.	Results may seem too ambitious for current needs.
Existing system or Competitor analysis	Effective means of identifying current problems, possible new features and acceptance criteria.	May lead to including too many new functions or make system too similar to a competitor's.
4. ENVISIONING & EVALUATING		
Brainstorm	Blank page approach allowing for rapid elicitation and innovative thinking.	Doesn't cover detailed design aspects.
Card sorting and affinity diagrams	Effective means of organising structure of a system e.g. a website.	Needs way to combine results if performed by individuals or groups separately.
Storyboards	Demonstrates software interactions and possibly user context simply and early in the development cycle.	Lacks interactive quality of prototyping.
Prototyping	Quick to build and refine. Allows early detection of usability issues in response to user feedback	Paper prototypes do not support evaluation of fine details. Throwaway software prototypes do but are time consuming to build.
Allocation of function and User cost benefit analysis	Identifies task concerns for the whole work process. Helps define fulfilling jobs and reduces risk of dissatisfied staff.	Needs good overview of whole system. Many allocation options can cause confusion. Cost benefits sometimes hard to estimate.
Design guidelines and standards	Draws upon established knowledge to assist design.	May be too general or constrain design.
Parallel design	Produces range of design ideas and solutions. Can pick best from each.	Requires certain amount of organisation to assemble design teams.

Table 2. **Comparison of user requirements methods (continued)**

5. REQUIREMENTS SPECIFICATION		
Task/function mapping	Way of selecting functions that are relevant to specific tasks. May be a way to avoid including too many functions.	Knowing when task definitions sufficient. Make include tasks to justify unnecessary functions.
User, usability and organisational requirements	Effective way to categorise user requirements. Covers user and organisational levels.	May be hard to decide which user requirements fall into which categories.
Prioritisation	Ensures that effort is put into the most important aspects of the system.	Poor management of user expectations may results in disappointed users.
Criteria setting	Way to determine if developed system has met the user requirements.	Not easily to define suitable criteria. Extensive testing of achievement may be resource intensive.

Table 2. Comparison of user requirements methods (continued)

7. CASE STUDIES

This section describes a series of case studies to show how the methods described in this paper support user requirements development. Normally a mix of methods and techniques is needed.

Development of intranet site. A study was carried out by HUSAT (Maguire & Hirst, 2001b) to evaluate and redesign an intranet site for a police service in the UK. Human Factors consultants performed the study working with a police officer who was project manager for intranet development, and a civilian co-ordinator with a knowledge of police procedures and human factors. Semi-structured interviews were performed with users and stakeholders covering: needs and aspirations regarding the intranet, how well the current system meets those needs, and possible improvements that could be made. Interviewees were given access to the intranet site so they could demonstrate their comments. They included a constable, sergeant, inspector, senior officers and non-police admin staff.

Following the user and stakeholder interviews, an expert review of the intranet pages was performed to establish the strengths and weaknesses of the current service. General recommendations for change were made following the expert evaluation. These were discussed with police representatives and different options for concept designs were proposed using storyboards and screen prototypes. These methods matched the requirement to create and discuss rapid prototypes within the design team. Having developed the design concept, several options for the graphic design for the site were produced as software prototypes to demonstrate both look and feel. A final design for the home page and secondary level content pages was then produced with web templates to allow the police service to install the new pages and maintain them in the future.

The project showed how a combination of methods can produce an acceptable new system design within a relatively short time (3 months).

Expert evaluation of training opportunities. An evaluation was carried out by HUSAT (Maguire & Hirst, 2001a) which provided information about business-related courses to SME's (Small and Medium Enterprises). This was part of a programme of work to develop user requirements for a web-based e-learning service or 'virtual campus'. An evaluation was performed by two Human Factors experts who spent time reviewing each of the main parts of the system from their own experience, a knowledge of typical tasks and usability principles. When providing comments on the system the aim was not to improve the current system but to identify features and implications for the new system. Inputs, from a usability perspective, were made to the user specification of the new virtual campus system. These included elements such as: the inclusion of functions to cover course providers as well as users (as this stakeholder had not previously been considered); suggestion for a mechanism to enter, modify and delete course information and course modules; and provision of typical scenarios of use by the users to make sure that the supplier and customer have the same 'vision' of the system. The project demonstrated how expert evaluation of a current system can provide useful feedback into the requirements specification for the new system.

Interviews to assess future requirements for financial services. Interviews were carried out by HUSAT with family groups to study their management of home finances (Maguire, 1999). Context of use information was gathered, supported by photographs taken of rooms where financial tasks were carried out. The interviews were held as a series of focus group sessions within each household to discuss how and where they performed financial tasks, how they would like to receive services in future and through which devices, e.g. TV, PC, or other domestic appliance. The sessions were video-taped and areas and devices in the home were photographed. The study showed where household devices were located and where family members performed current financial tasks. This provided a basis for identifying innovative ways to deliver future financial services to the home.

Survey to establish user needs for a climate change system. The EC IST EuroClim project (http://euroclim.nr.no) aims to develop an advanced climate monitoring and prediction system for Europe. Climate related data will be stored in digital form collected from a network of sites across Europe. The system will produce raster maps and datasets for scientists and public users showing changes in snow on land, glaciers, sea ice, and general climate trends. To understand the diversity of user requirements for data precision, metadata and data formats, a user needs survey was carried out with climate professionals and public users across Europe. Much effort was required to analyse all the different needs and to summarise them in a form that the design team could assimilate. User needs for data quality varied between users. Therefore charts were produced to show what proportion of users in the survey would be satisfied by different components of data quality i.e. resolution, accuracy and delivery delay. For a specialist system such as EuroClim, it is important to be able to trace the requirements back to the organisations that specified them so that clarification of user needs can be obtained. Based on the information gathered from the survey, a user interface mock-up is being developed to demonstrate the system concept and to 'prototype' the user requirements before the system specification is firmed up and development begins.

User centred design at IAI. Serco worked with IAI LAHAV to evaluate the benefits of applying user-centred methods on a typical project. The user centred design techniques recommended by TRUMP (Bevan et al, 2000) were selected to be simple to plan and apply, and easy to learn by development teams.

1. *Stakeholder meeting and context of use workshop* The stakeholder meeting identifies and agrees on the role of usability, the usability goals, and how these relate to the business objectives and success criteria for the system. The context workshop collects detailed information about the intended users, their tasks, and the technical and environmental constraints. Both events each last for about half a day.
2. *Scenarios of use* A half day workshop to document examples of how users are expected carry out key tasks in a specified contexts, to provide an input to design and a basis for subsequent usability testing.
3. *Evaluate an existing system* Evaluation of an earlier version or competitor system to identify usability problems and obtain measures of usability as an input to usability requirements.
4. *Usability requirements* A half-day workshop to establish usability requirements for the user groups and tasks identified in the context of use analysis and in the scenarios.
5. *Paper prototyping* Evaluation by users of quick low fidelity prototypes to clarify requirements and enable draft interaction designs and screen designs to be rapidly simulated and tested.
6. *Style guide* Identify, document and adhere to industry, corporate or project conventions for screen and page design.
7. *Evaluation of machine prototypes* Informal usability testing with 3-5 representative users carrying out key tasks to provide rapid feedback.
8. *Usability testing* Formal usability testing with 8 representatives of a user group carrying out key tasks to identify any remaining usability problems and evaluate whether usability objectives have been achieved.

IAI concluded that most of the techniques are very intuitive to understand, implement and facilitate. Practicing these techniques in the early stages of design and development ensures less design mistakes later on. All participants and developers thought that most of the techniques were worthwhile and helped in developing a better and more usable system. The techniques were assessed as cost effective and inexpensive to apply.

8. CONCLUSION

To ensure a successful outcome, the design team must satisfy the needs and wants of the user when the development is complete. To achieve this, user needs should not only be elicited by techniques such as surveys, focus groups, interviews etc., but they should also be reflected back to users via simulations in order to prototype the user requirements. The requirements will of course then evolve as the system develops and more formal user evaluation takes place.

9. REFERENCES

Andriole, S. J. (1989), *Storyboard prototyping: a new approach to user requirements analysis*, QED Information Sciences, Inc.

Bevan N (2001) International Standards for HCI and Usability. *International Journal of Human-Computer Studies*, 55, 4.

Bevan, N, Bogomolni, I, & Ryan, N (2000) *Cost-effective user centred design*, www.usability.serco.com/trump

Bevan, N. & Macleod, M (1994) Usability measurement in context. *Behaviour and Information Technology*, **13**, 132-145

Beyer, H. & Holtzblatt, K. (1998), *Contextual design: defining customer-centered systems*, Morgan Kaufmann Publishers.

Bruseberg, A. & McDonagh-Philp, D. (2001), New product development by eliciting user experience and aspirations, *International Journal of Human-Computer Studies*, **55**(4), 435-452.

Checkland, P. (1981), *Systems thinking, systems practice*, Wiley.

Cooper, A. (1999), *The inmates are running the asylum: why high tech products drive us crazy and how to restore the sanity*, Sams publishing.

Eason, K.D. (1988), *Information technology and organisational change*, Taylor and Francis.

Ericsson Infocom Consultants AB and Linköping University (2001), *The Delta method*. www.deltamethod.net/

Hackos, J. & Redish, J. (1998), *User and task analysis for interface design*, Wiley.

Hall, R.R. (2001), Prototyping for usability of new technology, *International Journal of Human-Computer Studies*, 55, 4, 485-502.

IBM (2002), *EZSort* http://www-3.ibm.com/ibm/easy/eou_ext.nsf/Publish/410

ISO (1997), ISO 9241: *Ergonomics requirements for office work with visual display terminals (VDTs), 17parts*, International Standards Organisation.

ISO (1999), ISO 13407: *Human-centred design processes for interactive systems*, International Standards Organisation.

ISO (2002), ISO/IEC 9126-4: *Software engineering – software product quality – Part 4: Quality in Use Metrics*, International Standards Organisation.

Kirwan, B. & Ainsworth, L.K. (eds.) (1992), *A guide to task analysis*, Taylor and Francis.

Macaulay, L.A. (1996), *Requirements engineering*, Springer Verlag Series on Applied Computing.

Maguire, M.C. (1998), *User-centred requirements handbook*. EC Telematics Applications Programme, Project TE 2010 RESPECT (Requirements Engineering and Specification in Telematics), WP4 Deliverable D4.2, version 3.3, May. http:www.lboro.ac.uk/research/husat/respect/rp2.html

Maguire, M.C. (1999), *NCR Knowledge Lab. Report on study of the management of domestic finances by family groups*, 7 May, RSEHF (formerly HUSAT), Loughborough University, Loughborough, UK.

Maguire, M.C. & Hirst, S.J. (2001a), *Usability evaluation of the LINK project TIGS website and feedback on OVC specification*. HUSAT Consultancy Limited, 2 March 2001. RSEHF (formerly HUSAT), Loughborough University, Loughborough, UK.

Maguire, M.C. & Hirst, S.J. (2001b), *Metropolitan Police Service redesign of corporate intranet pages*. HUSAT Consultancy Limited, 26 March 2001. RSEHF (formerly HUSAT), Loughborough University, Loughborough, UK.

Maguire, M.C. (2001c), Context of use within usability activities, *International Journal of Human-Computer Studies*, **55**(4), 453-484.

Mander, R. & Smith, B. (2002), *Web usability for dummies*, New York: Hungry Minds.

Nielsen, J. (2000), *Designing web usability: The practice of simplicity*, New Riders Publishing.

Nicolle, C. & Abascal, J. (eds.) (2001), *Inclusive design guidelines for HCI*, Taylor & Francis.

Olphert, C.W. & Damodaran, L. (2002), Getting what you want, or wanting what you get? - beyond user centred design, *Proceedings of the Third International Conference on Design and Emotion*, Loughborough, UK, 1-3 July 2002.

Preece, J., Rogers, Y., Sharp, H., Benyon, D., Holland, S. & Carey, T. (1994), *Human-computer interaction*. Addison-Wesley.

Robertson, S. & Roberston, T. (1999), *Mastering the requirements process*, Addison-Wesley and ACM Press.

Taylor, B. (1990), The HUFIT planning, analysis and specification toolset, In D. Diaper, G. Cockton, D. Gilmore & B. Shackel, (eds.), *Human-Computer Interaction - INTERACT'90*, 371-376. Amsterdam: North-Holland

Usability: Gaining a Competitive Edge
IFIP World Computer Congress 2002
J. Hammond, T. Gross, J. Wesson (Eds)
Published by Kluwer Academic Publishers

Specifying and Evaluating Usability Requirements using the Common Industry Format

Four case studies

Nigel Bevan
Serco Usability Services
nbevan@usability.serco.com

Nigel Claridge
Scandinavian Usability Associates
nigel_claridge@hotmail.com

Martin Maguire
Loughborough University
M.C.Maguire@lboro.ac.uk

Maria Athousaki
SIEM
siem@otenet.gr

Abstract: The Common Industry Format for usability test reports has been used to introduce usability into public and private contracts for the development of two web sites, acquisition of a travel management system and acquisition of travel agency software. Four pairs of supplier and consumer organisations worked with usability specialists to establish usability requirements and/or to evaluate whether the supplied system met the requirements.

Key words: usability, evaluation, requirements, procurement, standards

1. INTRODUCTION

Incorporating usability requirements in the procurement process can reduce the risk of failure when implementing a newly acquired system and increase ease of use and thus productivity and/or profitability.

- Lack of user performance requirements was a fundamental reason for the expensive costs and delays incurred when new passport issuing software developed by Siemens was installed in the UK (Public Accounts Committee, 1999).
- Two studies have shown that the user success rate in purchasing from current ecommerce web sites is in the range of 25-60% (Nielsen, 2001; Spool & Schroeder, 2001). Small improvements in user performance could lead to substantial increases in revenue.

A new Common Industry Format (CIF) for documenting usability results for use in the procurement process has been developed by a US-based group of companies coordinated by NIST (Bevan, 1999a; Blanchard, 1998). The format has been approved as American standard (ANSI/NCITS 354), and is intended to be submitted to ISO.

The EU-funded PRUE project (Bevan et al, 2001) has demonstrated the value of using the Common Industry Format in four case studies: public and private contracts for development of a web site, and acquisition of a travel management system and travel agency software.

Serco worked with the Italian Ministry of Justice to introduce usability requirements into the acquisition of a new legal information web site, and Scandinavian Usability Associates (SUA) worked with Ericsson to introduce usability requirements in the procurement of an office software product.

Loughborough University and SIEM used the CIF to evaluate the effectiveness of an existing system to assess its acceptability and the need for improvements as part of a contractual relationship with a supplier. Loughborough University assessed an online shopping website in the UK, and SIEM assessed travel agency software in Greece.

2. WHAT IS THE COMMON INDUSTRY FORMAT?

The Common Industry Format for usability test reports specifies the format for reporting the results of a summative usability evaluation. The most common type of usability evaluation is formative, i.e. designed to identify usability problems that can be fixed. A summative evaluation produces usability metrics that describe how usable a product is when used in a particular context of use (Bevan & Macleod, 1994; Macleod et al, 1997). The CIF report format and metrics are consistent with the ISO 9241-11 definition of usability:

> The extent to which a product can be used by specified users to achieve specified goals with effectiveness, efficiency and satisfaction in a specified context of use.

The type of information and level of detail that is required by the CIF standard is intended to ensure that:

- Good practice in usability evaluation had been adhered to.
- There is sufficient information for a usability specialist to judge the validity of the results (for example whether the evaluation context adequately reproduces the intended context of use).
- If the test is replicated based on the information given, it should produce essentially the same results.

- Specific effectiveness and efficiency metrics must be used, including the unassisted completion rate and the mean time on task.
- Satisfaction must also be measured.

It was envisaged that a supplier would provide a CIF report to enable a corporate purchaser to take account of usability when making a purchase decision. A purchaser could compare CIF reports for alternative products (particularly if a common set of tasks had been used). The purchaser might specify in advance to a supplier the required values of the usability measures (for example based on the values for an existing product).

The original motivation for the CIF came from usability staff in purchasing companies who were frustrated at purchase decisions made exclusively on the basis of functionality. These companies experienced large uncontrolled overhead costs from supporting difficult to use software (Blanchard, 1998).

The CIF format was agreed by a working group of usability experts from purchasing and supplying companies. It was based on collating good practice from the different companies, and aligning this with ISO 9241-11.

3. PURPOSE OF THE TRIALS

The main purpose of the PRUE project was to evaluate the business value of introducing the CIF into the purchasing and procurement process in a variety of contractual environments. There were four trials (Table 1).

One trial was for the originally envisaged role in the acquisition of corporate software (Ericsson/Electrolux). Another extended this to acquisition of a custom-designed web site (Ministry/SEMA). These trials both focussed on evaluating whether a new web-based system meets requirements established by prior evaluation of the existing text-based system.

The two other trials (in2netlogic/prezzybox.com and Robissa Travel/ExcelSoft) assessed the usefulness of the CIF in negotiating for improvements in a custom-designed system, by evaluating the usability of an existing product to establish requirements for an improved version. The in2netlogic/prezzybox.com trial was in the UK where usability is well-established as an issue, and Robissa Travel/ExcelSoft was in Greece where usability is less well recognised.

	Italian Ministry of Justice + SEMA	Ericsson Telecom + Electrolux	In2netlogic + prezzybox. com	Robissa Travel + ExcelSoft
Product	Web site: legal info	Travel expense reporting	Web site: ecommerce	Travel management
Users	Legal staff and public	Office staff	Public	Travel agent staff
Existing system	Traditional dial up	Text based	Existing web site	Existing product
New system	Web based	Web based	Improved version	Improved version
Contractual relationship	The Ministry will use CIF results as part of acceptance criteria	Ericsson will use CIF results as part of acceptance criteria	Basis for negotiation for improvements	Basis for negotiation for improvements
Consumer organisation benefits	Convenient and accurate legal info	Increased productivity and quality of travel info	Increased business	Increased office efficiency

Table 1. Summary of trials

4. ITALIAN MINISTRY OF JUSTICE/SEMA: LEGAL WEB SITE

PRUE has helped the Italian Ministry of Justice introduce usability requirements into the procurement of a new enhanced version of the existing dial-up ITALGIURE-FIND legal information service. This builds on previous work with Italian Public Administrations (Catarci, 2002; Catarci et al, 2000).

SEMA has a contract with the Ministry to produce a new system accessible from internet browsers and mobile phones. No information was previously available on the usability of the existing system, and there were no usability requirements in the contract (although the contract required ISO 13407 to be used).

PRUE planned three activities to introduce usability to the procurement process:

- A stakeholder meeting to identify the importance of usability and the intended context of use.
- An evaluation of the existing system to provide measures of usability as baseline requirements.
- An evaluation of a prototype of the new system to establish whether the requirements have been met.

The stakeholder meeting was attended by senior representatives of the Ministry, SEMA and other stakeholders. Two user groups were identified: expert users with legal knowledge need functionality to support fast and efficient searches, consistent with the natural logic of juridical research. The system will also be accessible to new users without any legal knowledge who should be able to carry out simple searches without training.

In the evaluation of the existing system, five experts and four non-experts attempted to complete different sets of typical tasks. Expert users successfully accomplished 63% of tasks in comparison with 52% of non-expert users. The evaluation also provided the opportunity for SEMA designers to observe real usage of the system.

An important objective was for the new system to at least equal and if possible improve on these success rates. If the measured success rates and user satisfaction scores are not acceptable, the Ministry could negotiate with SEMA to provide an improved system.

The trial has demonstrated several benefits of introducing summative usability testing into the procurement process:

- It provides a concrete benchmark for user performance and satisfaction, thus reducing the risk that the new system is more difficult to use (and therefore less successful) than the existing system.
- It highlights usability problems with the existing system that need to be addressed in the design of the new system.
- It provides specific goals for usability and gives developers the opportunity to become familiar with typical user task scenarios.
- It provides the framework for the more detailed usability work required by ISO 13407.

Summative evaluation results reported in the CIF format have thus been very useful in helping the Ministry understand the needs of different user groups, and in establishing usability requirements for the new system. The user testing has also clear benefits in helping the supplier (SEMA) better understand Ministry of Justice requirements.

5. ERICSSON/ELECTROLUX: TRAVEL MANAGEMENT SYSTEM

In order to support the procurement process, the Common Industry Format (CIF) for usability testing has been used to obtain usability metrics at Ericsson and Electrolux in Sweden. First, the current Ericsson system was tested using the CIF to obtain a baseline value for usability, which resulted in a usability requirements document. The document required information about the way in which the supplier had developed the product and detailed information about user performance and user satisfaction metrics. Secondly, the likely supplier of a new system called WEBRES developed by Electrolux was tested and the results compared to the requirements document.

Ericsson was investigating the purchase of a new interface to the existing travel management system - RES. The current text-based interface no longer supported users task demands and requirements effectively and it was not found easy to use. RES was used by about 25% of Ericsson employees although the goal was to increase this percentage significantly. It was a complete system that supported business travel management both nationally and internationally.

Ericsson did not wish to make significant changes to the underlying system. They looked to a number of potential suppliers who were able to provide a new interface, which would enhance the efficient and effective use of the existing system. At this time, the prime candidate supplier was Electrolux. They used essentially the same travel management system as Ericsson but had developed in-house interface solution - WEBRES. This interface was a possible replacement to the current RES interface.

At this time, Ericsson had not considered any usability issues during the purchase process. There was no objective data about user performance/subjective assessment using RES and there was no usability requirements document. The PRUE project was able to support the procurement process by conducting summative usability testing on RES using the CIF format. The objective was to obtain user performance and satisfaction metrics of the RES interface through formal user testing. The results from testing, which showed low satisfaction scores and a mean task completion rate of only 55%, led to a usability requirements document against which potential suppliers could be assessed. Subsequently, similar testing using the CIF was conducted on Electrolux's WEBRES. The test results were then compared and contrasted to the usability requirements document prepared by Ericsson.

PRUE has been of great value to Ericsson. Without PRUE, usability issues would not have been included in this procurement process. PRUE has resulted in a usability requirements document for a new interface to RES, which was regarded as a new and positive input to the Ericsson decision process when selecting a supplier organization. The usability requirements were regarded as a good complement to the existing functional and technical specifications. Further, there were benefits of increased understanding of user performance using the current system (poor performance is a large cost in time to Ericsson), an objective understanding of what users thought of the current system and what they require from the new.

From the supplier perspective, Electrolux have been able to understand the performance/ satisfaction related Ericsson requirements for WEBRES. The CIF for usability testing enabled them to assess how WEBRES compared to the Ericsson requirements, and it has provided a clear indication of what improvements need to be made to the interface design.

6. PREZZYBOX/IN2NETLOGIC: ECOMMERCE WEB SITE

This study was concerned with an online shopping website called *Prezzybox*. The site, developed by *in2netlogic*, offers a wide range of gift ideas for purchasers to select and have delivered, either to themselves, or to a friend or relative. The website was evaluated by the PRUE partner - the Research School of Ergonomics and Human Factors (RSEHF) at Loughborough University (which incorporates the former HUSAT).

The main objective of the user test was to obtain user performance and satisfaction metrics for Prezzybox along with user comments to highlight any problems with the site. Testing was carried out with 12 users who were all experienced with the Internet and interested in buying from the Prezzybox site. Users were asked to make a real purchase from the site - this being their payment for taking part. Thus the evaluation was designed to test the success of users in completing an online purchase - a crucial success factor for any online shopping site.

The result of the evaluation was a CIF report that documented user performance and satisfaction with the site. This showed that 2 out of the 12 users failed to make a purchase. If the consumer organisation could capture those two users, their sales would increase by 20%!

These performance results were also supported with user satisfaction ratings. The levels of satisfaction recorded were in general around just 'satisfactory' representing clear scope to improve the 'user experience' when using the site.

Evaluator comments and recommendations for change to the site were also included, highlighting features that could be changed to help improve user success in making a purchase.

The CIF benefited the consumer organisation (Prezzybox) by enabling it to:

- Find out how successful consumers will be in making a purchase from their site i.e. what percentage can actually make a purchase?
- Provide a benchmark for user performance and attitude, which can be used for comparison with the shopping site when it is revised.
- Obtain insights into any problems that users face when using the site (to complement the summative results) and to receive suggestions for improving the site.

The CIF benefited the supplier organisation (in2netlogic) by enabling it to:

- Obtain objective feedback on the success of the design they produced.
- Identify the most important usability issues that will enable the shopping site to support more successful purchases – and therefore improve the profitability of the site for the consumer organisation.
- Negotiate a new contract to improve the site, based on the test results and the comments and suggestions for improving the site.

Currently the Prezzybox site is being refined based on the feedback. A second round of usability evaluation is planned so that the consumer and supplier organisations can receive concrete evidence that the site has been improved. It is also hoped to show that this usability activity has enhanced the site from the user's point of view.

In summary, the evaluation approach of the CIF is recommended for other online shopping providers in order to test what proportion of users actually make a purchase from their site. It also sets a baseline against which new versions and upgrades to the site can be compared, while also highlighting the problems that need to be fixed if the site is to achieve a greater number of online sales.

7. ROBISSA TRAVEL/EXCELSOFT: TRAVEL AGENT SOFTWARE

In the context of the PRUE Project, SIEM, in cooperation with a software development company and a representative client (Robissa Travel, a travel agency), planned and carried out a usability test for a software application (Global Travel) that supports the management tasks of a travel agency. All the steps of the evaluation procedure, as well as the final results were recorded and reported using the CIF format. The procedure that was followed included the following steps:

1. Definition of the product to be tested
2. Definition of the context of use
3. Specification of the usability requirements
4. Specification of the context of the evaluation
5. Design of the evaluation
6. Performance of the user tests and collection of data
7: Report and analysis of the collected data

The benefits for both participating organizations (i.e., the supplier and the consumer) were considerable:

- The supplier, through a standardised and valid test procedure obtained a concrete and objective measure of the usability of the tested product in order to demonstrate its quality but also spot potential problems.
- Additionally, the evaluation data (usability problems, new user requirements, ideas, etc.) that were collected will be useful as input for the design of a future version of the product.
- The consumer was able to judge the usability of the supplier's product, through the evaluation process as well as the extent to which the specific product caters for his/her particular needs.
- Another expected benefit was that the consumer's opinion and needs, highlighted during the whole process, will be taken into account for the design of the next version of the product.
- Additionally, the process helped the consumer identify his / her real needs, state them to the developers in an organised and understandable way, and produce a document for common reference.
- Finally, since, on the one had, the supplier will be able to take into account the consumer's needs by using a well-documented and objective procedure, and, on the other hand, the consumer will have an objective process (the CIF report) for judging the extent to which this was accomplished, it is clear that there is a unique opportunity for the creation of a close and mutually beneficial relationship between them. The results of such a relationship can be for the supplier: a loyal customer, and for the consumer: software products of higher quality, productivity and usability.

In conclusion, the study proved that the CIF format can provide real added-value to a software project, because it is a structured and well-defined process. Both the consumer and the supplier considered it as an efficient, effective and worthwhile activity that had positive results for both. The extra resources (time and effort) required are well justified and spent, and both organizations are positive to using again the CIF format in the future. Of course it has to be noted that in order for the whole process to be resource-effective but also valid and productive, an organization that has high expertise in usability engineering is required, since both the wording and the process of the CIF format require a theoretical background, but also a considerable amount of concrete previous experience, in the field.

8. CONCLUSIONS

Much early usability work used summative methods (Whiteside et al, 1988), but was not always supported by other user centred design activities. It therefore gained the reputation for being an expensive way to identify problems when it was too late to fix them! So the emphasis moved to formative evaluation (so-called "discount" usability methods) that could be used earlier in development (Nielsen, 1993). It is essential to introduce usability early in the development process, but without subsequent summative testing, it is difficult to judge the effectiveness of the usability work (Bevan, 1999b).

Summative usability testing using the CIF has advantages to both consumer and supplier organisations during procurement. It is one of the most effective ways to enrich the consumer's requirements document with objective user performance and satisfaction metrics (based on the existing system/product used). It provides a platform on which to evaluate potential competitive products from a number of supplier organisations during the procurement of a new system/product. By using the CIF test structure, suppliers are able to demonstrate that their product complies with the usability metrics defined in the requirements document.

The adoption of the format as an international standard should provide a strong case for the wider use of summative testing reported in the Common Industry Format. The PRUE case studies provide strong evidence for the benefits of this approach.

9. ACKNOWLEDGEMENTS

The work with the Italian Ministry of Justice was carried out in conjunction with Tiziana Catarci (Universita' di Roma "La Sapienza"), Giacinto Matarazzo (Fondazione Ugo Bordoni) and.Gianluigi Raiss (AIPA, Rome).

10. REFERENCES

Bevan, N. (1999a) Industry standard usability tests, in S. Brewster, A. Cawsey & G. Cockton (eds.) *Human-Computer Interaction – INTERACT '99 (Volume II), British Computer Society*, pp 107-108.

Bevan, N. (1999b) Quality in use: meeting user needs for quality, *Journal of Systems and Software*, **49**(1), pp 89-96.

Bevan, N. and Macleod, M. (1994) Usability measurement in context. *Behaviour and Information Technology*, **13**(1), pp.32-145.

Bevan, N., Bogomolni, I. & Ryan, N. (2001) *PRUE: Providing Reports of Usability Evaluation*, www.usability.serco.com/prue

Blanchard, H. (1998) Standards for usability testing. *SIGCHI Bulletin*, **30**(3), pp.16-17.

Catarci, T. (2002) Driving usability into the Italian public administration, submitted for publication.

Catarci, T., Matarazzo, G., and Raiss, G. (2000) Usability and Public Administration: Experiences of a difficult marriage, in *Proceedings of the 1st ACM international conference. on universal usability*, ACM Press, pp.24-31.

ISO 9241-11 (1998) *Ergonomic requirements for office work with visual display terminals (VDT)s - Part 11 Guidance on usability.*

ISO 13407 (1999) *User centred design process for interactive systems.*

Macleod, M., Bowden, R., Bevan, N. & Curson, I. (1997) The MUSiC Performance Measurement Method. *Behaviour and Information Technology*, **16**, pp 279-293.

Nielsen J (1993) *Usability Engineering*, Academic Press.

Nielsen J (2001) http://www.useit.com/alertbox/20010819.html

Public Accounts Committee (1999) *Improving the Delivery of Government IT Projects* http://www.publications.parliament.uk/pa/cm199900/cmselect/cmpubacc/65/6502.htm

Spool, J. & Schroeder, W. (2001) Testing Web Sites: Five Users is Nowhere Near Enough. *Proceedings of ACM SIGCHI 2001.*

Whiteside, J., Bennett, J. & Holzblatt, K. (1988) Usability engineering: our experience and evolution, in M. Helander (ed.), *Handbook of Human-Computer Interaction,* Elsevier.

Usability: Gaining a Competitive Edge
IFIP World Computer Congress 2002
J. Hammond, T. Gross, J. Wesson (Eds)
Published by Kluwer Academic Publishers

Formal Usability Testing of Interactive Educational Software: A Case Study

Darelle Van Greunen and Janet Wesson
University of Port Elizabeth, South Africa
csadvg@upe.ac.za, csajlw@upe.ac.za

Abstract: As the amount and variety of interactive educational software grows, so does the need to assess the usability of the software. The usability of educational software can be defined as the extent to which the software can be used to achieve specified learning outcomes effectively, efficiently and with user satisfaction. This paper discusses the evaluation of the usability of interactive educational software and proposes a method for formal usability testing of such software that has been successfully used at the University of Port Elizabeth (UPE). After describing the method, it presents a case study to illustrate the implementation of the proposed method.

Keywords: Usability testing, usability methodology, usability, empirical evaluation.

1. INTRODUCTION

The usability of educational software such as tutorial programs is closely related to how much a person learns from using the software. Usability of educational software can be defined as the extent to which the software can be used to achieve specified learning outcomes with effectiveness, efficiency and satisfaction in a specified learning context (Geisert and Futrell, 1995). In this context, effectiveness and efficiency are measures of learner performance. Satisfaction can also affect learning outcomes indirectly, as poorly motivated learners do not use educational software to the best effect (Geisert and Futrell, 1995). These performance measures are best measured by allowing learners to use the educational software. The more they learn from using the software, the more effective it is. The quicker they learn, the more efficient it is. Satisfaction is a more subjective measure, but still important as satisfaction and motivation are closely related. Standard questionnaires such as Questionnaire for User Interaction Satisfaction (QUIS^{TM}) can be used to assess the users' satisfaction with software generally (HCI Laboratory University of Maryland, 2000).

When evaluating educational software, it is important to specify usability objectives that are target levels of effectiveness, efficiency and satisfaction for the particular software package. Usability experts or consultants can assess the usability, but such assessments are rarely as reliable and meaningful as evaluations involving the actual users themselves (Barnum, 2002). There is, however, a lack of expertise in usability testing in South Africa. Most tertiary institutions in South Africa lack usability testing facilities to formally or empirically evaluate system usability. No standard or suggested guidelines currently exist for usability testing in South Africa. This paper will briefly review formal usability testing and discuss a method for conducting a successful formal usability evaluation in a usability laboratory. After describing the formal usability evaluation method, a case study is presented to illustrate the implementation of the method. This case study involved a formal usability evaluation of an educational software package developed at UPE, called Interactive Learner (IAL).

2. INTERACTIVE EDUCATIONAL SOFTWARE

The usability of educational software is heavily dependent on the context in which the software is used (Squires and Preece, 1996). Therefore educational software that is well matched to one learning context may be poorly matched to another context, depending on who the learners are and what their learning objectives are. The environment in which they will learn and the equipment they will be using also play a role.

There are general design guidelines for educational software (based on research in Human-Computer Interaction) that can be applied in a variety of contexts (Squires and Preece, 1996). A key technique is to get feedback from prospective learners and users during the development of educational software (Alessi and Trollip, 2001). Testing prototype educational software with users can be a particularly useful way of getting feedback about usability. To get good feedback, you need a reliable means of assessing and measuring usability.

3. MEASURING USABILITY OF CAL SOFTWARE

A Computer Assisted Learning (CAL) package is both a software artefact and a piece of courseware (Gagne et al., 1992). From its original conception to its production and in-service maintenance, the team working on CAL courseware moves through the lifecycles of both courseware design and software production.

Alessi maintains that CAL software may be evaluated from different perspectives (Alessi and Trollip, 2001). These relate to the different needs of the stakeholders in a CAL system: developers, tutors and students. Usability of educational software can be assessed by measuring each of its components, namely effectiveness, efficiency and satisfaction (Squires and Preece, 1996). Testing the educational software with a group of users and measuring their learning progress via assessments are good ways to measure these. The more users learn from working through the educational software, the more effective it is. The quicker they learn, the more efficient it is. Satisfaction is a more subjective measure, but no less important in assessing educational software since satisfaction and motivation are closely related to achievement of lasting learning outcomes.

4. FORMAL USABILITY TESTING

Formal usability testing is an empirical method that requires the design of a formal usability experiment that is undertaken under controlled conditions in a usability laboratory (Faulkner, 2000). Evaluators give a user a specific task to perform within specific timeframes (Barnum, 2002). The laboratory shown in Figure 1 is typical of those in use today.

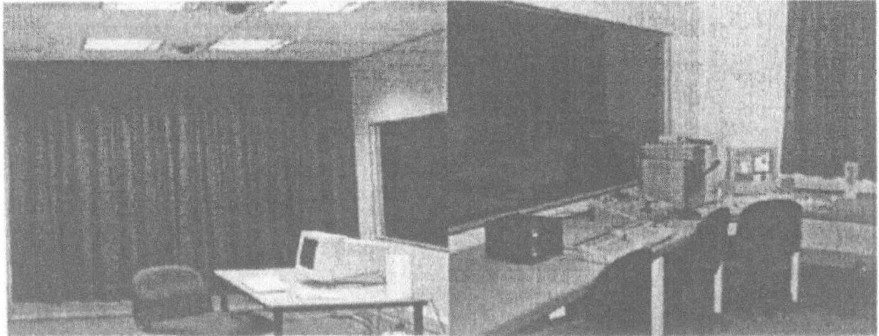

Figure 1. The Participant Room (left) and the Observer Room (right) of the UPE Usability Laboratory

The UPE laboratory consists of two rooms, divided by one-way window in the wall between the two rooms. One room provides a place for the user to perform the tasks required of the test.

The other room, where the test administrator or observer records the activities on videotape for later review, is typically called the observer room.

Evaluators observe the problem(s) the user has, videotape the session and what is happening on the user's computer screen, and then analyze the observational logs and videotapes. Essential components of such an evaluation include a usability laboratory with special-purpose hardware and software; a test plan for the usability experiment; a methodology or technique to conduct the usability experiment and the analysis of the results obtained from the experiment. The results of formal usability testing can provide essential empirical information for the software design process.

5. EVALUATION METHODS

Several guidelines exist in the literature on how to conduct a formal usability evaluation (Rubin, 1994). Most of these are, however, very general and do not give specific guidance on how to conduct the evaluation.

The overall process is simple; get some users and find out how they work with the product. Usually you observe individual users performing specific tasks with the product. You collect data on how they are doing, for example, how long do they take to perform a task, whether they can complete the task successfully, or how many errors they make. Then the data from all the experiments is analysed with the aim of looking for trends.

The above is, however, only a very high-level description of how to conduct a formal usability evaluation and does not represent a complete methodology. Our research into usability testing has shown that an evaluation methodology is needed to successfully design a formal usability evaluation. A decision was made, therefore, to use the methodologies as suggested by Faulkner (Faulkner, 2000) and Rubin (Rubin, 1994) and to supplement these with the additional detail suggested by Dumas and Redish (Dumas and Redish, 1993). Certain aspects of the Common Industry Format Report for Usability Testing were included to present a more detailed, step-by-step descriptive methodology for formal usability testing (Common Industry Format for Usability Test Reports, 2001). An overview of the proposed methodology is given in Table 1 below.

Step	Description of Step
1	Formulate an overall goal of the product to be tested.
2	Formulate objectives for the usability test.
3	Formulate research hypotheses.
4	Determine specific evaluation metrics.
5	Establish the user profile.
6	Select the tasks to be performed.
7	Determine how to analyse the results.
8	Formulate and write the test plan.
9	Create the post-test questionnaire.
10	Select representative participants.
11	Conduct a pilot test.
12	Conduct the usability test.
13	Organise and collate the data.
14	Analyse the findings.
15	Draw evaluation conclusions.
16	Report the results.

Table 1. **Basic steps of the proposed methodology**

The next section discusses a case study to illustrate the application of this methodology to do a formal usability evaluation of an educational software package at UPE. As discussed above, a test plan is an essential element of such a formal usability evaluation. The following sections are extracts from the test plan.

6. CASE STUDY: INTERACTIVE LEARNER

For the purpose of this research, we did a formal usability evaluation of an educational software package called Interactive Learner (IAL). This tutorial was developed at UPE in 1998 in order to teach and test certain basic computing skills, including keyboard and mouse skills. IAL also produces a simple categorization of the computer expertise of the user as novice, intermediate or expert, based on the time taken by the user to complete the tutorial and the frequency of user errors. IAL is currently being used as part of a model to derive a user classification framework for prospective students at UPE (Streicher et al., 2001).

The usability objectives of IAL were not clearly defined during the development of the tutorial package, but could be summarized as follows:

- Users should achieve the outcomes of being able to successfully use a mouse and keyboard after having completed the tutorial. This could be regarded as a measure of effectiveness of the tutorial.

- It should take users no longer than 25 minutes to achieve the outcomes as mentioned before. This is a measurement of efficiency of the tutorial.
- Satisfaction can be determined by means of questionnaires relating to whether users enjoyed using the tutorial package.

A heuristic evaluation and user observation revealed that IAL contained several usability problems that could affect the user performance. This heuristic evaluation was based on Nielsen's ten usability heuristics (Nielsen, 1994). The key findings of the heuristic evaluation indicated moderate usability problems relating to the visibility of the system status and the use of language in IAL. Johnson defines "unprofessional writing" as "Inconsistent, unclear, and difficult to understand terminology" (Johnson, 2000). Unprofessional writing was used in IAL, which forced the user to reread instructions and text. High usability problems were identified with regard to consistency and standards, as well as error prevention. Inconsistent error messages caused confusion and uncertainty and the user was not always clear how to proceed after the occurrence of a message. The problems revealed by the heuristic evaluation were used as a basis for the planning of the formal usability test.

6.1 The goal of the test

The goal of the usability test was to determine if there were any specific usability problems with IAL that would negatively affect the students' performance. Representative users were asked to complete the tutorial, and measures were taken of effectiveness, efficiency and satisfaction.

6.2 Research Hypotheses

Our research hypotheses were as follows:

H_0: No usability problems exist with IAL.

H_1: Any usability problems that may exist will not affect user performance in IAL.

H_2: Any usability problems that may exist will not affect the different user groups (novice, intermediate, expert) differently.

6.3 User Profile

Background questionnaires were distributed to 350 potential participants who were first-year students at UPE. This questionnaire was used to categorise the potential participants into three different groups based on a user classification model as developed by Streicher et al (Streicher et al., 2001). This grouping was done on a basis of the different ability groups (i.e. novice, intermediate and expert). Once this grouping was done, a random selection of 7 participants per user group was then made (see Table 2).

	User group	**Home Language**				**Gender**		
		Afrikaans	**English**	**Xhosa**	**Total**	**Male**	**Female**	**Total**
1	Novice	0	3	4	7	0	7	7
2	Intermediate	3	3	1	7	4	3	7
3	Expert	0	7	0	7	6	1	7
	Total	3	13	5	21	10	11	21

Table 2. Profile of the participant population

A total of 21 participants were tested. The participants were divided into three groups based on the background questionnaire as follows:

- **Novices:** 7 participants were computer novices. These participants represented the least competent (novice) user who will use IAL.
- **Intermediate:** 7 participants had previous computer experience. Participants in this group had the following characteristics:
  - Work with a computer on a regular basis;
  - Use keyboard keys, cursor keys and mouse; and
  - Spend the majority of computer usage performing word processing tasks.
- **Expert:** 7 participants who had advanced computer experience. Participants in this group had the following characteristics:
  - Work with a computer on a regular basis;
  - Use keyboard keys, cursor keys and mouse;
  - Are familiar with checkboxes and radio buttons; and
  - Spend computer usage time performing tasks ranging from word processing to spreadsheets to desktop publishing tasks.

The above user classification was made based on the intended user population of IAL, as well as the student population at UPE.

6.4 Data Collection

Data was collected and calculated by means of:

- Video recordings with the purpose of capturing the test session (live) on tape so that it could be evaluated at a later stage.
- A preference questionnaire was used to gather feedback and usability metrics using a modified version of the Questionnaire for User Interaction Satisfaction (QUIS™).
- Monitoring of tasks.

7. TEST PLAN

7.1 Performance test

The performance test consisted of the completion of the tutorial within the allocated time period of 25 minutes while being observed.

7.2 Participant debriefing

After the tutorial was completed, the test facilitator debriefed each participant. The debriefing included the following:

- Filling out a brief preference questionnaire pertaining to the usability and aesthetics of IAL.
- Participant's overall comments about his or her performance.
- Participant's responses to probes from the test facilitator about specific errors or problems during the test, e.g. repeating exercises.

7.3 Test environment and equipment requirements

The UPE usability laboratory was used as the test environment with a personal computer (PC) connected to the LAN and loaded with the IAL software and a mouse connected to the PC.

7.4 Evaluation metrics

The objectives of the usability test relate to the measurable goals of the test (Barnum, 2002). These are also called the evaluation metrics and are used to gather information about the performance of the user.

Efficiency:

- **Amount of time spent reading of information on the screen**. This metric involved measuring the time taken to open/enter a screen and then read the instructions/text on the screen before executing the first action.
- **Real-time events**. This metric involved monitoring and filtering events such as the push of a key, click of a mouse or the use of the arrow keys per screen.

Effectiveness:

- **Amount of time spent on an exercise**. This metric consisted of monitoring the time a user spent on reading the instructions for an exercise prior to completing the exercise. This also included the time spent on the exercise, as well as the number of iterations per exercise.

- **Completion of events.** This metric consisted of monitoring the successful completion of different events on different screens.
- **Error rate and recovery.** This metric consisted of monitoring the number of errors made by the user, as well as the number of errors from which the user could not recover.

Satisfaction:

- **User satisfaction.** This metric was measured using a subjective ratings scale and the modified version of Questionnaire for User Interaction Satisfaction (QUIS^{TM}), at the end of the session. The following five factors were measured: overall satisfaction, screen design, terminology and system information, learnability and system capabilities. Each of the specific interface factors consisted of a main question followed by related sub-questions. Each item was rated on a scale from 1 to 5 with 1 representing a negative response and 5 representing a positive response. In addition, "not applicable" was listed as a choice.

8. RESULTS

The first step in evaluating the data was the analysis of the post-test questionnaire. The questionnaire was analysed statistically using MS-Excel and Statistica (Statsoft, 2001). A t-test analysis was performed to analyse the results in the different categories.

The second step in evaluating the data was the analysis of the videotapes taken during the session. The focus here was on the general understanding of the instructions and tasks to see whether the test participants could determine how to complete the tasks. Data from the videos was analysed using the Elementary Statistics function of the Observer Video Pro package (Noldus Technology, March 2001).

8.1 Questionnaire results

The results of the modified version of Questionnaire for User Interaction Satisfaction (QUIS^{TM}) were analysed using a t-test analysis. In general, the majority of the responses were positive and only one significant difference in overall user reactions was identified between novice and expert users. This section of the questionnaire posed questions regarding the user's overall reaction to the tutorial, the effectiveness of the tutorial and whether the tutorial tested the users' skills adequately.

8.2 Performance results

The mean extent to which each task was completely and correctly completed, was scored as a percentage. In addition to data for each task, the combined results show the total task time and the mean results for effectiveness and efficiency metrics. These results are discussed in more detail below.

Task Completion: All participants completed the tutorial successfully, but with significantly different completion times. The expert users, as expected, had the shortest mean completion time (10.76 min); followed by the intermediate users (13.29 min) and the novice users (15.47 min). Further analysis of these results was restricted to two groups of users only, namely expert and novice users. The reason for this was that the results of the intermediate user group and the novice user group were very similar (99% significance).

Incidence of errors: In general, very few errors were recorded. The novice user group had one occurrence of an error, whilst the expert user group had two occurrences.

Recovery from errors: All user groups managed to recover from their errors in a very short space of time. They completed the exercises successfully.

Speed of performance: An analysis of the speed of performance is contained in Figure 2. Despite significant differences in actual time spent, it was noted that both novice and expert users spent approximately 45% of their time reading instructions on the various screens of the tutorial. Since the primary goal of IAL is instructional, this can be regarded as acceptable (Alessi and Trollip, 2001).

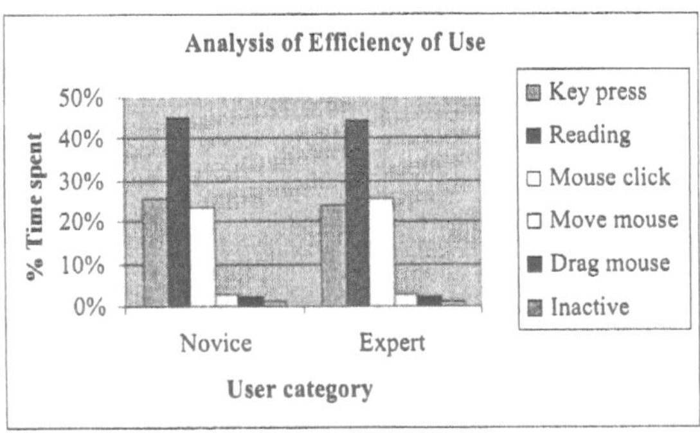

Figure 2. Analysis of user performance

Ease of use: IAL displays a reminder message after a specific time delay to guide the user in navigation between different screens. Both expert and novice users received several reminder messages. Novice users received considerably more reminder messages (93%) than the expert users.

Task closure: IAL displays the message "You have completed the exercise" on the screen on completion of an exercise. The user can, however, continue with the exercise. When the users do continue because they do not recognise or realise that the exercise is completed, a reminder message is displayed which reminds the users how to navigate forward. The frequency of these messages indicates that the task closure for completing an exercise is incorrect and that users should be prevented from redoing an exercise.

9. ANALYSIS OF RESULTS

This section examines the results obtained from an analysis of the performance of the different user groups. No significant usability problems were identified in the post-test questionnaire. The video analysis identified certain specific usability problems (see Table 3). These usability problems identified, were as follows:

Frequency of Reminder Messages			Mean time on screen (in min)			
Screen	Expert users	Novice users	Expert users	Novice users	Mean	StdDev
2	0	1	0.00	10.00	5.00	7.07
3	6	4	3.26	11.96	7.61	6.15
4	1	4	1.08	2.64	1.86	1.10
5	0	1	0.00	2.96	1.48	2.09
6	1	2	4.27	0.78	2.53	2.47
7	0	1	0.00	1.20	0.60	0.85
9	1	4	0.84	3.53	2.19	1.90
10	0	3	0.00	4.84	2.42	3.42
11	1	2	8.80	2.12	5.46	4.72
12	1	0	3.04	0.00	1.52	2.15
13	3	4	6.13	4.39	5.26	1.23
15	1	3	3.08	5.02	4.05	1.37

Table 3. Frequency of Reminder Messages on different types of screens

- The screen titles did not contain a clear classification of the different screen types. IAL consists of 4 different types of screens, namely

General, Information, Exercise and Question screens. The only type of screen that is labeled is the Exercise type screen. Considerable time is spent on the task of reading text and instructions on the screens of IAL (see Figure 2). The main reason for this was determined to be that the user was not always clear what was expected on a particular type of screen. This had a negative impact on the overall speed of performance of not only the novice users but also the expert users.

- Navigation between screens appeared to be a problem together with a lack of task closure at the end of an exercise. This is evident in the fact that both an Exercise Completed message, as well as a Reminder message was often displayed simultaneously on the screen.
- Unprofessional writing resulted in long, unclear and inconsistent lines of text and instructions (Johnson, 2000). This had a negative impact on the overall speed of performance of users as a considerable amount of time was spent on the task of reading and understanding the text and instructions (see Figure 2).
- Inconsistent Error, Reminder and Exercise Completed messages caused users to wonder whether different words or actions meant the same thing. Platform conventions for user interface design were not followed making it difficult for the user to recognize the different messages.
- The system did not always keep the user informed about what was going on. Feedback occurred, but not necessarily within a reasonable time period.

Screens 3, 4, 9 and 13 exhibited specific usability problems. The frequency of Reminder Messages on these screens for both novice and expert users indicated that there were some usability problems. These problems included those mentioned above, but related more specifically to unprofessional and unclear writing and no titles on the screens. The frequency of Reminder Messages indicated that both novice and expert users were unclear as to what was expected of them. This correlates strongly with the usability problems identified in the heuristic evaluation, specifically visibility of system status.

Several usability problems with IAL were therefore identified. We can thus reject H_0 (see Research Hypotheses). Likewise, we can reject H_1 since these usability problems were seen to negatively affect the speed of performance of the users. The increased frequency of reminder messages for novice users is an indication that novice users were affected more than expert users, and thus we can also reject H_2.

10. DESIGN CHANGES

As a result of the formal usability evaluation, the following design changes were proposed:

- All screens must be labeled according to the type of screen they represent. This will enable users to recognize what is expected of them on a particular screen (Visibility of system status).
- All exercise screens must contain a clear task closure and not allow the user to continue with the exercise. This will enable the user to recognize that the exercise has been completed (Error prevention).
- The speed of performance could be improved by rewording the instructions/text displayed on the screens taking into account guidelines on how to shorten text in a graphical user interface (Johnson, 2000). By limiting the instructions and text to the essentials only, the user will not have to spend an excessive amount of time on reading.
- All messages (Error, Reminder and Exercise Completed) should be reworded and designed according to Johnson's guidelines. Messages should be redesigned to adhere to platform conventions (Consistency and standards).
- To improve feedback to the user, the time delay before a message is displayed should be reduced from 25 sec to 5 sec after the user has completed a specific action (Johnson, 2000).

A further usability evaluation was conducted after the suggested changes were implemented to IAL. The test was conducted with 7 participants who were computer novice users (see User Profile in Table 4).

Novice user group	Mean completion time (min)	StdDev (min)
Initial design	15.47	2.6
Improved design	13.96	2.6
% Improvement	9.8 %	

Table 4. Comparison of Efficiency of IAL

Task completion: The mean completion time of the novice user group was reduced from 15.47 minutes to 13.96 minutes. All 7 participants completed the tutorial successfully within the allocated 25 minutes.

Incidence of errors: No instances of error messages were recorded.

Ease of use: In the improved system, Reminder Messages and Exercise Completed Messages were combined into one message that appears at the end of an exercise assisting the student with navigation. The time delay between the completion of an exercise and the message appearing on the screen was reduced from 25 sec to 5 sec. No Reminder Messages appeared on screen, neither were there any instances of user errors.

Task closure: As task closure was implemented, users could not continue with exercises once these were completed. A user could only repeat an exercise from the beginning if he/she felt the need to do so.

Speed of performance: In some instances, there were significant differences between the two novice user groups. Group 1 (Novice users in initial test) spent approximately 45% of their time reading instructions on the various screens of the tutorial, whilst Group 2 (Novice users in second test) spent only 37% of their time reading instructions on the various screens. Group 2 also spent less time on key presses than Group 1. The percentage time spent on mouse clicks increased by approximately 14% with Group 2 spending 37% of their time on mouse clicks as opposed to the 23% of Group 1. One can thus conclude that as the novice users of group 2 made more use of the mouse than the keyboard, their overall completion time would be significantly reduced. This conclusion is based on the typical times for different operators in the Keystroke-Level Model as proposed by Card, Moran and Newell (Dix et al., 1999).

11. FUTURE RESEARCH

For the purpose of this paper, we only concentrated on formal usability testing of one case study in educational software, i.e. IAL. In order to validate the proposed methodology further, more case studies in formal usability testing will have to be conducted. Such an evaluation should comprise both an evaluation of the methodology and a formal usability evaluation of the software products. The nature of the case studies should be different. The case study in this paper is typical of many interactive educational tutorials. The usability of other types of educational software packages still remains to be fully investigated.

12. CONCLUSIONS

There is no doubt that formal usability evaluation can provide significant results for assessing the usability of interactive software. In addition, there is also a growing need to assess the usability of educational software. In this paper we have discussed a methodology for the formal usability evaluation of interactive educational software packages such as tutorials. The formal usability testing methodologies reviewed were found to give very high-level descriptions of how to conduct a formal usability evaluation and did not represent a sufficiently complete methodology. The proposed methodology as discussed in this paper, uses the methodologies as suggested by Faulkner (2000) and Rubin (1994) and is supplemented with the detail suggested by Dumas and Redish (1993). Certain aspects of the Common Industry Format Report for Usability Testing were included to produce a more detailed, step-by-step descriptive methodology for formal usability testing.

The case study included a detailed formal usability test of Interactive Learner (IAL) tutorial. The results obtained from the formal usability evaluation of the IAL software highlighted several usability problems and were used to propose several design changes. These design changes resulted in significant improvements in usability. Whilst more research is still necessary, we can conclude that the method developed at UPE can be successfully used to conduct formal usability evaluations of interactive educational software.

13. REFERENCES

Alessi, S. M. and Trollip, S. R. (2001), *Multimedia for Learning: Methods and Development,* Allyn & Bacon.

Barnum, C. M. (2002), *Usability testing and research,* Pearson Education, United States.

Dix, E., Abowd, F. and Beale, J. (1999), *Human-Computer Interaction, Second Edition,* Addison-Wesley.

Dumas, J. S. and Redish, J. (1993), *A Practical Guide to Usability Testing,* Intellect, England.

Faulkner, X. (2000), *Usability Engineering,* Macmillan Press.

Gagne, R., Briggs, L. and Wagner, W. (1992), *Principles of Instructional Design,* Harcourt Brace, Jovanovich.

Geisert, P. G. and Futrell, M. K. (1995), *Teachers, Computers and Curriculum,* Allyn and Bacon, Boston.

HCI Laboratory University of Maryland (2000), Questionnaire for User Interaction Satisfaction (QUIS), http://www.cs.umd.edu/QUIS/index.html

Common Industry Format for Usability Test Reports (2001), Document No. ANSI/NCITS-354-2001, http://www.usability.serco.com/prue/summary.htm

Johnson, J. (2000), *GUI Bloopers,* Morgan Kaufmann.

Nielsen, J. (1994), http://www.useit.com/papers/heuristic/heuristic_list.html

Noldus Technology (March 2001), The Observer [R], 4.0, http://www.noldus.com/products/index.html?observer/index

Rubin, J. (1994), *Handbook for Usability Testing,* John Wiley & Sons Inc, New York.

Squires, D. and Preece, J. (1996), Usability and Educational Software Design Seminar, King's College, London, http://www.icbl.hw.ac.uk/~sandra/uesd/

Statsoft (2001), Statistica, 6.0, http://www.statsoft.com

Streicher, M., Wesson, J. L. and Calitz, A. P. (2001), The Development of a User Classification Model for a Multicultural Society, *Proc. of the Annual Conference of the South African Institute of Computer Scientists and Information Technologists*, (Eds. Renaud, K., Kotze, P. and Barnard, A.) Unisa Press, Pretoria, 25-28 September.

Usability: Gaining a Competitive Edge
IFIP World Computer Congress 2002
J. Hammond, T. Gross, J. Wesson (Eds)
Published by Kluwer Academic Publishers

EQUAL:Towards an Inclusive Design Approach to Novice Programming Languages and Computing Environments for Native Users

Basawaraj Patil, Klaus Maetzel and Erich. J. Neuhold
Fraunhofer Institute for Integrated Publication and Information Systems, Dolivostrasse 15, 64293, Darmstadt, Germany {patil,maetzel,neuhold}@ipsi.fraunhofer.de

Abstract: In the current textual programming languages (conventional, novice, etc.) and programming paradigms (e.g., procedural, declarative, functional etc.), the programming constructs, semantic concepts, and syntactic elements are based on English paradigm and implemented using ASCII character sets, seriously limiting the universal access to programming and computing skills. Especially, non-English speaking native users (students, adults etc.) from non-English speaking geographical regions, including visually challenged users, encounter serious cognitive, semantic and syntactic difficulties in understanding and translating their programming plans into the syntax and semantics of English based paradigm of a programming language. Authors have developed an inclusive, universal design framework with flexible cognitive, semantic and syntactic, and cultural adaptations in the textual languages and their compilers/interpreters to satisfy the computing requirements of native users.

Key words: native users, novice programming, universal access, universal design, textual languages, and universal usability.

1. INTRODUCTION

In the evolving Information Society, programming, computing and IT skills are becoming important in educational, professional and personal endeavours. With globalisation and rapid developments in IT, the majority of Internet users do not use English. Native users' issues may become serious because the vast majority of the world's population who do not, and will not in the foreseeable future speak English will be excluded from the Information Society. Students and people lacking programming and computing skills may become a serious individual and social problem (Dyson, 1997) and in the worst case, may lead to – *Internet Apartheid* (Shneiderman, 2000). Native users referred to here include users, such as students (e.g., primary and high schools, colleges and universities), adults, indigenous societies, linguistic minorities, including people with special needs, from non-English speaking geographical regions (e.g., Asia, the Middle East, Europe, Africa and South America). In particular, millions of native students, for perhaps political, social, economical reasons are compelled to learn in their native medium, and have no learning opportunities to acquire programming skills. We use the generic term textual languages to cover a broad spectrum of textual information structures, command and macros, query and programming languages that inherently textual in nature. Lack of appropriate technologies that support Universal Access (UA) to linguistic and cultural content, textual languages and vernacular computing resources have been a serious impediment to the development of computer literacy skills and programming expertise. Thus, Universal Access to textual languages and programming languages (e.g., novice, conventional), constitute a major step towards an *Inclusive Society* and helps in reducing *Digital Divide gap.*

In teaching and learning of programming languages and computing skills with English as *programming paradigm* will seriously limit universal access to programming and computer literacy skills. Because of historical reasons, the majority of novice programming languages, such as LOGO, BASIC, conventional programming languages such as C, C++, Java and programming paradigms, declarative, procedural, functional, object oriented are mainly based on English semantics and syntax and implemented using ASCII character sets. Native students and adults, whose medium of education and instruction is in their native medium and socio-cultural environments, encounter enormous linguistic, cognitive, semantic, syntactic, and cultural difficulties in understanding and translating their programming plans into English-based semantics and syntax of a programming language. In the new technology adaptation for *Educational Computing and Learning*, non-availability and non-accessibility of programming languages and computing environments and language processors (e.g., interpreters, compilers, translators) constitute major stumbling block to harness the power of IT technologies (Rogers, 2000).

In this paper, we focus on our research work related to the universal usability issues of textual languages as found in programming languages, language processors and, computing environments from native users' perspectives with more emphasis on semantics and syntax i.e., notational aspects of programming languages and programming constructs. We also discuss a universal, inclusive design methodology of textual information structures and programming languages, language processors and computing environments. Furthermore, it will contribute to the better understanding of native user requirements, universal design of programming languages and computing environments, and implications to scaffolding and teaching tools.

2. NATIVE USERS: A PROFILE AND THEIR COMPUTING REQUIREMENTS

Research studies on needs and computing requirements of native users are scarce and poorly understood. In-house studies on universal usability textual languages, novice programming languages and programming paradigms were conducted with the help of researchers, HCI experts, native users and students with diverse multilingual and multicultural backgrounds. From these preliminary studies, we may characterise computing requirements of native users as follows:

- A majority of native users are novices and lack English knowledge. They prefer native language-like constructs and interactions in programming and computing tasks and vernacular computing environments. They want to learn basic skills of programming and computing and do not intending to become professional programmers. These native users need *enabling mechanisms, processes and technologies* to enable them to acquire the basic skills of programming and computing.
- A majority of native users, especially students with good mathematical background would like learn basic and advanced programming skills, and intend to become professional programmers. These native users need special *scaffolding mechanisms, processes and technologies* to make a effective transition from native computing to the main stream of computing.
- A majority of native users have special needs. For example, native visually challenged users prefer to interact and program in native Braille (e.g., Asian, European, and African Braille) or native voice interactions. These users need *assistive mechanisms, processes and technologies* to avail new opportunities, facilities and services to enhance their quality of life.

3. USER HCI MODEL AND PROGRAMMING LANGUAGE ISSUES

Programming is a complex activity and programming languages make the task more difficult than necessary because, the programming languages are designed without serious considerations of human factors and HCI issues (Pane et al., 2001). In general, programming is the task of mapping the mental plans and program compositions into language constructs, i.e., semantics and syntax of a computer language to achieve a particular computing task. For historical reasons, the majority of programming languages and programming paradigms are derived from English semantics and syntax, and implemented using ASCII character sets. A HCI model of interaction and communication between the programmer and the computer for programming tasks can occur at conceptual, cognitive, cultural, semantic and syntactic levels, as follows.

- **Conceptual Level:** The *meaning* of the task model should match the native user's world model and because this is where the concepts of programming, programming language features, relationships, and operations reside. At the *conceptual level,* the new technologies, complex concepts, unfamiliar metaphors, unnatural programming paradigms, lack of pedagogical concerns constitute a serious conceptual gap for the majority of native users. Native users make it more complicated because of their lack of knowledge and misunderstanding and misconceptions about computing tasks (Bayman & Mayer, 1983; Boulay, 1989; Coombs et al., 1982; Mayer, 1981).
- **Semantic Level:** The ideas from the conceptual level are represented by means of a programming language placed in the context of a computing task. The abstract operations from the conceptual level are fully defined in terms of objects, functions and programming constructs of a programming language. At the *semantic level*, the semantics of programming do not match well with the natural semantics of native users' languages. In novice programming studies, it is observed in (Bonar & Soloway, 1985; Ebrahimi, 1994; Dyck & Mayer, 1985) that, the majority of semantic errors arise due to the semantic mismatch and novice users relaying on preconceived knowledge and translating the programming plans using their natural language semantics.
- **Syntactic Level:** At the *syntactic* level, the *grammar* of the programming language is defined, including the arrangement of valid programming elements and program construction. At the *lexical* level, the primitive elements such as tokens, programming

vocabularies and literals of a programming language are used to write a program to achieve a computing task. The grammar at the *syntax* level is highly inflexible and the ASCII-based lexical tokens at the *lexical* level do not cover the majority of writing systems, complex scripts and diacritics.

- **Cognitive Level:** Cognition plays a vital role in computer programming. Each programming construct has its own cognitive load. Most programming languages use grammatical cues such that subject precedes the verb. These grammatical cues have diverse interpretations in other natural languages and cultures (e.g., Arabic, Hebrew, and Indian). These mismatching grammatical cues in programming languages introduce cognitive loads and have serious implications to programming constructs.
- **Cultural Issues**: Cultural factors, locale conventions and standards, bi-directional display of textual languages are not supported in the current programming languages and computing environments. These cultural factors help to motivate the users and enhance end user acceptability.

4. EQUAL UNIVERSAL DESIGN AND DEVELOPMENT METHODOLOGY

Visual programming systems, programming by demonstration, intelligent tutors and form-based programming may address some of the native users programming issues by providing native *customised* graphical programming environments. Visual languages for programming may help, but highlight only a few aspects of programming and manipulation of textual information structures. But, it is observed in (Gilmore & Green, 1984; Green & Petre, 1992) that the textual languages are more useful in learning the skills of programming such as comprehension, creation, documentation, modification and debugging and learning programming.

Universal Design or *Design for All* is a design methodology that recognises, respects, values and attempts to accommodate the broadest range of human abilities, skills, requirements and preferences in the design of all computer based products and environments. With about 6000 languages spread across some 200 countries, design of universally accessible textual information structures, programming languages and computing resources with diverse needs and preferences, requirements, a wide range of human capabilities, including native users with special needs is a difficult and a challenging task. EQUAL (Easy, Quick, Universal, Accessable Language) is a user-centred, universal design methodology that has been explicitly developed to support native users' requirements in the domain of textual languages (Patil et al., 2001a; Patil et al., 20001b). The EQUAL system provides a design and development environment that supports an universal usability engineering cycle with goals satisfying a broad range of the universal usability attributes such as availability, learnability, understandability, accessibility, and acceptability of textual programming languages and interactions.

The EQUAL universal usability engineering process and methodology consists of comprehensive set of guidelines on linguistic, cognitive, semantic and syntactic, cultural aspects of programming languages and computing resources. A basic guiding principle *speak native users' language* is exploited at language features, in compiler/interpreter components, and in editor and programming environment.

In general, there has been a conscious effort to make programming languages as natural as possible. It is observed that natural language-like constructs and commands are effective in the design of user interactions with the computer systems (Ledgard et al., 1980; Miller, 1981; Landauer et al., 1983; Biermann et al., 1983). Even recent studies (Pane et al., 2001) demonstrate the concept of "natural programming". Natural programming does not mean that native users should use their natural languages for programming, but the languages of programming and interactions should be as natural as possible and able to mentalize the computations and operations, learn quickly and use effectively the programming skills.

The empirical studies in (Carroll, 1978; Teasley, 1994) have demonstrated that meaningful variable names improved program comprehension and facilitate learning. Both formal and informal observational studies (Landauer et al., 1983; Rosenberg, 1982) repeatedly identified names, naming and structural contexts, and commands as an important practical problem The general interpretation of statement termination symbols, separators, programming cues, string constants (e.g., ';' is used for question mark in Greek, «string constant» in French, „string constant" in German) have diverse representations and interpretations in various languages and cultures. These notational representation and semantics of operators (e.g., relational, logical) are quite confusing and discouraging to many native users. A majority of native users misinterpret the meaning of relational operators and it is mainly due to lack of knowledge of Boolean algebra.

Cognitive processes and structures, program constructs play a vital role in problem solving, programming and comprehension (Hoc & Nguyen, 1990; Rogalski & Samurcay 1994). Control strategies and looping constructs are difficult concepts and demand high cognitive loads (Soloway et al., 1983). It may be observed that, just by providing equivalent controls and looping constructs in native programming language constructs may be insufficient and inadequate, and some time quite misleading and confusing from preconceived knowledge (Bonar & Soloway, 1985). In IF-THEN statement and its variants, it is observed that (Pane et al., 2001) end-users use THEN for "sequencing" which contradicts the meaning of "consequently" in the formal languages. In REPEAT or WHILE control constructs, native users fail to understand the terminating or exit conditions. Such an understanding would lead to better programming languages whose syntactic structure more closely reflects internal semantic structures thereby easing the process of programming.

EQUAL universal design framework supports these notational flexibility and adaptations, and enhances easy comprehension and facilitates effective learning. Simple adaptations will reduce cognitive loads, avoid unnecessary frustrations and motivate native students to learn programming skills. The EQUAL design process may also be suitably transcribed into various native Braille codes. The universal design process consists of the following major steps.

- **Collect Native User Requirements:** The native user requirements, needs, and preferences, skill levels are collected and stored in the database as user profiles.
- **Specify HCI Specifications:** HCI experts can specify the human factors (e.g., linguistic, cultural, cognitive) and locale standards information, that play vital role in textual information structures, programming constructs and vernacular computing environments.
- **Specify Language Design Constraints:** The grammar of the EQUAL language may be expressed by regular expressions (RE) or extended BNF (EBNF) notations by the language designers. Each context-free grammar generates language, which is a set of strings of terminal symbols from the production rules. By changing the grammar, it is possible to incorporate different computing paradigms (e.g., declarative, procedural).
- **Generate Language and Compiler Components:** From the specifications generate (automatic or semiautomatic) the language and its compiler components such as scanners, lexical analysers and parsers. Special morphological data and language engineering skills are necessary to deal with complex writing systems and scripts.
- **Evaluate Language and Compiler Components:** After generating a language and its compiler components, the HCI experts, language designers and native users can test and evaluate the programming language and compiler components.

We illustrate how linguistic, cultural, syntactic and semantic specifications and constrains are used in the EQUAL design space and are integrated into the EQUAL design and development process cycle. From a language designer's perspective, a syntax tree of grammar G is an ordered label tree such that:

- the terminal nodes are labelled by terminal symbols;
- the non-terminal nodes are labelled by non-terminal symbols;
- each non-terminal node labelled by N has children, represented by $X_1, X_2, .., X_n$ such that $N ::= X_1, X2,..,X_n$ is a production rule.

A phrase grammar G is a string of terminal symbols labelling the terminal nodes of a syntax tree. A sentence of grammar G generated is an S-phrase where S is a start symbol. Since, the concrete syntax has no influence on the semantics of the language, this feature is exploited thoroughly to map various linguistic and cultural notations in a flexible manner. The guiding principle is to separate syntactic elements or vocabularies and semantic concepts and represent them in native users' language independent, culture neutral forms in the design space. The EQUAL design process is a multilevel, iterative process and modelled with a set of production rules. The production rules fire an action, when all the necessary universal usability criteria are satisfied. Any inconsistent or conflicting design decisions are reported to the designers. Any modifications and recommendations may be incorporated in the design-evaluate-redesign cycle of EQUAL universal design methodology. The majority of programming statements (e.g., assignment, input, and output) has a generic format: *<verb>* *<operator>* *<variable>* *<terminator>*. These generic formats have different representations and diverse interpretations in native languages and cultures. In localising these programming statements, the verb may be represented by one or more words and depends on number of variables, gender and polity. The terminating symbol may be represented by locale conventions and standards used in general communication.

In novice programming environments, it is observed (Eisenstadt, 1983; Witschital, 1994) user-friendly programming environment and visualisation of operations and computations helps in learning. The diagnostic and visualisation information may be used in feedback, tracers, debuggers or intelligent tutorials (Soloway et al., 1981; O'Shea & Monk, 1981). The EQUAL programming environment provides this visual feedback and helps to acquire operational details of programming constructs.

Even simple literal translation or transliteration process of textual languages is difficult to cover all languages and cultures and may serve the following purposes:

- Helps in generating localised programming languages and computing environments for un-represented native users. (e.g., Pascal in Shona or Arabic).

- Offers deeper insights into the universal usability issues of textual languages and helps in universal usability studies.
- Enables generation of equivalent representation in conventional programming languages, i.e. programming constructs in native languages and standard languages (e.g., Pascal in Arabic and English) and helps in scaffolding and learning.

5. EQUAL SYSTEM ARCHITECTURE AND IMPLEMENTATION

The majority of functional components are implemented using Java and exploit its internationalisation features and XML technologies. The EQUAL system supports Unicode standards that cover major scripts, symbols, and Unicode Braille patterns. The major functional components of the EQUAL system architecture are shown in Figure 1.

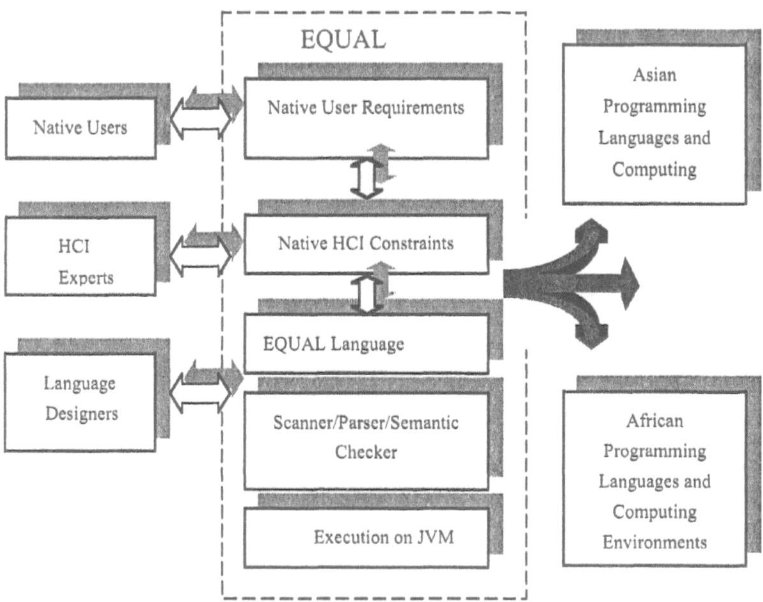

Figure 1. Architectural components of EQUAL design and development environment.

The components consist of:

- **EQUAL Grammar Specifier:** Regular expressions or EBNF notations may express the grammar of the language by the language designers. Each context-free grammar generates language, which is a set of strings of terminal symbols. The concrete syntax is important to the implementers to check the syntactically well-formed programs. But the concrete syntax has no influence on the semantics of the program and used to represent the grammar in a flexible way. It may be observed that by changing the production rules, different programming paradigms may also be incorporated in the design process.
- **EQUAL Database:** The universal usability guidelines are stored in the relational database in the form of production rules. The database also includes the syntactic elements or vocabularies, and compiler components. A XML language is used to represent the metadata about the user profiles, cultural and linguistic factors, compiler components, and syntactic and semantic specifications. This metadata is used extensively at various stages of EQUAL development cycles of language design and generation of compilers and interpreters. The database may be extended and enriched by the HCI experts and language designers.
- **Compiler/Interpreter Components:** These components (e.g., lexical analyser, parser) are mainly concerned with the scanning or lexical analysis in which the source program written EQUAL is transferred into the streams of tokens and executed on a Java virtual machine.

6. NATIVE USER COMPUTING ENVIRONMENT

The user interfaces to systems for programming and computing environment can critically influence the development of programming skills. The EQUAL computing environment is similar to a conventional integrated programming environment consisting of multiple windows, GUI interface for programming, editor and language compiler/interpreter are localised to the computing requirements of native users. The native users can write EQUAL programs using Unicode compatible text editor and submit them for the compilation. The syntactic and semantic errors are displayed in the *Error Window* with necessary information to facilitate easy correction. In case of an error-free program, the interpreter/compiler will execute the program on Java Virtual Machine (JVM). The *Input Window* expects the inputs to the program and generates the outputs in the *Output Window*. Simple EQUAL programs are shown in Figure 2 supporting imperative style in Arabic or procedural i.e. PASCAL-like in Zimbabwean.

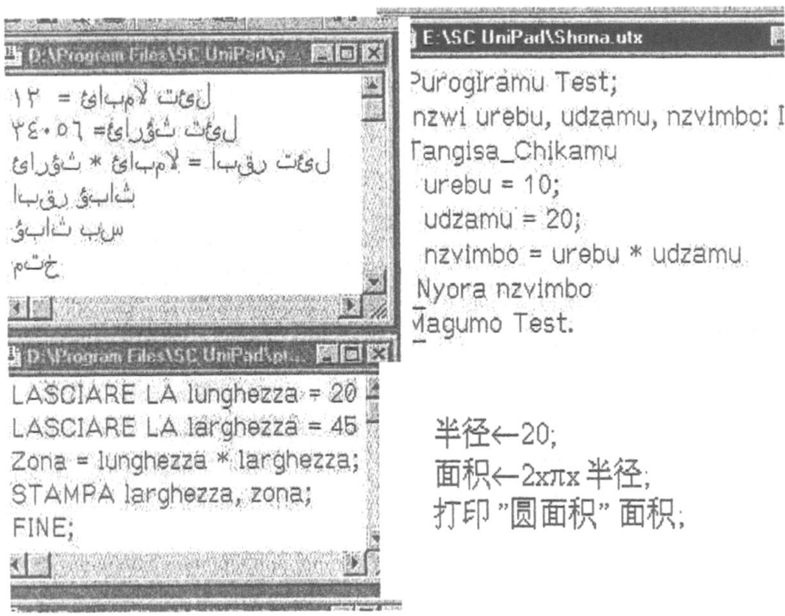

Figure 2. Cropped screen shots of EQUAL programs in Arabic, Zimbabwean (Shona) Italian and Chinese.

Online help and documentation are available in the *Help Window*. The error messages, dialogues, training and learning material are stored as resource bundles. The programming environment also generates the equivalent programs in English and native language and used for scaffolding.

The EQUAL language and computing environment uses Unicode for encoding to cover a majority of writing systems, cultural conventions, scientific and communication symbols. The majority of EQUAL language features and compiler/interpreter components are implemented using Java, and exploits its internationalisation and localisation features to support vernacular computing. These functional components may be deployed as standalone application or client-server model and helps in distribution and dissemination of learning resources for programming.

7. CONCLUSIONS AND FUTURE WORKS

In this paper, we have discussed the universal usability issues of textual languages, novice programming languages and computing environments. We have discussed the universal design framework that can accommodate linguistic, cognitive, cultural, semantic and syntactic requirements of native programming languages and vernacular computing. Availability of native programming languages and computing resources is a pre-requisite attribute of universal usability and EQUAL fulfils availability of resources, by developing native textual languages and computing resources. We have shown the feasibility of the EQUAL language and its computing environments in a few representative nativised languages and computing environments. We believe that, the EQUAL language and EQUAL programming environment provides scaffolding mechanisms and offer unique opportunities to the native users to learn programming and computing skills. The EQUAL rapid prototyping environment helps in conducting universal usability studies in textual languages. Universal usability studies related to learnability, scalability, understandability, transfer of programming competence and critical evaluations are planned in the future work.

8. REFERENCES

Bayman, P. and Mayer, R.E. (1983). A Diagnosis of Beginning Programmers' Misconceptions of BASIC Programming Statements. *Communications of the ACM*, 26(9), 677-679.

Biermann, A.W., Ballard, W.B.W. and Sigmon, A.H. (1983). An Experimental Study of Natural Language Programming. *International Journal of Man-Machine Studies*, 18, 71-87.

Bonar, J. and Soloway, E. (1985). Pre-Programming Knowledge: A Major Source of Misconceptions in Novice Programmers. *Human-Computer Interaction*, 1, 133-161.

Boulay, B. (1989). Some Difficulties of Learning to Program. In *Studying the Novice Programmer*, Soloway, E. and Sphrer, J.C (Eds.). New Jersey: Lawrence Erlbaum Associates.

Carroll, J.M. (1978). Names and Naming*: An Interdisciplinary Review*. IBM Research Report RC 7370, 1978.

Coombs, M.J., Gibson,R. and Alty, J.L. (1982). Learning a First Computer Language: Strategies for Making Sense. *International Journalof Man-Machine Studies*, 16, 449-486.

Dyck, J.L, and Mayer, R.E. (1985). BASIC Versus Natural Language: Is There One Underlying Comprehension Process? *Human Factors in Computing Systems – II, Proceedings of the CHI'85*, San Francisco, USA,221-223.

Dyson, E. (1997). Education and Jobs in the Digitial World. *Communications of the ACM*, 40(2), 35-36.

Ebrahimi, A. (1994). Novice Programmer Errors: Language Constructs and Plan Composition. *International Journal of Human-Computer Studies*, 41, 457-480.

Eisenstadt, Marc. (1983). A User-friendly Software Environment for the Novice Programmer. *Communication of the ACM*, 26(12), 1058-1064.

Gilmore, D. J. and Green, T.R.G. (1984). The Comprehensibility of Programming Notations. *HCI-Interact'84: Proceedings of the IFIP Conference Organised by Task Group on HCI*, London, U.K, 461-464.

Green, T.R.G. and Petre, M. (1992). When Visual Programs are Harder to Read than Textual Programs. *Human-Computer Interaction:Tasks and Organisation, Proceedings of ECCE-6 (6th European Conference on Cognitive Ergonomics)*, van der Veer, G.C, Tauber, M.J., Bagnaroa, S. and Antavolts, M. (Eds.), Rome, Italy.

Hoc, J.M and Nguyen-Xuan.A (1990). Language Semantics, Mental Models and Analogy. In *Psychology of Programming*, Hoc, J.M, Green, T.R.G, Samurcay, R and Gilmore, D.J (Eds.). London:Academic Press.

Landauer, T.K., Glotti, K.M. and Hartwell, S. (1983). Natural Command Names and Initial Learning: A Study of Text Editing Terms. *Communications of the ACM*, 26, 495-503.

Ledgard, H., Whitehead, J.A., Singer, A. and Seymour, W. (1980). The Natural Language of Interactive Systems. *Communications of the ACM*, 23, 556-563.

Mayer, R.E. (1981). How Novices Learn Computer Programming. *Computing Surveys*, 13(1), 121-141.

Miller, L.A. (1981). Natural Language Programming: Styles, Strategies and Contrasts. *IBM Journal*, 20(2), 184-215.

O'Shea, Tim. and Monk, John. (1981). The Black Box Inside the Glass Box: Representing Computing Concepts to Novices. *International Journal of Man-Machine Studies*, 14, 237-249.

Pane, J.F, Ratanamahatana, C.A. and Myers, B.A (2001). Studying the Language and Structure in Non-programmers's Soultions to Programming Problems. *International Journal of Human-Computer Studies*, 54(2), 237-264.

Patil, Basawaraj., Maetzel, K. and Neuhold, E.J. (2001a). Design and Implemenation of Universal End-User Commands, Interfaces and Interactions. *UAHCI, 2001, New Orleans, USA, 516-520.*

Patil, Basawaraj., Maetzel, K. and Neuhold, E.J. (2001b). Native End-User Languages: A Design Framework. *13th Annual Workshop on Psychology of Programmng, Bournmouth, UK, 113-126.*

Rogalski, J. and Samurcay, R. (1994). Acquisition of Programming Knowledge and Skills. In *Psychology of Programming*, Hoc, J.M.,Green, T.R.G., Samurcay, R. and Gilmore, D.J (Eds.). London: Academic Press.

Rogers, P.L. (2000). Barriers to Adopting Emerging Technologies in Education. *Journal of Educational Computing Research*, 22(4), 455-472.

Rosenberg, J. (1982). Evaluating the Suggestiveness of Command Names. *Behaviour and Information Technology*, 1, 370-400.

Shneiderman, B. (2000). Universal Usability. *Communications of ACM*, 43(5), 85-91.

Soloway, E., Bonar, J., and Ehrlich, K. (1983). Cognitive Strategies and Looping Constructs:An Empirical Study. *Communications of the ACM*, 26(11), 853-860.

Soloway, E., Wolf, B., and Barth, P.(1981). MENO-II: An Intelligent Tutoring System for Novice Programmers. *Proceedings of the Seventh International Joint Conference on Artificial Intellegence*, Vancouver, 975-977.

Teasley, B.E. (1994). The Effects of Naming Style and Expertise on Program Comprehension. *International Journal of Human-Computer Studies*, 40, 757-770.

Witschital, Peter. (1994). TRAPS – An Intellgent Tutoring Environment for Novice Programmer. In *Cognition and Computer Programming*, Karl F. Wender, Franz Chmalhofer and Heinz-Dieter Böcker (Eds.). New Jersey: Ablex Publishing Corporation.

Usability: Gaining a Competitive Edge
IFIP World Computer Congress 2002
J. Hammond, T. Gross, J. Wesson (Eds)
Published by Kluwer Academic Publishers

MouseLupe

An Accessibility Tool for People with Low Vision

Luciano Silva[1], Olga R. P. Bellon[2], Paulo F. U. Gotardo[2] and Percy Nohama[1]
[1]*CPGEI - CEFET/PR - Curitiba-PR, Brasil.*
[2]*Universidade Federal do Pararå - Curitiba-PR, Brasil.*

Abstract: This paper presents a new accessibility tool developed to help people with low vision disabilities. The tool was initially designed to aid in Web navigation, but it can also be useful in other applications. First, we describe the importance of the Web as a source of information and knowledge and explain the main difficulties that disabled people have in accessing Web pages. We present relevant software applications for accessibility of people with low vision and explain their features and limitations. The developed tool named, *MouseLupe*, its characteristics and main contributions are presented in detail. Finally, we show a comparison of the developed tool with other related applications highlighting its efficiency and usefulness.

Key words: web navigation, usability, low vision disabilities, magnifier lens

1. INTRODUCTION

The World Wide Web has become the largest source of information, knowledge and entertainment in recent years, used mainly by people involved in teaching activities, scientific research and electronic commerce. Originating in the academic world, it is already considered an indispensable work tool for researchers in many different areas.

Although there is a ready access to many subjects provided on the Web, this does not avoid the common situation that a simple search for specific information may be a quite difficult task. Frequently precious time is wasted finding and visualizing significant content on some Web sites. For people with visual disabilities, the problem may be worse than that and practically unbearable.

Initially, Web pages had only text and their evolution to complex pages with images, sounds, graphics, and animations provided great benefits for many users. However, they also created difficulties for people with disabilities and have become practically inaccessible for the disabled (Head, 2000; Taucsher, 1997).

Even with the complex and constant transformations of Web organization, the number of disabled people using computers has surely been increasing (Paciello, 2000).

The World Wide Web Consortium (W3C) (Berners, 2000), an organization interested in all aspects of the Web, sponsors the most extensive set of programs and initiatives devoted to the issue of Web accessibility for people with disabilities. The W3C has created the Web Accessibility Initiative (WAI, 2000). It has published many documents and provided a single most comprehensive and useful set of resources for Web designers who wish to make their sites more accessible to people with disabilities.

There are four main categories of disabilities that affect a person's ability to use the Web:

- Mobility, including inability to move, insufficient dexterity to operate a mouse or a keyboard, inability to control unwanted movement, and lack of limbs.
- Hearing, ranging from inexact hearing, or diminished hearing, to no hearing at all.
- Cognition and learning, including various difficulties in reading, understanding, staying focused, remembering, and writing.
- Vision, including blindness, low vision and colour-blindness.

For people with mobility disabilities, there are several hardware devices and software applications that provide Web navigation and make computer usage possible: mouth devices to control cursor movements, Web cameras to capture eye or head movements and guide the cursor movements, speech recognition software to write words, execute commands, and others. Using these devices, people with mobility disabilities can access every Web page (Carter et al, 2001).

Sounds created as part of Web pages are normally irrelevant in the page's context except when they are songs or speeches. People with hearing impairments usually have easy access to the Web because most of the Web pages do not contain sound information.

Cognition and learning problems are very complex. Many researchers have been studying the relationship between the structured content of a Web page and people with these disabilities in order to propose efficient solutions and accessibility rules for designing Web pages. It is known that a page with a simple and intuitive interface, with clearly formulated text, and a consistent navigational scheme between pages can facilitate access to those disabled people (Paciello, 2000).

Vision disabilities are considered a permanent concern in the research and development of accessibility tools. Many research groups have been concentrating on this subject and proposing new alternative techniques to aid those people.

Screen-magnification software and high contrast displays are commonly used by people with low vision and help them to read the text and interpret the images on websites. Such software improves the readability of small text, but limits the visible area of a document. Enlarged graphics that contain text may be difficult to read.

People who are blind do not use the screen display or mouse. Instead of reading Web pages or viewing images, they listen to the Web through software that acts as a screen reader. These screen readers convert text into synthesized speech and are unable to interpret the graphical content of images. Because of that, some pages may be very difficult or impossible for a blind person to understand or navigate.

In the United States approximately 3.5% of the population have low vision and only 1% of these uses a computer. If we consider this equivalent percentage for the whole world population, probably the percentage of people with impaired vision that use computers will be even smaller (Paciello, 2000).

Today, the knowledge about biological vision is extremely limited. Some research groups in computer vision have been proposing systems using procedures similar to human vision processes to explain its properties and to develop new computer vision applications (Cutzu, 1998; Georgeson, 1998). Projects are being developed to insert accessibility tools in many computer applications or in widely used computer operating systems such as Microsoft Windows and more recently LINUX (LINUX, 2001).

Section 2 of this paper discusses related works on accessibility tools for low vision disabilities. In Section 3 the developed tool is described and shown through the number of examples. The conclusion is presented in Section 4.

2. RELATED WORK

There are many accessibility tools for each disability category. In this paper, we highlight and compare just those accessibility tools for people with low vision, not for blind people. For blind people, we would have, for example, IBM's software named, *Home Page Reader*, a text reader that uses the company's *Via Voice Out loud* text-to-speech synthesizer.

A visually impaired user can use the IBM software to speak text, describe images, and other fields of Web pages (IBM, 2000). Accessibility tools for people with low vision are dedicated to help people in visualizing the content of a computer display more easily, as well as to aid in Web navigation.

Apple is an important company that develops a number of products for people with disabilities to view websites, including screen-magnification software, text-to-speech synthesis, voice recognition, and so on (Apple, 2000).

Most of the accessibility applications for people with low vision make zoom amplification of a certain area of the computer display to facilitate the visualization of its content. These applications are commonly named as screen magnification and generally the centre of the amplification area is the mouse cursor position. The zoomed area is shown in a different window of the computer display, overlapping other application windows. Whenever the user moves the mouse, the amplification screen is refreshed automatically.

In the most recent versions of its Windows operating system, Microsoft added an application named *Magnifier* (Microsoft, 2000), (Figure 1) that divides the computer screen horizontally in two parts. The top half, composed generally of 20% of the total screen area, is used for the amplification and the other is used for the Windows desktop.

Figure 1. Example of the Microsoft Magnifier application.

Because of the restriction on the amount of viewable area of the screen, a large, high resolution monitor is required for the screen magnification software to effectively increase the viewable area on the screen.

The main problem of this application is that, besides the reduced display area, the user can be confused when moving the cursor in the applications window, while looking at the magnified part of the screen. That is because of the difficulty in identifying the relative mouse position in the amplification window and its relationship to the application window. This problem is worse when the application is a Web browser with which the user reads the content of a Web page and moves the mouse to continue reading. In this case, the user may become disoriented and waste time to find the required position again.

In many applications, the option of changing the size of the text characters (font size) is considered an accessibility option. However, to enable this option, a disabled person initially needs the help of another person. In Microsoft Windows, there is an accessibility wizard (Windows, 2000), which guides the user through a series of Windows appearance options. These include adjustments to the font size, screen resolution, scroll bar size, icon size, colour scheme, mouse cursor appearance and mouse cursor blink rate.

The *Loupe* (Loupe, 2001) shown in Figure 2, is a small utility that displays a magnified view of whatever is beneath the mouse cursor, much like a jeweller's or printer's loupe. The captured image can be pasted into any graphics program and most word processors. The *Loupe* also includes options to monitor a specific area of the desktop instead of normal mouse tracking.

Figure 2. The Loupe application applied on Microsoft Windows Desktop.

The *BIGSHOT* (Bigshot, 2001), see Figure 3, is a screen magnification program that enables users working with large monitors and high screen resolutions to quickly magnify part or the whole screen to display small pictures, icons and text in a more comfortable way.

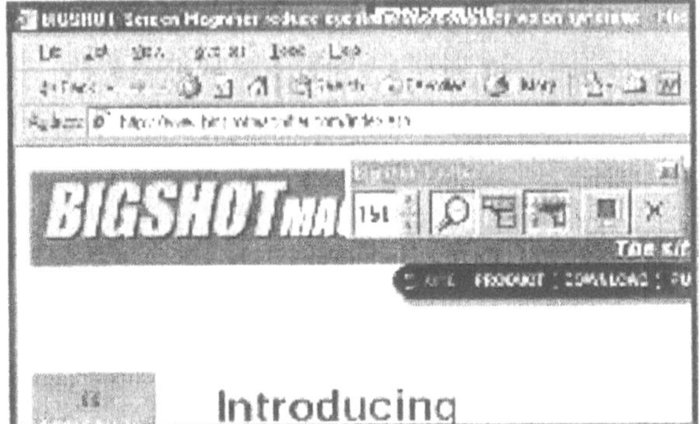

Figure 3. The BIGSHOT applied on a Web browser.

The *Lunar* (Lunar, 2001) is a software magnification system that magnifies the screen from 2 to 32 times, at any screen resolution and colour depth. It allows horizontal and vertical magnification to be adjusted separately, and incorporates image smoothing, to make characters more readable particularly at higher levels of magnification.

The *ZoomText Xtra* (Xtra, 2001) software combines screen magnification software with a built-in document reader and is supplied in modular form, where level 1 provides magnification and level 2 adds speech output using any sound card. A speech synthesizer can also be used to provide the speech output (Figure 4).

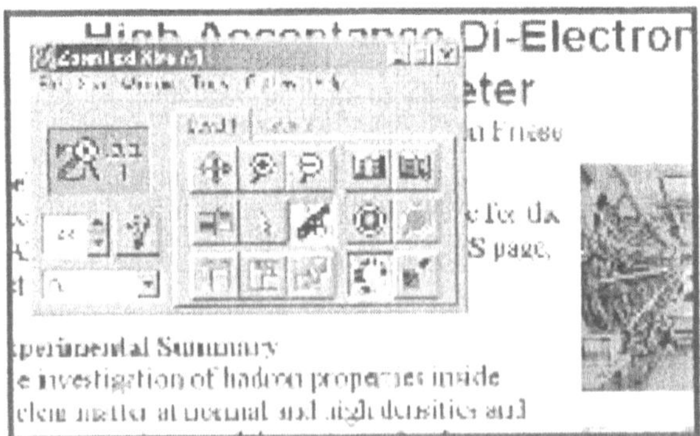

Figure 4. Example of the ZoomText Xtra application.

Most of the available accessibility software is for Windows. There are some LINUX packages of accessibility tools for example, the *gmag* and *xlupe* (LINUX, 2001). The *gmag* is a screen magnification software similar to the *Magnifier* of Microsoft Windows. The *xlupe* software is a simple application that has a window of variable size which shows the amplification image of the region where the mouse cursor is. Software for LINUX is in its greater part open source, free software, which means no acquisition cost.

The main limitations of these applications and their implications for the user are:

1. The amplification window limits the useful display area.
2. The windows overlapping may hide significant parts of an application.
3. The user's attention is focused in a small region covered by the amplification window.
4. The user can be disoriented when visualizing the relative position of the mouse cursor in the amplification window.
5. The user may not have a perception of the global aspect of the application because they are always visualizing the small amplification window whose location is fixed.
6. In most of the applications in which it is possible to change the font size, there is no way to change the font size of the toolbars or option menus. In this case the user has to requests the help from another person.
7. The change of the amplification level is a difficult task when this option is on the amplification window.

Following this initial study of the current accessibility applications, and their limitations and their virtues, we have proceeded to develop a new and more efficient accessibility tool.

3. DEVELOPMENT OF THE MOUSELUPE ACCESSIBILITY TOOL

We had difficulties obtaining a specification of the Microsoft Windows window manager. Thus, we decided to develop the *MouseLupe* for the LINUX operating system. As LINUX distributions have no acquisition cost, the adoption of this operating system made it possible to develop accessibility applications at an insignificant cost.

Our objective was to develop a tool like the traditional screen-magnification software, but not having a static window. The application needed to be fast and dynamic and show quickly whatever the user would like to enlarge.

We envisaged a tool integrating the mouse cursor movement and the displacement of the amplification window. The result was the development of *MouseLupe*, see Figures 5 and Figure 6.

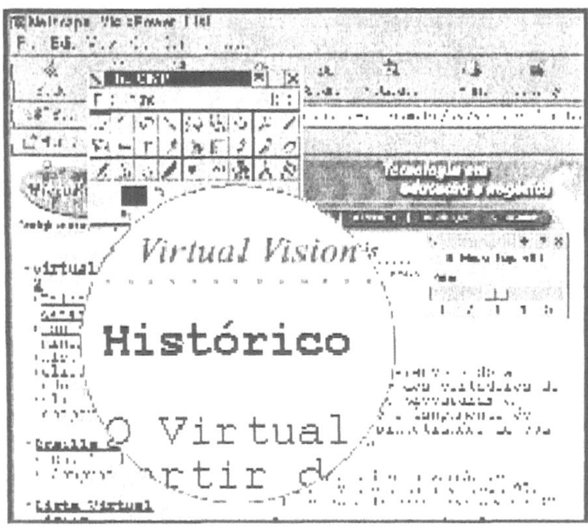

Figure 5. Example of the MouseLupe amplification result over the Netscape browser.

MouseLupe is an original tool that simulates perfectly a magnifying glass (Lupe) guided by the mouse movement. It preserves the functions of the mouse buttons allowing a common Web navigation (Figure 5). It makes a great general purpose screen magnification utility for computer users with sight impairments.

The development guides of *X Window System* were used in this work (Nye, 1992a; Nye, 1992b) and made it possible to consult all the sub-routines of the *X window server*, mainly the window and mouse events. The *X* controls the graphic interface of LINUX and a window manager is executed as a first X client application, for example *WindowMaker, KDE, IceWM*, and so on.

When *MouseLupe* starts, it initially creates a transparent window, without borders, to contain the magnifying glass. The window borders of an application are attributes of the window manager. In order to create a window without its borders we needed to use the resource *OverrideRedirect* of *X*. This resource makes the application answer only to the *X server* commands and not to the window manager ones. This way, the window is directly controlled by the *X* events.

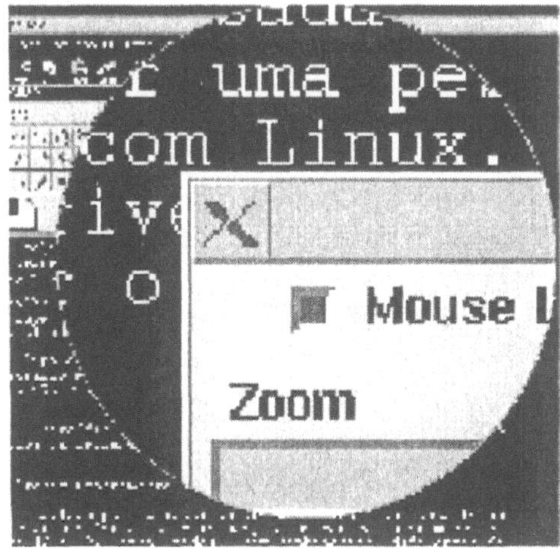

Figure 6. Example of the MouseLupe with high amplification result (zoom 8x).

The mouse and window events, obtained by the *XQueryPointer* and *XMoveWindow* methods, were used to move the amplification window following the mouse cursor position. The methods *XUnmapWindow* and *XMapWindow* were used to quickly remove the amplification window, copy the content of the display on the mouse position, and show the amplification window again. When doing that, a blink in the magnifying glass is noticed, facilitating the *MouseLupe* identification on the screen.

A circle of 2 pixels wide in a light green colour was added to the border of *MouseLupe* to improve its limits identification in the screen. The *MouseLupe* content is refreshed every 5 seconds by default configuration, however the refreshing time may be decrease to allow the visualization of image animations shown in a Web browser. The size of the glass magnifying region is proportional to the amplification factor and its shape is a circle.

There is a 1-pixel hole in the centre of *MouseLupe* circle to allow mouse clicks to function. The mouse events are applied in the window below the *MouseLupe*.

The *MouseLupe* was tested by several users that checked its efficiency not only for people with visual impairments but also for people that need to magnify regions of its applications in a fast and dynamic way. The users' main comment was that they found this tool to be an efficient screen magnification tool that could be used in most computer applications.

The developed tool was compared with the other accessibility tools and the results showed the efficiency of the *MouseLupe* tool. The test was accomplished equally for each accessibility tool. A group of 20 users of different ages (between 20 years and 50 years) was consulted. Testers were asked to rate each tool on 8 different criteria between 1 (very unsatisfied) and 5 (very satisfied).

The chosen criteria for the test were:

1. Easiness for web navigation.
2. Easiness to start and stop the tool.
3. Easiness to change the tool configurations (e.g. zoom factor).
4. Easiness in the use of the interface.
5. Increase of the productivity in the use of the computer.
6. Time for adaptation with the tool.
7. Graphic quality.
8. Number of tool options.

Figure 7 presents a graph of the comparative results of the tools with the average of the evaluations.

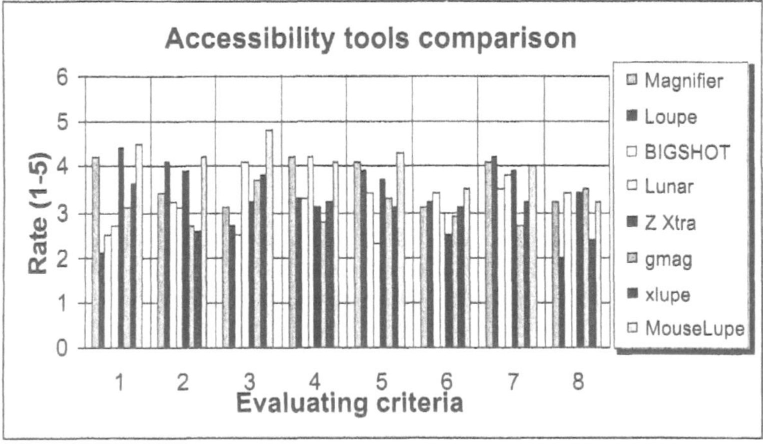

Figure 7. Comparative results.

The *Mouselupe* tool is efficient and simple and it does not require any resource of special hardware. In this first version, the only requirement is a computer with a LINUX operating system.

The main advantages of the *MouseLupe* in relationship the other tested applications are:

1. It eliminates the overlapping window of traditional screen-magnification software.
2. It eliminates user confusion when the screen is split in 2 windows as is shown in the Microsoft Magnifier application.
3. It allows normal mouse functions, move and button clicks.

4. It is possible to see an animated Web page because of the continuous refresh, even when the mouse cursor is not moving.
5. It is possible to move the mouse and quickly see an amplified region of the screen quickly.
6. The user can change the *MouseLupe* configurations using their own *MouseLupe* magnifying region to see the configuration options enlarged.

In the next version, other features are being developed for *MouseLupe*. These are:

- **Colours reduction mode** to reduce the number of colours shown in the amplification window.
- **High contrast view mode** to show the amplification image in high contrast colours.
- **Voice command recognition** to allow changes of magnification level, or Lupe window shape, or to enable or disable the *MouseLupe*.
- **Lupe window shape** to allow different shapes of the *MouseLupe*, such as a circle, cube, rectangle, Lupe, and so on.
- **Text mode** so that the image on the amplification window has only white or black pixels.
- **Image smoothing** to make characters more readable particularly at higher levels of magnification.

4. CONCLUSION

In this paper, we have reported on the results of our research on accessibility tools to aid people with low vision to access computer applications, mainly Web navigation ones. We have also developed an accessibility tool, named *MouseLupe*, for people with low vision. This tool allows disabled users to access the Web in a more comfortable and pleasant way, stimulating their social inclusion and improving their access to information and, thus, their quality of life.

The *MouseLupe* is an original tool that simulates perfectly a magnifying glass (Lupe) guided by the mouse movement and preserves the functions of the mouse buttons allowing a common Web navigation. It makes a great general purpose screen magnification utility for computer users with sight impairments.

For our future work, we intend to finish the new features of *MouseLupe* and make it available for other operating system platforms, including the Microsoft Windows versions.

5. REFERENCES

Apple (2000), Apple Computer, Inc., Disability resources, Apple Computer Website, http://www.apple.com/education/k12/disability

Berners, L. T. (2000), Web accessibility initiative, World Wide Web Consortium, http://www.w3.org/WAI/

Bigshot (2001), The BIGSHOT screen magnification software, http://www.bigshotmagnifier.com

Carter, J. & Markel, M (2001), Web Accessibility for People With Disabilities: An Introduction for Web Developers. *IEEE Transactions on Professional Communication*, (44)4:225-233.

Cutzu, F. & Edelman, S. (1998), Representation of object similarity in human vision: psychophysics and a computational model, *Vision Research*, (38):2229-2257.

Georgeson, M.A. (1998), Edge-finding in human vision: a multi-stage model bas

ed on perceived structure of plaids, *Image and Vision Computing*, (16):389-405.

Head, M. & Archer, N. & Yuan, Y. (2000), World Wide Web navigation aid, *International Journal of Human-Computer Studies*, (53):301-330.

IBM (2000), The voice of the world wide web, http://www-3.ibm.com/able/hpr.html

LINUX (2001), The blind LINUX project, http://leb.net/blinux/

Loupe (2001), Loupe package for accessibility of people with low vision, http://www.gregorybraun.com/Loupe.html

Lunar (2001), The Lunar magnifier, http://www.dolphinuk.co.uk

Microsoft (2000), Microsoft Corporation, Accessibility policy and strategy, http://microsoft.com/enable/microsoft/policy.htm

Nye, A. (1992a), Xlib Programming Manual, vol. 1., OReilly and Associates, Inc.

Nye, A. (1992b), Xlib Reference Manual, vol. 2., OReilly and Associates, Inc.

Paciello, M. (2000), People with disabilities can't access the Web, http://www.webable.com/mp-pwdca.html

Tauscher, L. & Greenberg, S. (1997), How people revisit Web pages: empirical proceedings and implications for the design of history systems, *International Journal of Human Computer Studies*, (47):97-137.

WAI (2000), Policies relating to Web accessibility, http://www.w3.org/WAI/

Xtra (2001), The "ZoomText Xtra" application, http://www.aisquared.com

Usability: Gaining a Competitive Edge
IFIP World Computer Congress 2002
J. Hammond, T. Gross, J. Wesson (Eds)
Published by Kluwer Academic Publishers

A Framework for Rapid Mid-Fidelity Prototyping of Web Sites

Daniel Engelberg and Ahmed Seffah
Human-Centred Software Engineering Group, Concordia University, Canada
dan.engelberg@sympatico.ca; seffah@cs.concordia.ca

Abstract: This paper presents a prototyping framework situated mid-way between low fidelity and high fidelity. The framework is used after requirements definition and early design but before development. The approach provides a solution to the classical trade-off between the ease of production associated with low-fidelity approaches and the realism associated with high-fidelity techniques. Within this framework, we present a generic mid-fidelity prototyping method supported by a tool, MS-PowerPoint, which we have found well adapted for mid-fidelity prototyping.

Key words: rapid prototyping, PowerPoint, low fidelity, medium fidelity, high fidelity, Internet, web sites, user-centred design.

1. MOTIVATION

Our purpose in presenting this paper is to share a rapid prototyping method we initially developed for our own use, over the course of about 5 years of application in industrial projects. The framework grew from a desire to prototype the interactive and navigational aspects of user interfaces as quickly as possible, with a minimum investment of learning time and with no programming skills. This is not the case with many current prototyping tools.

2. LOW, MID AND HIGH FIDELITY TOOLS

Only two levels of fidelity of rapid prototypes are commonly recognized in the literature: low fidelity and high fidelity (e.g. Isensee & Rudd, 1996; Virzi et al., 1996). Unfortunately, low and high fidelity are loosely defined and each covers a broad range of fidelity levels, leading to confusion in comparing different tools. For example in the traditional classification, two different "low-fidelity" tools could create prototypes of radically different fidelity.

Therefore, we have found it useful to define an intermediate "mid-fidelity" category, which has properties distinct from the two extremes. There are no formal references in the literature to this intermediate category, apart from two studies referring to the use of medium-fidelity prototypes for flight simulators and pilot training (Metalis, 1993; Becker & Hamerman-Matsumoto, 1989).

Table 1 summarizes the characteristics of these proposed fidelity levels.

Fidelity	Appearance	Optimal uses	Advantages	Limitations
Low	Rough sketch; highly schematic and approximate. Little or no interactive functionality.	Early design: conceptualizing and envisioning the application.	Low cost: useful communication vehicle; proof of concept.	Limited usefulness after requirements established; limitations in usability testing
Mid	Fairly detailed and complete but ob-jects are presented in schematic or approximate form. Provides simulated interactive func-tionality and full navigation.	Designing and evaluating most interactive aspects, including navigation, functionality, content, layout and terminology.	Much lower cost and time as com-pared to high fidelity; detail is sufficient for usability testing; serves as a reference for the functional specification.	Does not fully communicate the look and feel of the final product; some limitations as a specification document.
High	Lifelike simulation of the final product; refined graphic design. Highly functional, but the back end might be simulated rather than real.	Marketing tool; training tool; simulation of advanced or highly interactive techniques.	High degree of functionality; fully interactive; defines look and feel of final product; serves as a living specification.	Expensive to develop; time consuming to build.

Table 1: Comparison of different levels of prototype fidelity

They represent a continuum from low to high. In our three-level framework:

- Low-fidelity prototyping tools and methods are used for early design just after requirements analysis, to help conceptualize and envision the interface at a high level. These tools often support rough sketching of interface screens by freehand drawing with a mouse or tablet pen.
- Mid-fidelity prototyping tools are used after early design, for the purposes of detailed design and usability validation. They present detailed information about navigation, functionality, content and layout, but in schematic ("wireframe") or approximate form.
- High-fidelity prototyping tools permit the creation of a lifelike simulation, normally for marketing purposes or sometimes for user tests, before the final version has been developed. High-fidelity prototyping tools tend to target developers, and are often general-purpose development tools. Due to the efforts required, high-fidelity prototypes are usually not "rapid"; nevertheless the expression RAD (rapid application development) is widely used in the field.

A re-classification of existing tools into our proposed three levels of fidelity is beyond the scope and purpose of the current paper. Therefore in the following overview of existing tools, for the moment we wish to sidestep the issue of whether they are low, mid or high fidelity in the new framework. We therefore refer to existing tools under their originally defined fidelity level in the two-level system.

Under the original two-category framework, low-fidelity tools proposed for the early design of graphical interfaces have ranged from simple pen and paper (Landey, 1995; Rettig, 1994) to scripting-based prototyping tools such as Visual Basic and HTML. SILK (Landay & Myers, 1995) and PatchWork (van de Kant et al., 1998) have been suggested as intermediate solutions for early design. Based on the SILK approach, DENIM offers another dedicated tool for the early design of Web sites (Lin et al., 2000).

For high-fidelity prototyping of Web sites, Jung and Winter (1998) summarize CASE (Computer Aided Software Design) tools, including Microsoft FrontPage, Adobe PageMill, Aimtech's Jamba, W3DT, and application development tools such as Sun Microsystem's Java Workshop, Microsoft's Visual J++, Symantec's Visual Café, Rational Rose and Oracle Designer. In addition, Graphical User Interface (GUI) builders such as Visual Basic and Borland Delphi, and their associated user interface toolkits such as MFC and JDK, provide direct manipulation for visually combining and organizing the basic GUI widgets onto screens and windows. Although very powerful, these high-fidelity tools require considerable learning time and technical support, and offer considerably more functionality and detail than necessary for the purposes of usable design.

As explained by Myers et al. (2000), it is difficult to find a user interface software tool which is both easy to learn and highly functional. Tools that are easy to learn and use tend to have basic functionality and low versatility, and tools offering advanced functionality and high versatility tend to be hard to master and use effectively.

Our solution to this trade-off lies in the use of mid-fidelity tools such as PowerPoint. A well-designed mid-fidelity tool can simultaneously offer ease of production and versatility, by focusing on what is essential for prototyping a usable design, and by supporting detailed design through direct manipulation without programming.

3. PROTOTYPING METHODS

There is little detailed reference to any structured methodology for user interface prototyping in the literature. This lack of detail is probably in part because most design methodologies are still in their early stages, and perhaps also because prototyping methods are seen as contextual to the tool. As explained by Isensee and Rudd (1996) and still applicable today, "...the optimum methods of prototyping have not yet been agreed on." One of our motivations for this paper was therefore to document a generalizable prototyping method.

Wilson and Rosenberg (1988) were among the first to define the major classes of prototyping method. Their main categories are the top down approach and the bottom up approach.

Top down approaches define the interface progressively in increasing levels of detail, starting with the task analysis and conceptual design and proceeding through to the detailed design. These approaches are especially appropriate for projects where the functional requirements are known in advance, which should be the case with most user-centred approaches.

Bottom up approaches are not strongly based on a needs or task analysis, and are therefore more highly iterative than top-down approaches. These approaches start by creating a "best guess" design and then by progressively changing and refining that design until it meets the usability requirements. This trial-and-error approach is appropriate when it is impossible to clearly know the functional requirements in advance. Although this context is rare, it could occur in the design of a radically new tool that supports a task that does not yet exist.

Our own method, described in Section 5, is largely top-down, but incorporates iterative loops allowing for bottom-up feedback.

4. BENEFITS AND VALIDITY OF RAPID PROTOTYPING

Rapid prototyping is known to offer many advantages across all levels of fidelity. The following summarizes the most important benefits of rapid prototyping (Isensee & Rudd, 1996; Rudd, Stern & Isensee, 1996; Wilson & Rosenberg, 1988):

- Cost savings in the total life cycle
- Improved usability and quality of the final application
- Permits usability testing before coding
- Improved communication of the design concept to the client and end-users, and communication of the functional specifications to graphic designers and developers.

In several controlled experimental studies (Virzi et al., 1996; Wicklund et al., 1992; Virzi, 1989), it was found that "low-fidelity" prototypes (probably mid-fidelity according to our classification scheme) are as effective as high-fidelity prototypes for validation with users. In other words, rapid prototypes are able to capture almost all of the usability issues that could be communicated in a fully developed system.

5. THE GENERIC MID-FIDELITY PROTOTYPING FRAMEWORK

In this section we present our generic rapid prototyping method for mid-fidelity prototypes. The generic method is presented separately from its application using PowerPoint. This separation allows the method and tools to be evaluated separately and facilitates reuse of the method with other tools.

The method is used after sketching a preliminary design or vision. The method itself does not provide a cookbook recipe for usable design; rather it provides a framework within which designers can easily create usable prototypes, assuming some prior familiarity with the principles of usability. The main steps of the method are described in Figure 1.

The current description uses menu-based architectures as a typical design assumption, since this is the most common type of system designed today for the Web.

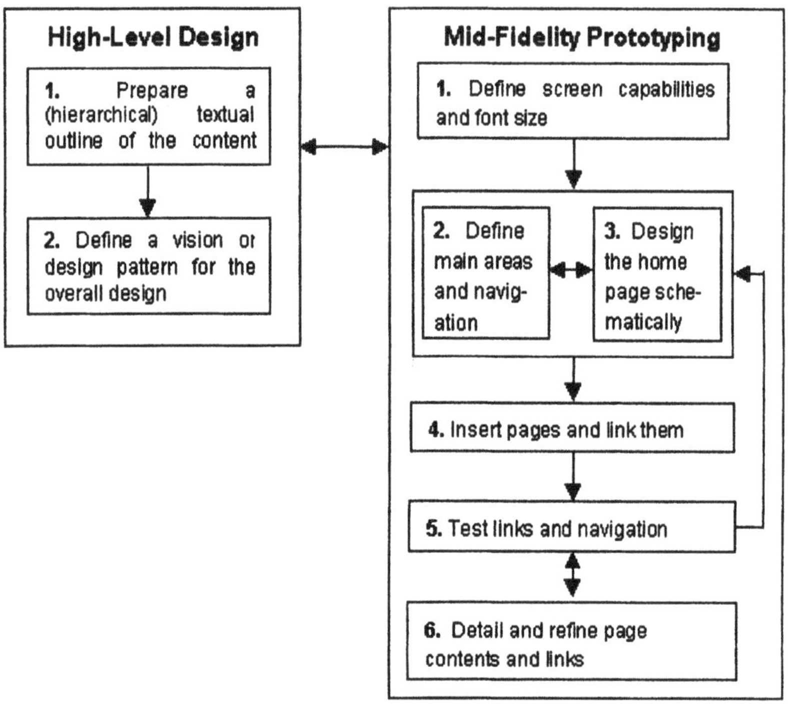

Figure 1: Main steps of the method

Before starting to create the mid-fidelity prototype, it is important to prepare a preliminary (high-level) design. This stage of design is described by Torres (2002) as "Conceptual design and architecture". Early design tools such as Patchwork and DENIM can be very useful at this stage, but pen and paper sketches are adequate. Two steps are involved:

1. A hierarchical (tree-format) outline of the content and functionality of the information architecture is created (Rosenfeld & Morville, 1998). The outline serves as a reference to help structure the early stages of defining menus, navigational structure and page content. The outline accelerates the graphical prototyping and ensures that crucial elements are not forgotten.
2. A rough overall design is sketched, including the general navigation scheme (Mayhew, 1999; Torres, 2002). Solutions can be drawn from design patterns in order to accelerate this step (Borchers, 2001). This step is inherent to usable design but is considerably more complex than can be explained in this paper.

5.1 Define screen capabilities and font size

The prototype should simulate the screen resolution and screen size at which the final site will be viewed. Some prototyping tools allow the user to set the screen resolution, but in other tools it is necessary to approximate font size by "eyeballing" (trial and error tests) in full-screen mode. If the prototyping tool does not allow the designer to specify screen resolution, the use of a smaller font will simulate the increased space available at higher screen resolutions.

The font size affects how much space a menu requires, how much information will fit into the content zone, and how many top-level items can fit into a horizontal menu. The main fonts to define are for menu items, page titles, subtitles, textual content, field labels and buttons.

5.2 Define main areas and navigation strategy

This step is performed in parallel with the definition of the home page. Figure 2 provides an example.

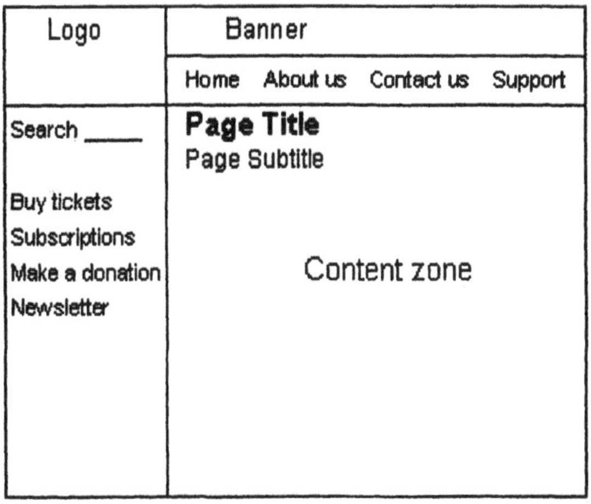

Figure 2: An example of definition of main zones and navigation approach

This step consists of defining the page layout and basic behaviour, in particular for the elements listed in Table 2.

In a first step, the designer places repeating elements (such as menus) in a dedicated and normally fixed-size zone. Some prototyping tools such as PowerPoint have a "page background" or "master" function that allows users to identify elements that repeat on all pages.

The general navigation approach (menus and any other tools) should be defined at this point, by referring to the architecture and navigation needs described in the textual outline prepared in the first step. Normally menus are placed horizontally at the top and/or vertically at the left.

Finally, the menu content is defined (i.e. the specific items to be used in the menus), by referring to the textual outline.

Graphical element (zone)	Main properties to define
Repeating header	Location, dimensions
Menus (horizontal and vertical)	Location, dimensions, number of embedded levels, behaviour, font
Main content area	Location, dimensions, font
Adjunct content areas	Location, dimensions, font
Promotional information areas	Location, dimensions, font
Additional navigation tools	Location, dimensions, behaviour
Page title	Location, dimensions, font
Page subtitle (if relevant)	Location, dimensions, font

Table 2: Main graphical elements to define

5.3 Design the home page schematically

This step is performed in parallel with defining the main zones and the navigation approach. It consists of inserting a page into the prototype for the home page, and defining the page schematically, in particular for the menu and navigation system.

5.4 Insert pages and link them

Firstly, a destination page in the prototype is inserted for each main link on the home page (e.g. menu elements), and for linked items on secondary pages. The most important thing at this point is to place a title on the secondary page immediately as a reminder of its purpose. The blank page is mainly a placeholder for linking to the page from hyperlinks elsewhere in the prototype. It is not yet necessary to start designing the detailed contents of each page.

Secondly, if not performed automatically by the prototyping tool, the menu defined on the home page can be added to each secondary page, opening the appropriate configuration of sub-levels as needed. Some secondary pages might of course use menus that are different from the home page.

Thirdly, if not performed automatically by the prototyping tool, menu items can be provided with hyperlinks and other links to the target pages.

Finally, schematic content is added to the pages. At this point it can be sufficient to indicate the main zones by drawing text boxes or rectangles with descriptive titles.

5.5 Test links and navigation

After a navigation structure has been created, the prototype is tested informally by navigating with the hyperlinks through typical paths. This step helps the designer determine whether the navigation is fluid and efficient. Afterward, links and pages can be changed or added if necessary.

Since the design process is iterative, it is possible that at this step, or at any other step, issues will arise that will require reconsidering the general approach or some specific element of the design. If so, it is possible to return to this previous design step and loop back through the same sequence of procedures, adjusting the prototype as necessary.

5.6 Detail and refine the page contents

Once the "skeleton" or navigational framework of the design has been completed in the previous steps, the page contents and interaction are refined. In forms and interactive dialogues, field labels and sample field are also added. Graphics may also be useful. Objects can be aligned at any stage. This is the time to fine-tune the alignment of objects and zones. See Figure 3 for an example of the results of this step.

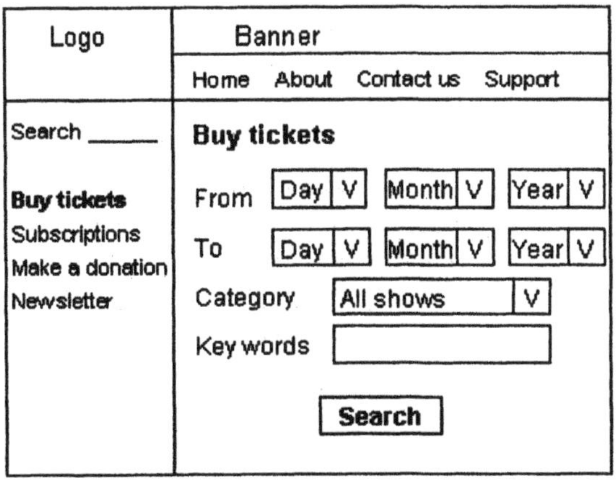

Figure 3: An example of detailed contents

5.7 General techniques

The following additional methods apply across all of the prototyping steps:

- Because the goal of a mid-fidelity prototype is simply to communicate the concept and create the illusion of the target system, it is usually not essential to model every single page in the target site. Particularly for large sites, the designer can put less detail in the less important sections and pages. Where the same page format repeats across a large number of pages, a single page can be provided as an example.
- It is possible to simulate virtually any interaction technique using simple approaches. For example, complex database architectures can be simulated simply by providing sample data in the fields. The prototype does not need to actually use advanced technology to present advanced techniques – it only needs to paint the picture of how the results would look.
- In addition to the prototyping process itself, it is important to validate the prototype before sending it out to the developers, in the following steps:
  1. The prototype is compared to the textual or graphical outline to ensure that it correctly implements the vision and definition of needs.
  2. All links are tested.
  3. The prototype is validated with the client.
  4. Usability tests are performed with target users.

6. APPLYING THE METHOD WITH POWERPOINT

The following refinements of the generic design steps take into account technical aspects specific to PowerPoint functionality.

In the first step (Defining type fonts): PowerPoint does not inherently define a screen resolution, so the designer must adjust the font and object size to simulate different resolutions and screen sizes. To simulate a screen resolution of 800x600 pixels, a font size of about 12-14 points is used for content and menu items, and other objects are sized in proportion. To simulating a target resolution of 1024x768, the standard text size for content and menus should be about 10-12 points.

In the second step (Define main zones areas and navigation approach): Repeating elements are put in the slide master. The slide master is a valuable functionality in PowerPoint. It allows the designer to enter elements that will be repeated on all pages. Normally the master is used for the horizontal header bar at the top with the company's logo and a repeating horizontal menu. The master can also be used for a one-level repeating vertical menu, but it cannot be used for dynamically expanding vertical menus using a simple text-link approach, because the master allows for only a single configuration of elements.

If the design uses a dynamically expanding vertical menu at left, then the menu is copied and pasted into every page, expanding different sub-sections as appropriate for the context. It is best to copy and paste a version of the menu where the menu hyperlinks have already been defined, so as to avoid having to re-program them on each page.

In designing menus, a text box is used for menu items, normally without an outline. A separate text box is used for each item, rather than putting all the menu items in a single text box. It is important to use separate text boxes so as to allow different hyperlinks for each menu item.

In the fifth step (Testing links and navigation): Links and navigation can be tested in PowerPoint by entering Slideshow mode. Links are active in this mode, but not in editing mode.

General techniques: In addition to the above step-specific techniques, we have found the following techniques to be useful:

- Repeating elements can be copied and pasted from other slides. In copying elements from one slide to another, PowerPoint automatically aligns pasted elements to the same position as on the slide from which they were copied.
- Sequences of slides can be animated, using the "Slide Transition" function in the Slide Show menu, to model certain types of interactive effects.
- Collaborative approaches: PowerPoint can be used in real time in a conference room for collaborative design sessions, brainstorming, and design validation sessions.

6.1 Benefits and weaknesses of PowerPoint

Based on our experiences in industrial projects, PowerPoint provides the following benefits as a mid-fidelity prototyping tool:

- The tool takes only a few hours to learn for the purposes of prototyping, and does not require any technical or programming expertise.
- Prototypes can be developed very quickly, often close to the same amount of time that it would take to draw the screens by hand.
- The tool can simulate virtually any type of graphical interaction quickly, easily and directly.

Although PowerPoint is a very solid and versatile prototyping tool, we have found from experience that it has some weaknesses. In particular, as the prototype becomes larger, it becomes increasingly more difficult to modify globally. This is partly due to the fact that there are no global utilities for managing links. In addition, there is no inherent functionality for creating dynamic menus; therefore each different configuration of a menu needs to be drawn by hand on a different page. Finally, it is difficult to prototype pages that extend beyond one screen length. Nevertheless, the benefits of PowerPoint outweigh the weaknesses.

7. CONCLUSION

The framework for mid-fidelity prototyping described here presents a simple, easy-to-apply structured method for rapid prototyping. This framework consists of a generic method for Web application prototyping supported by the PowerPoint tool. PowerPoint fits well into the gap between low-fidelity and high fidelity prototyping tools.

Although the generic method can be applied with a broad range of prototyping tools, we have found that PowerPoint supports this process well, reducing the possibility of the traditional tradeoff that occur between ease of use and functionality. PowerPoint is especially well adapted for rapid mid-fidelity prototyping, allowing designers to quickly translate their ideas onto the screen, while also permitting interactive content and high-quality page layout.

In future research we will test this framework empirically with usability specialists and Web designers. This will help us refine the method and define elements for improving PowerPoint's adaptation to mid-fidelity rapid prototyping.

8. REFERENCES

Becker, C.A. & Hamerman-Matsumoto, J. (1989), The Use of Low-Cost Microcomputers as Medium-Fidelity Simulators for Prototype Development, Training and Research, in *Proceedings of the Human Factors Society 33rd Annual Meeting 1989*, v.2, 1068-1071.

Borchers, J. (2001), *A Pattern Approach to Interaction Design*, Wiley.

Isensee, S. & Rudd, J. (1996), *The Art of Rapid Prototyping*, International Thomson Computer Press.

Jung, R. & Winter, R. (1998), Case for Web Sites, in *Proceedings of the 1998 ACM Symposium on Applied Computing*, Atlanta, Georgia, United States, 726-731.

Landay, J.A. & Myers, B.A. (1995), Interactive Sketching for the Early Stages of User Interface Design, in *Proceedings of CHI '95: Human Factors in Computing Systems*, Denver, Colorado, 43-50.

Lin, J., Newman, M.W., Hong, J.I. & Landay, J.A. (2000), "DENIM: Finding a Tighter Fit Between Tools and Practice for Web Site Design," *CHI Letters: Human Factors in Computing Systems, CHI 2000*, 2(1): 510-517.

Mayhew, D. (1999), *The Usability Engineering Lifecycle*, Morgan Kaufmann Publishers.

Metalis, S. A. (1993), Assessment of Pilot Situational Awareness: Measurement via Simulation, in *Proceedings of the Human Factors and Ergonomics Society 37th Annual Meeting*, v.1, 113-117.

Myers, B., Hudson, S.E. & Pausch, R. (2000), Past, Present and Future of User Interface Software Tools, *ACM Transactions on Computer Human Interaction (TOCHI)*, 2000, 7(1): 3-28.

Rettig, M. (1994), Prototyping for tiny fingers, *Communications of the ACM*, 37(4): 21-27.

Rosenfeld, L. & Morville, P. (1998), *Information Architecture for the World Wide Web*, O'Reilly.

Rudd, J. Stern, K. & Isensee, S. (1996), Low Vs. High-Fidelity Prototyping Debate, *Interactions*, 3(1): 76-85.

Torres, R.J. (2002), *Practitioner's Handbook for User Interface Design and Development*, Prentice Hall.

Van de Kant, M., Wilson, S., Bekker, M., Johnson, H. & Johnson, P. (1998), Patchwork - A Software Tool for Early Design, in *Proceedings of CHI '98 Conference Companion: Human Factors in Computing Systems*, Los Angeles, California, 221-222.

Virzi, R. (1989), What can you learn from a low-fidelity prototype? In *Proceedings of the Human Factors Society 33rd Annual Meeting, HFES*, Santa Monica, California, 224 - 228.

Virzi, R., Sokolov, J.L. & Karis, D. (1996), Usability Problem Identification Using Both Low- and High-Fidelity Prototypes, in *Conference on Human Factors in Computer Systems (CHI 96)*, Vancouver, Canada, 236-243.

Wiklund, M., Thurrott, C. & Dumas, J. (1992), Does the fidelity of software prototypes affect the perception of usability? In *Proceedings of the Human Factors Society 36th Annual Meeting, HFES*, Santa Monica, California, 399 - 403.

Wilson, J. & Rosenberg, D. (1988), Rapid Prototyping for User Interface Design, in M. Helander (ed.), *Handbook of Human-Computer Interaction*, North Holland, 859-873.

Usability: Gaining a Competitive Edge
IFIP World Computer Congress 2002
J. Hammond, T. Gross, J. Wesson (Eds)
Published by Kluwer Academic Publishers

Keep on Trying:
Online Securities Trading Sites

Dmitri Morenkov
Allied Testing LLC (Moscow team), Russia

Abstract: This paper focuses on sites analysis in two usability categories: 'Navigation', and 'Help and Advice'. We have compared 24 on-line securities trading sites and 22 shopping sites. Several areas in these two usability categories demonstrated significantly lower performance of the on-line brokers compared to the on-line retailers. This paper looks in detail into these deficiencies.

The research is based on the Allied Testing Usability Assessment Questionnaire consisting of 200 questions that cover categories essential for web usability: Navigation, Bugs-free functionality, Information Accessibility, Transaction Processing and Speed, Help and Advice, Viewing Options, and Visual Design and Wording.

Key words: usability, web, site, trading, e-broker, e-shop, navigation, help, testing

1. INTRODUCTION

The Allied Testing Company has been researching web usability features in different categories of e-commerce sites for the last two years, collecting statistical data and identifying key features. In this paper, we look at website usability features that may affect business objectives of on-line trading companies.

We were interested in researching the usability features from the point of view of two specific groups: potential new customers (people not yet in the on-line securities trading industry but very interested), and on-line securities traders who are not satisfied with the services offered by their current broker and search resources in order to change it. We suggested that what these people see during their first clicks at a new site is very important.

According to Cawthon (2001), 'usability, customer service and personalization are the most important elements' of financial sites. There is, however, another statement (Mauro, 2001), which says that financial sites lack usability features: "On absolute terms, all financial service sites tested for usability ... were near the bottom in terms of usability and customer satisfaction." Our findings support this statement.

2. RESEARCH METHODOLOGY

Allied Testing, registered in Delaware, USA, is a distributed company, which allows us to perform 24 hours testing and produce the test results quickly. It is a dynamic team of testers who test a client's on-line applications remotely over the web.

Allied Testing's usability evaluation of a website is based on the usability analysis, and consists of four activities:

a) The use of the AT Usability Assessment Questionnaire with about 200 questions, covers the following categories or principles essential for usability of a website:
   1. Navigation
   2. Bugs-free functionality
   3. Ability to find and access information
   4; Transaction Processing and Speed
   5. Help
   6. Viewing Options
   7. Visual Design and Wording

b) The automated tools execution aimed to check spelling, load time, and the presence of broken/dead links.

c) The research of the users' experience from visiting sites through their comments and interviews with them conducted in the process of dynamic site evaluation.

d) The internet resources documentary research, the industry statistics data and ratings evaluation, and an average customer-oriented analysis of the received data.

In this paper, we used data from two of a total of seven categories of our questionnaire: 'Navigation' and 'Help and Advice'. These two sections are vital for attracting first-time visitors.

An individual securities trader is likely to have previous experience of using e-shops, which have enjoyed much attention and feedback both from individual visitors and the mass media in recent years. This is why comparing e-brokers with e-shops may bring positive results.

Regardless of the nature and particularities of a business, 'Navigation' and 'Help and Advice' features are critical for commercial websites. Thus, instead of performing a commonly used comparison within an industry, we compared the assessment results obtained from brokerage sites with retail shopping sites. Our goal was to discover those usability issues, that show significant differences in performance and usage.

Ten questions out of the entire question set were selected, dwelling on the fact that these questions show a significantly lower performance of securities trading sites, in comparison with assessed sites from the neighboring e-shopping industry. Other questions returned results that were similar (with 1% to 4% difference) for both e-brokerage and e-trading sites. These are outside the scope of this paper and are not discussed here.

All web sites selected were analyzed during September-October 2001, using its usability testing technology allowing competitive speed and cost-efficiency of usability evaluation. The standard way of usability evaluation includes finding from 2 to 50 people who agree to try and use the web site (which takes some time and money, but seldom touches the target audience), and a system of analysis of their activities. The Allied Testing system of training allows its staff testers to imitate user behavior, which allows sites to be evaluated in eight hours. While this method may mean greater deviation, it is 50-150 times faster and 20-100 times less expensive than the former.

2.1 On-Line Securities Trading Sites

We selected 24 of the most accessible on-line securities trading sites on the Internet by checking out large financial sites, such as Cbs.marketwatch.com, Thewallstreetjournal.com, e-Signal.com, as well as banners, advertisements and articles about on-line trading services. These search strategies are likely to be used by inexperienced traders without any particular on-line trading habits and preferences who want to start on-line securities trading, as well as by on-line traders who search resources in order to change their broker.

On-line securities trading sites (also called e-brokerages, online brokers, etc) are web sites allowing traders to access securities market via the Internet. They provide access to securities market information and the software that allows orders to be placed on the securities market. The following sites were used for our on-line securities trading sites list:

www.accutrade.com, www.ameritrade.com, www.bidwell.com, www.blackwoodtrading.com, www.brokerageamerica.com, www.brownco.com, www.castleonline.com, www.castletrading.com, www.CSFBdirect.com, www.cybertrader.com, www.datek.com, www.edreyfus.com, www.etrade.com, www.fidelity.com, www.geeksecurities.com, www.jboxford.com, www.ml.com, www.protrader.com, www.quickandreilly.com, www.schwab.com, www.scottrade.ru, www.stocktrade.net, www.tdwaterhouse.ca, www.terranovaonline.com

2.2 On-Line Shopping Sites

A total of 22 shopping sites (Department, Music, Books and Toys stores) were analysed. We used the same principle of selection as for e-brokerage sites. The following sites were used for our on-line shopping sites list:

www.allbooks4less.com, www.amazon.com, www.areyougame.com, www.belk.com, www.bestbuy.com, www.bloomingdales.com, www.BN.com, www.booksamillion.com, www.booksinprint.com, www.boscovs.com, www.emusic.com, www.hearthsong.com, www.macys.com, www.milesofmusic.com, www.music.com, www.samgoody.com, www.sears.com, www.sonymusicdirect.com, www.totallyfuntoys.com, www.twec.com, www.urbanq.com, www.vstore.com

The selected websites were assessed according to the Allied Testing Usability Assessment questionnaire in the 'Navigation' and 'Help and Advice' categories. For some questions, such as broken/dead links, automated tools were used. Each question, when applied to a particular website, was rated as follows:

100% - if the feature existed on the site and its performance was good
50% - if the feature needed enhancements
0% - if the feature did not exist or did not work as it was supposed to.

If the question was not applicable, it was not included in the average percentage calculation. For example, "Can Help be printed?" is not applicable if there is no Help section on the site. The figures were then used to calculate the average percent for the sites representing the industry. The results are shown in Table 1.

Table 1 gives figures of the assessment evaluation results. The following sections of this paper explore every issue in detail.

Category and Question	Average percent for RETAIL E-SHOPS	Average percent for E-BROKERAGE S
NAVIGATION		
Are all links working properly?	79%	64%
Are external and download links accompanied by a clear description of what is available at the next click?	83%	73%
Does the site have a clear reference to Home from all pages?	95%	85%
Do the navigation bars remain visible if a long/large page is displayed?	88%	77%
Are Terms and Conditions, as well as the privacy policy pages, easily accessible from the main browsing pages?	100%	92%
HELP AND ADVICE		
Does the site offer dynamic Help facilities?	73%	33%
Does microhelp text exist for the site's main enabled fields & buttons?	60%	29%
Is the help text legible? (all forms of Help)	100%	95%
Does a clear link to Help exist on each page?	88%	77%
Can Help be printed?	92%	86%

Table 1. The average rating for e-shops and e-brokers.

3. FINDINGS

3.1 Questions relating to Navigation

Successful navigation encourages customers to stay on a website. The majority of websites have similar navigation bars, structure, paths and titles, which makes site navigation easy. When the user visits a site for the first time, his/her previous site navigation experience gained from visiting similar sites comes in handy. We used 24 questions to explore site navigation possibilities.

In general, the e-brokerages tend to structure information better, provide menus, and tables of contents in a clearer way and more often than the retailers. On the other hand, most e-shops pay more attention to supporting details, such as links 'To the Top' on their long pages, references to their Home page, etc. The Allied Testing team investigated these particular features as part of usability requirements.

The following selection makes obvious that, being generally very good in terms of issues of their website navigation, a significant part of on-line brokers lose to e-retailers on issues specific to the Web.

3.1.1 Assessment question: Are all links working properly?

Priority of the feature: Links are extremely important features. The presence of broken links indicates a lack of maintenance and might be a reason for customers to leave the site.

E-Brokers	64%
E-Retailers	79%

Table 2. Are all links working properly?

Finding: Brokerage web sites seem to be less concerned about the issue of whether their site links work well. Their score for the 'Yes links work correctly' was 13% lower than that of the on-line retailers.

Examples: When testing Terranovaonline.com, we discovered that the site failed to provide active links at the upper navigation bar from the site's "search results" page, while its support staff were reporting that the navigation bar was working for them. There are most probably several servers that support the site in different ways, and the site tested by an administrator may not work for some external users that are connected to a server other than the one this administrator uses.

3.1.2 Assessment question: Are the external and download links accompanied by a clear description of what is available at the next click?

Priority of the feature: Medium. To make service competitive, it is generally recommended that site developers clearly state download size and functions of software they offer to download, as well as operating requirements. External links are only applicable if they are necessary, and customers may wish to understand why they are necessary. As technology features change every day, a customer may not be acquainted with the downloads offered. Therefore, a clear description is highly recommended.

E-Brokers	73%
E-Retailers	83%

Table 3. Are the external and download links accompanied by a clear description of what is available at the next click?

Finding: The on-line brokers under-performed compared to the on-line retailers. The brokers do not give as much information (such as description, size and operating requirements for downloads) about partner sites or downloadable software they link to, as retailers. This is surprising, because external links and downloads would seem to be more important for brokers than for most retailers. Downloads are often supporting tools at shopping sites, while at on-line trading sites they are primary products enabling users to trade.

Examples: Schwab.com provides a positive example in terms of a detailed description of Schwab's trading software, the modem speed required to use the software, etc. An example of how external links were misused may be Brownco.com. It has an external link at its main page to the site where the citation it refers to cannot be found. Another example was Stocktrade.net, providing links to several sites where users can obtain trading software for download. However, the site failed to explain that these are links to external sites, and to outline the differences between the links.

3.1.3 Assessment question: Does the site have a clear reference to Home from all pages?

Priority of the feature: High. The home page is the page that gets most visitors, and, in most cases, it is the starting page of any site navigation. It was observed that users may feel lost if they are more than 3 clicks away from the Home page (Telerise, 2000). A link to the site's main menus should be provided on every page.

E-Brokers	85%
E-Retailers	95%

Table 4. Does the site have a clear reference to Home from all pages?

Finding: Visitors cannot return in one click to the point where they started surfing through a broker's site.

Examples: The importance of a link to Home page seems to be realized by some on-line retailers, such as Amazon.com or CDNow.com. Some positive examples can be found among the on-line brokers too. Schwab (Schwab.com) would be one of them.

3.1.4 Assessment question: Do the navigation bars remain visible if a long/large page is displayed?

Priority of the feature: High. First-time users may feel disoriented when browsing through long web pages. Permanent users may feel uncomfortable too, as they have to use scroll bars to get back to the menu – an excessive action they may see as unnecessary. Moving a scroll bar up and down long web pages can be annoying. Moreover, the navigation speed – a feature especially important on e-brokerage sites, due to the industry's specifics - is lost.

E-Brokers	77%
E-Retailers	88%

Table 5. Do the navigation bars remain visible if a long/large page is displayed?

Finding: The on-line brokers' web sites tend to have exceedingly long pages that neither have a link to "top of page", nor the main menu copied at the bottom, which complicates navigation. To illustrate this, we refer you to Castletrading.com and Castleonline.com.

Examples: Castleonline.com is an example of how long pages may confuse site developers themselves. The site's long FAQ page contains a list of questions with quick links to their explanations provided on the same page, but does not have either "back to top" links or answers to several questions placed at the top of the page.

3.1.5 Assessment question: Are terms and conditions and privacy policy pages easily accessible from the main browsing pages?

Priority of the feature: Medium to high. At any time, these sections (or even some of their subsections) may become crucial for a serious trader when he/she needs to make a decision. The inability to reach them in one click irritates the user. Terms and conditions, as well as Privacy Policy (including the terms of collecting personal information), contain important disclosures and regulatory information regarding Services offered by the company. There is a considerable amount of detail listed in these sections. The availability of this information may become a pivotal point of a user's decision-making process. Users should be able to find answers to their questions immediately.

E-Brokers	92%
E-Retailers	100%

Table 6. Are terms and conditions and privacy policy pages easily accessible from the main browsing pages?

Finding: The retail sites have links to "terms and conditions" and "privacy policy" at every applicable place, which is not characteristic of the on-line brokerage sites.

Examples: Two companies tested, eTrade.com and ML.com, made a notable effort to provide enhanced navigation features. We have discovered that easy navigation to the 'terms and conditions' and 'privacy policy' pages is also provided by the smaller sites, such as Protrader.com.

3.2 Questions relating to Help

The size and complexity of sites make Help tools availability a requirement. Customer service cannot be underestimated in e-trading, and its priority might be even higher in e-shopping. Securities traders often select a given brokerage company's site, in hopes of establishing a long-term relationship, based on how much advice and help they can get.

In order to test help and advice tools available on the shopping and brokerage sites, Allied Testing used a set of 15 questions. We found that the majority of sites in either category offered help facilities. We approached Help from the point of view of its context, functionality and accessibility. Retailers, as opposed to brokers, meet a specific group of requirements more accurately. The Allied Testing team thoroughly examined the difference in the area of help accessibility.

3.2.1 Assessment question: Does the site offer dynamic Help facilities?

Priority of the feature: High. Customers (96%) stated that "If a company's customer service department or website is responsive to my questions, I am more likely to trust that company". This statement is shared by a large number of people (Taylor, 2001). The number of people who are satisfied with on-line chat is likely to grow significantly in the future, as it is currently one of the most popular forms of Internet contact among young people. There are also households that have a single phone line connection, so some clients are not able to use the 1-800 telephone number while they are connected to the Internet. We assume that some traders are attracted by the Internet securities trading, because it allows being in control of the securities market from any place in the world, including those where "1-800 number" is not toll-free. The trading session is a fast interactive process, and real-time contact is crucial for it.

E-Brokers	33%
E-Retailers	73%

Table 7. Does the site offer dynamic Help facilities?

Finding: Most brokerage sites do not provide any tools for customer-staff interaction. However, some brokerage sites, such as Schwab.com, do offer help via e-mail, message boards and/or phone numbers. In this respect, interactivity is understood narrowly as availability of real-time on-line response from the company's support staff via company's website (chats/message boards).

Examples: The most obvious functional match for this question is the real-time Internet chat. This feature is represented well on such sites as eDreyfus.com and Castleonline.com, where the chat area is easily accessible from the site's main page and does not require registration. There are also problems associated with chat support: brokerage firms need trained customer support personnel, who are able to be there for people who want advice via chat on a 24hour and 7day a week schedule. Users often complain that the availability of chat and messages areas on the site does not guarantee feedback from the customer support staff. The Allied Testing team experienced difficulties with loading the Terranovaonline.com chat, as well as their customer support responding only in two cases out of three tests made during the standard session on various days.

3.2.2 Assessment question: Does the microhelp text exist for the main enabled fields & buttons?

Priority of the feature: Medium. Regular visitors of the site may not need it; new users may positively need it, as the on-line brokerages have developed a variety of frequently used industry-specific terms and functionalities at their websites.

E-Brokers	29%
E-Retailers	60%

Table 8. Does the microhelp text exist for the main enabled fields & buttons?

Finding: Less than 1/3 of the brokerage sites tested use microhelp text for the main enabled fields and buttons. Microhelp is understood as either a small text next to an object (entry box, selection box, etc.) or the so-called "balloon help" - a local clue right on the page. There are, however, good examples of microhelp availability among the brokerage sites: the site Brownco.com has an appropriate amount of microhelp in corresponding locations (especially in the 'Site tour' section, provided specifically for new visitors).

Examples: It is not always easy to identify the basic Help sections, as there is no separate Help section; or there is a variety of titles for educational resources and the trading education information. The section called the 'Learning Center' at Schwab.com, at ML.com's web page Askmerrill.ml.com is called 'Financial Education'. However, there is no combined section like that at Fidelity.com. Instead, the site's several separate 'Education' sections can only be accessed at third level pages and cannot be seen as a single list of contents.

3.2.3 Assessment question: Is the help text legible?

Priority of the feature: Medium. The text can easily be made larger by using the Text size function in any Internet browser, except for those rare cases when the font sizes are fixed.

E-Brokers	95%
E-Retailers	100%

Table 9. Is the help text legible?

Finding: We have found that the developers of 5% of the brokerage sites tested seem to have considered the issue of whether the Help text is legible a smaller priority. Some sites customized for viewing in 800x600 resolution or lower fail to provide text of legible size in a larger resolution. This becomes evident in areas, where large amounts of text are displayed, as is the case in the Help section.

Examples: At Terranovaonline.com, they use fixed font sizes, thus disregarding the interests of users with poor eyesight. On the other hand, Schwab.com provides a positive example with its large fonts that can be enlarged in the browser, despite the fact that the site is operable at resolution as low as 640x480. However, other problems may be revealed when changing the font size: by enlarging the text size, failures in design layout may become evident, as is the case at JBOxford.com.

3.2.4 Assessment question: Does a clear link to Help exist on each page?

Priority of the feature: High. The first-time visitor may need advice or basic information at any time he/she uses the site, and they should be available in one click. If Help is hard to find, the user is likely to leave the site. This issue is closely tied with both customer psychology and navigation. Some users may feel lost at a site even if helpful sections, like the Site Map, are available: please refer to ML.com , where the site map is very large and features varied domain names, thus making it harder for a visitor to find a starting helpful topic.

E-Brokers	77%
E-Retailers	88%

Table 10. Does a clear link to Help exist on each page?

Finding: Our research has shown that 23% of the brokerage sites we tested do not have links to Help or FAQ at some of their pages.

Examples: A failure to provide Help as an easy-to-access single section is evident at the smaller sites we tested, such as blackwoodtrading.com . However, we found the same problem even on some advanced sites, such as ML.com. Some sites have easy-to-use Visitor sections, like Ameritrade.com's 'Tell me more'. There is also an example of how the issue of the Help section availability is solved at the larger sites: at Schwab.com , the Help section is placed at the bottom of every page.

3.2.5 Assessment question: Can Help be printed?

Priority of the feature: High. This issue is very important for the brokerage sites, as their business targets only the customers that use one brokerage service for a long period, unlike most retail shops. The amount of money spent by the trader can greatly vary from the money spent by the on-line shopper. Some customers may wish to have their brokerage site's 'Help' printed to read it offline. Any user may wish to read 'Help' offline and navigate the site at the same time to save time.

E-Brokers	86%
E-Retailers	92%

Table 11. Can Help be printed?

Finding: We discovered that 'Help' couldn't be printed adequately by clicking the Print button of a user's browser at 14% of the brokerage sites we tested. Some of them have a large margin (a navigation bar) to the left of the 'Help' section, which causes the 'Help' text to be cut off on the right hand side when printing. Some web pages have frames (which, in fact, rarely occurs on brokerage sites) containing navigation bars that are printed, while the Help text itself is omitted.

Examples: The Allied Testing team has evaluated the Help and FAQ sections at JBOxford.com as 'an example to be followed', not only from the point of view of its readiness for being printed, but also as far as its overall

'Help' section performance is concerned. Helpful topics are best used when presented in two ways: their "normal" format and the "printer-friendly" one.

4. CONCLUSION

Inside the primarily offline industry of securities trading, some of services and features offered, such as the amount of commission, may be more important for customer decision-making than certain Internet performance features. However, as the securities trading firms struggle to build more competitive websites, they may wish to use the experience of other industries that have established themselves on the Web. We decided that the comparison with the Internet shops used in our research may be productive: not only have some of them felt competitive pressure over the last few years, but they have also been discussed in various on-line and offline periodicals, and other kinds of feedback from experts and regular users in Web forums and newsgroups. This feedback has benefited them in several ways and has enabled them to provide a more user-friendly interface.

The set of questions we used to examine 'Navigation' shows that brokerage companies may wish to pay more attention to the Internet technologies. Poor site maintenance and failure to check the site for basic performance on the Web, which lead to dead links, and the lack of description for downloads, do not add to the sites' reputation. Navigation may be slowed down by the abundance of long pages, as well as the absence of clear 'Home page' and 'Terms of Use' links that traders require.

Our assessment of the 'Help and advice' area has shown that, generally speaking, the 'Help' areas are consistent. However, there are requirements to their presentation that should be met more accurately. They include the user's ability to read and print Help-related topics and the availability of links to 'Help' section. Due to the interactive nature of the trading process, the trading sites' owners should feel obliged to provide the user with dynamic help tools. The nuances of the industry's terminology are often not adequately supported with microhelp hints.

The on-line brokerages may wish to consider sufficient improvements at their sites to be able to meet the users' requirements and stay competitive. There is still a great need in development of special usability guidelines for securities trading sites, and we believe this paper is a small step forward in developing them.

5. REFERENCES

Cawthon, R. (2001), Taking Financial Websites to the Next Level. A new study questions the conventional wisdom in *Bank Technology News*, Forrester Research Inc., June 2001 [http://www.banktechnews.com/btn/articles/btnjun01-7.shtml (as of 11/25/2001)]

Telerise (2000), DIY website design, In Information sheets - TelecomsAdvice

[http://www.telecomsadvice.org.uk/infosheets/diy_website_design.htm (as of 4/30/2002)]

Mauro, Ch. L. (2001), Usability and on-line financial services: big losses in *ViewPointz*, MauroNewMedia July 25, 2001

[http://www.taskz.com/Usability_financial_indepth.htm (as of 11/25/2001)]

Taylor, H. (2001), Why Some Companies Are Trusted and Others Are Not: Personal Experience and Knowledge of Company More Important than Glitz, in The Harris Poll #28, June 20, 2001

[http://www.harrisinteractive.com/harris_poll/index.asp?PID=237 (as of 11/25/2001)]

Usability: Gaining a Competitive Edge
IFIP World Computer Congress 2002
J. Hammond, T. Gross, J. Wesson (Eds)
Published by Kluwer Academic Publishers

User Satisfaction, Aesthetics and Usability

Beyond Reductionism

Gitte Lindgaard & Cathy Dudek
Carleton Human Computer Interaction Institute
Carleton University, Ottawa, Ontario, Canada
gitte_lindgaard@carleton.ca , cdudek@chat.carleton.ca

Abstract: Results from a series of web site studies suggest that the concept of user satisfaction comprises more than perceived aesthetics and usability. Satisfaction was repeatedly found to be a complex construct comprising 'emotion', 'likeability', and 'expectation' as well. A web site very high in appeal but low in usability scored highly on user satisfaction when first encountered. However, when faced with serious problems in a usability test, users' overall level of satisfaction dropped considerably, but perceived aesthetics remained unchanged. Given the known importance of the first impression for subsequent judgments, our results suggest that user interface designers of e-commerce sites would be well advised to design pretty and usable sites. Designing for user efficiency and effectiveness alone is not enough unless the products and services offered on a web site are unique in the world.

Key words: satisfaction, aesthetics, appeal, usability, emotion

1. INTRODUCTION

According to the ISO 9241-11 standard, user satisfaction is supposed to contribute to usability along with effectiveness and efficiency (ISO, 1997). Among the plethora of usability assessment techniques, with few exceptions (Kirakowski, 1996), hardly any concern, or include, measures of user satisfaction. This is understandable when the goal is to make users more efficient and effective. Indeed, many measurements of user satisfaction tend to be limited to assessing "what users think of [a given application]" (Macleod, Bowden, Bevan & Curson, 1997). Fewer still are concerned with the emotional impact of an interface (Kim & Moon, 1998). Apparently, it is assumed that users will like and accept a highly usable application that enables them to do their job quickly and efficiently. This is a form of usability reductionism, where joy (or even satisfaction) is merely a by-product of great usability (Hassenzahl, Beau & Burmester, 2001). The assumption that productivity enhancement automatically fosters satisfaction may be justified in traditional office applications where a person's livelihood, a company's profit, public well-being or safety may depend on just that. However, even if we accept that assertion, it still does not follow that satisfaction is a component of usability – satisfaction may result primarily from usability issues.

In this paper we argue that satisfaction may be a by-product of great usability in traditional office environments, and that satisfaction can be defined in terms of efficiency and effectiveness. However, on the World Wide Web where users choose to spend their leisure time finding information, seeking entertainment, or shopping, and where the next competing site is but a click away, we suspect that users employ quite different criteria in evaluating their experience. We also believe that this evaluation depends upon users' needs and goals. In order to widen the notion of user satisfaction beyond efficiency and effectiveness of the user experience, researchers must start to think of usability as part of a satisfying user experience. In exploring the satisfaction construct, we consulted research in Human Computer Interaction (HCI), neurophysiology, and marketing.

Research in the consumer and marketing literature has shown that consumers readily recall the emotional content of customer service encounters and that they use semantically different words to describe their experiences with different industry sectors (Edwardson, 1998). The literature has also found that 'satisfied' customers are just as likely to defect as those who are neutral or mildly dissatisfied (Jones & Sasser, 1995). That is, unless customers are 'highly satisfied' with a company's goods and services, the company cannot take customer loyalty for granted. If user satisfaction is motivated by different criteria and if the questions phrased in 5-point or 7-point scales asking them to judge 'appeal'/'attraction' or 'pleasantness' of the interactive experience fail to capture the essence of user satisfaction in a given context, then we may be misled in our interpretation of satisfaction scores. The research we report here is motivated by a need to 'unpack' the notion of user satisfaction in the context of e-commerce web sites by listening to what users tell us about their interactive experience. Increasing attention to user satisfaction, however, does not mean that we can afford to neglect the performance-related aspects of usability that we have traditionally measured. We also need to learn how satisfaction relates to user effectiveness and efficiency. User Interface (UI) designers working within strict budgetary and time constraints need guidance on how best to divide resources to satisfy both and balance aesthetics with efficiency factors in their designs. As well as understanding how to measure user satisfaction, our aim is therefore ultimately to derive valid design guidelines for a wide range of interactive technologies.

Our concern with satisfaction arises from very robust findings in the neurophysiological literature where researchers constantly find that emotional responses are strikingly immediate, occurring within 3-4 milliseconds of a stimulus being shown (Bornstein, 1992; Zajonc, 1980). Thus, according to this research, emotional responses are pre-attentive and precede cognitive ones. The implications for web design are obvious and pervasive: if users decide that they dislike what they see in less than five milliseconds, then they may click onto the next site even before they have taken in any information it offers. The strength of the 'first impression', characterized by what psychologists call a 'primacy effect', has long featured very prominently in the psychological literature, (Anderson, 1981; Anderson, 1982) even in areas involving expert judgement such as diagnostic medicine (Lindgaard, 1985). Basically, judgments are overwhelmingly based on the first impression. Where a primacy effect occurs, the stimulus presented or detected first receives a disproportionate amount of attention. The subsequent search for evidence to substantiate the judgment already made is biased in favour of searching exclusively for confirmatory evidence while ignoring contradictory evidence, giving rise to the so-called 'confirmation bias' (Mynatt, Doherty & Tweeney, 1977). So, if users have already decided they dislike a site, they will interpret virtually all information as being more negative than if their first impression were positive.

A recent study by Tractinsky, Katz & Ikar (2000) investigated the extent to which "the initial perceptions of aesthetics-usability relationships hold after a period of system use, and whether these perceptions are affected by the interface's perceived aesthetics and/or by the actual usability of the system" (p.131). They found that judgments of interface aesthetics were not affected by traditional usability factors. Using an array of ATM interfaces with identical content but varying in layout and in appeal, as determined in the pre-experimental phase, they introduced several usability problems to which the 'low usability' but not the 'high-usability' group was exposed. While this manipulation affected the task-completion times, judgments of interface aesthetics did not change and neither did judgements of perceived usability. The researchers concluded that the relationship between usability and satisfaction is not orthogonal, which lead to their provocative claim that "what is beautiful is usable". Their findings suggest that the two concepts are correlated. One may regard this as a form of design reductionism, where joy of use can be brought about by aesthetics alone, even in the face of usability problems (Hassenzahl et al, 2001).

By contrast, studies performed in our laboratory suggest that usability may be judged independently of interface aesthetics when users are confronted with severe usability problems (Lindgaard & Dudek, 2002). For example, one site perceived to be extremely high in aesthetics but very low in usability scored substantially lower on usability, but as highly on satisfaction as another site perceived to be high in both usability and aesthetics. However, Tractinsky et al.'s (2000) subjects undertook tasks as in a traditional usability test, our results were based on retrospective self reports obtained in interviews immediately after subjects had inspected the site for 10 minutes. Subjects were instructed to verbalize their experience of the interaction. In the absence of a requirement to complete a set of usability tasks designed to test the extent to which usability flaws get in the user's way, it is quite possible that our subjects' experiential descriptions were based entirely on the first impression of the site. This begs the question of the strength and duration of the first impression in a web environment.

Much of the psychological literature on the primacy effect suggests that it is paramount and may determine any judgmental outcome (Anderson, 1982; Slovic & Lichtenstein, 1971), presumably including a judgment of 'satisfaction'. By the same token, the so-called 'mere exposure effect' suggests that the strength of the initial (emotional) impression starts to wane once the exposure time exceeds 50 milliseconds (Bornstein, 1992). A strongly negative first impression could be commercially damaging to a company aiming to increase its online sales, particularly if it competes with many others offering the same goods and services. To ensure a positive first impression, a greater proportion of the usually limited UI design resources may thus have to be devoted to interface aesthetics, perhaps even at the expense of some usability factors. If, however, the emotional first impression does fade as quickly as research into the mere exposure effect suggests, site visitors may well hang around long enough to consider the merits of the information/services/products offered on the site even if the first impression does not evoke a 'wow' effect. In that case, UI designers would be quite justified in their continued quest to create usable sites at the expense of making them strikingly 'beautiful'. In Tractinsky et al.'s (2000) study, users did not change their mind after completing tasks in which they encountered usability problems. The experiment reported here was designed to test the robustness of these authors' finding when users are exposed to more serious usability problems.

2. FRAMEWORK OF THE STUDY

A web site offering exclusive writing utensils was used. In an earlier experiment, this site was found to be significantly higher in appeal and lower in perceived usability than several other sites using the same method of investigation and different groups of subjects (Lindgaard & Dudek, 2002). In contrast to several of the other sites employed in the same series of experiments, all of which were typical shopping sites, the pen site contained no prices on goods or monetary transaction modules. Its purpose was thus apparently to market rather than sell goods. The present study proceeded in two phases. In Phase 1, an heuristic evaluation was conducted to identify the nature, location, and severity of usability problems in the web site. The outcome of this evaluation served as a basis for selecting and designing user tasks to be performed in the subsequent usability test. Phase 2 comprised the usability test enabling a comparison with an earlier study of the same web site, as follows:

Present study: Browse site (10 min) → unstructured interview → usability test → unstructured interview

Previous study: Browse site (10 min) → unstructured interview

2.1 Heuristic Evaluation

The heuristic evaluation revealed some 157 instances of moderate (n = 45) to severe (n = 112) usability problems. By our definition, a moderate problem gets in the user's way but does not prevent progress towards accomplishing a goal, whereas a severe usability problem does. As can be seen in Table 1 below, the majority of the problems involved navigation (n = 77). Some 29 of these concerned hyperlinks (e.g. looks like a hyperlink but is not; does not look like a hyperlink but it is; does not behave like a hyperlink). The remaining 48 were due to unusual, unpredictable, inconsistent navigation rules or awkward navigation operations. For example, menus were 'floating' in and out of view, forcing the user to select an option very quickly, and the active area surrounding a point on a map was tiny, requiring such fine motor movements that it was almost impossible to point precisely. Another group of problems (n = 33) concerned visibility and comprehension of text/objects, being marred by confusing or misleading vocabulary, contrast problems, or text displays that were partly obscured by overlapping graphics. Some (n = 24) were due to inconsistent system behaviour or display rules, e.g. information displayed in the topmost screen position in one screen was at the bottom of the next, or text would move while the user was reading it. The remainder (n = 23) were unique problems not falling into any of the above categories.

Nature of problem	N
Navigation, not including hyperlinks	48
Hyperlinks	29
Visibility & comprehension	33
System behaviour/display rules	24
Other	23
Total	**157**

Table 1. Number of usability problems by category

2.2 Selection of User Tasks

Upon loading, the site played an animated introduction taking several minutes with accompanying soft music matching the rhythm of the colourful, entertaining animation. This introduction looked more like a TV commercial than an e-commerce site. The site comprised three main sections, each of which was sub-divided into several sub-sections with these sub-dividing further to a maximum of four levels. The eight user tasks were selected to satisfy two objectives: (1) all three main sections were represented and, (2) they represented different levels of difficulty and number of clicks to the target information. Tasks appeared straight-forward, for example, asking subjects to find out when the company was established, whether the company had any job openings, and to find the nearest retail outlet.

2.3 Procedure

Twenty subjects, 10 males and 10 females, were recruited from around the University Campus in a semi-random fashion, ensuring that English was their first language, that they were regular Internet users (2-10hrs/week), and that they had no UI design or evaluation experience. Subjects first inspected the site for 10 min, having been told to concentrate on their interactive experience and pretending they were looking for a gift for a special person to send as an apology. At the end of the 10 minutes, an unstructured interview was conducted to elicit as many experience-related statements as possible. Next, they completed the eight usability tasks, given to all subjects in the same sequence, beginning with the easy tasks, and ending with more difficult tasks. This was done to give subjects a sense of success and motivate them to work through all the tasks, as we expected some of the searches to be unsuccessful. All subjects attempted all tasks, and there were no time- or accuracy constraints. Subjects were allowed to give up if they were unable to retrieve the information needed to complete the task. At the end of the usability test another interview was conducted in the same manner as before to learn whether the initial impression remained constant or whether appeal was attenuated compared with the first interview. Subjects were tested individually in sessions lasting up to 1.5 hours. They were paid $15 Canadian for their time.

2.4 Data Analysis

Interviews were audio taped. Data were transcribed ad verbatim and submitted to a content analysis. Statements were divided into 5 categories: aesthetics, emotion, expectation, likeability and usability. Aesthetics-type statements all referred to visual qualities of the interface (too much blue, too much white space, bright, pretty, pleasing to the eye). Emotion statements, defined in terms of Russell's Circumplex Model of Affect (Russell, 1980), were those that could finish the sentence "It was [made me feel]…." (uplifting, relaxing, calming, frustrating) and represented a concept that could reasonably have been contained in Russell's (1980) Model. Expectation statements expressed thoughts about components that the subject was surprised to find in the interface, thought would be there, or should have been there. In some cases, they used the word 'expected' in the statement; in others their expectation could be derived from what was said. For example, "I would have thought they would put all the pens together" reflected an unmet expectation. Likeability statements were overall judgements about the site or comparisons with other sites (better than, I like it, it's okay, fine, not as good as). Finally, usability comments were those that referred directly to efficiency or effectiveness, for example, 'there is no back button'; 'I could not click on that', and 'the choices are not logically displayed'. Statements in which subjects merely read aloud screen content were eliminated. Statements were counted once only regardless of the number of times a given word was repeated in an interview.

3. RESULTS

In this section, the data from the first interview (before usability test - Experiment 2) are compared with those obtained in the earlier experiment (browsing only – Experiment 1), details of which are reported elsewhere (Lindgaard & Dudek, 2002). The data comparing the 'before' and 'after usability test' conditions are reported in section 3.2. First, we wanted to explore whether people would have more or less to say about their experience when they expected to complete a usability test, so a two-tailed t-test was performed for the total number of statements. Participants had more to say when they were expecting to complete a usability test (Experiment 2) than when they were just browsing the site (Experiment 1) with no particular purpose in mind. (t(38)=-2.24, p<.05), as shown in Figure 1. Looking next to see if the strength or quality of the experience differed, the proportion of positive statements each group made are displayed in Figure 2.

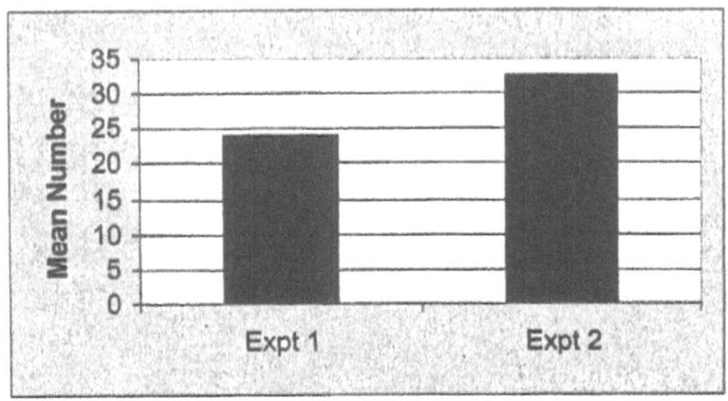

Figure 1. Mean number of all statements.

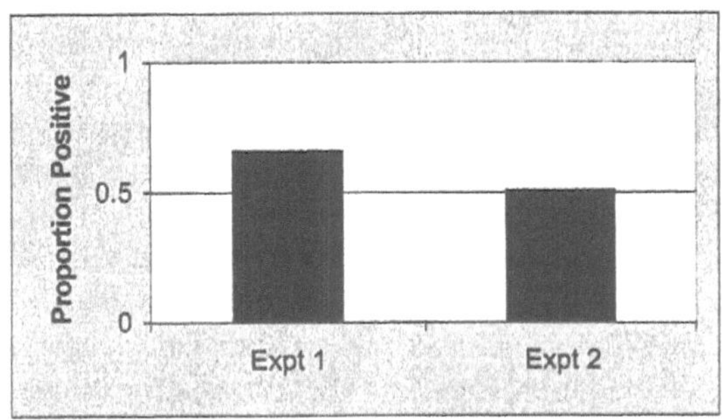

Figure 2. Proportions of all types of statements.

A two-tailed t-test comparing the proportion of positive statements in both experiments showed that the experience of 'just browsing' subjects was more positive than that for subjects who were preparing to complete a usability test (t(38)= 1.99, p<.05). Observation of subjects during the browsing session in both experiments showed that 'browsing only' subjects tended to move around the site in an ad hoc fashion. By contrast, those who knew the usability tasks would follow set out systematically to look through as much of the site as they could in the 10min browsing time. These latter subjects saw more of the usability problems owing to the sheer difficulty of navigating the site. This difference in browsing behaviour probably accounts for the difference in positive statements.

Consistent with earlier findings, statements fell into the categories mentioned earlier (likeability, emotion, aesthetics expectation and usability).

The mean number of statements in each category differed between experiments as shown in Figure 3. These results show that people had more to say in the second experiment than the first, particularly about likeability ($t(32)=-2.50$, $p<.05$), and aesthetics ($t(26)=-2.75$, $p<.01$). The mean number of emotion, expectation and usability statements did not differ ($p>.05$) from the first to the second experiment.

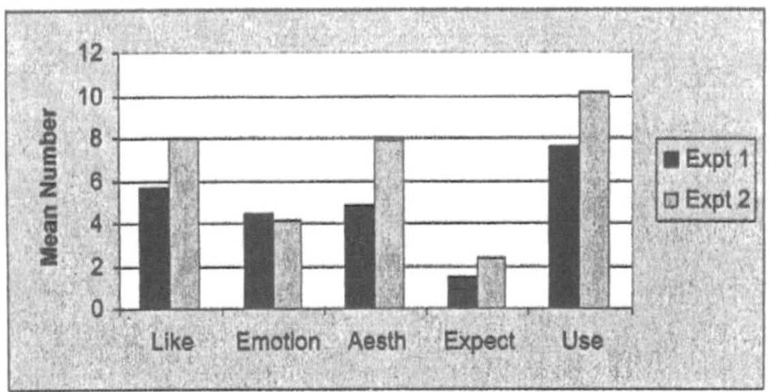

Figure 3. Mean number of all types of statements.

3.1 Usability Test

Of the 160 tasks attempted across all subjects, only 79 (49.38%) were completed successfully. The average success rate was 3.95 of the eight tasks. No one completed all eight tasks successfully, and none of the tasks were completed successfully by all subjects. Only one was completed successfully by more than 15 subjects. Three tasks were completed successfully by 10-15 subjects, and another three by 5-10 subjects. The remaining task was not completed successfully by a single subject. The number of clicks to success exceeded the optimal number in all tasks, ranging from 100% to 2800% above the optimum for successfully, and from 100% to 8650% for unsuccessfully completed tasks. Thus, when subjects did give up, it was only after trying hard. This allowed us to conclude that they took the tasks seriously. These data also confirm that the level of usability was very low.

3.2 Comparison of First and Second Interview

Now comparing the 'before' and 'after usability test' interviews, the data suggest that the user experience changed from the first to the second interview. Although we expected the number of statements to be lower in the second interview because the subjects had already said all that they wanted in the first interview, a one-tailed t-test for paired samples showed that the total number of statements did not differ (p>.05). This is shown in Figure 4.

As before, the proportion of positive statements was calculated. These are shown in Figure 5. A two-tailed t-test for paired samples showed that participants made significantly fewer positive statements after the usability test (t(19)=4.60, p<.001). Thus, although the total number of statements did not change from the first interview to the next, the user experience was apparently more negative after than before the usability test.

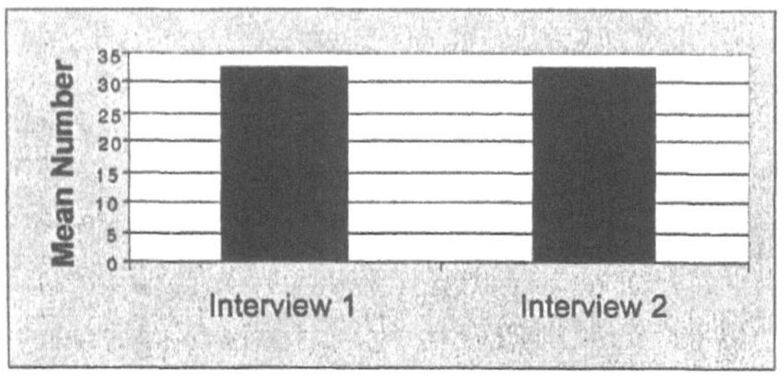

Figure 4. Mean number of all statements.

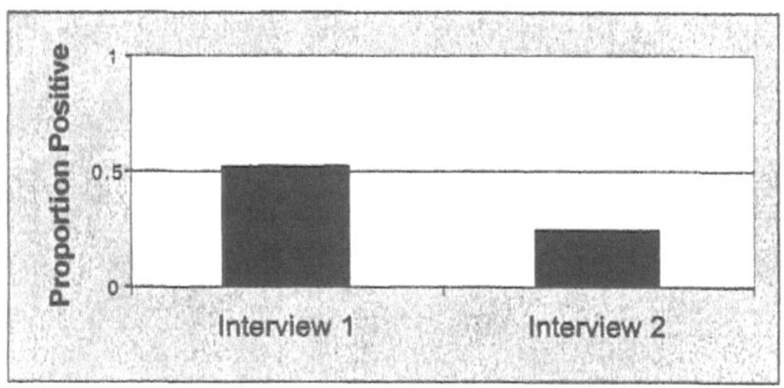

Figure 5. Proportion of positive statements.

Breaking down the statements by category as before showed that there were dramatic changes in some of these. This is shown in Figure 6.

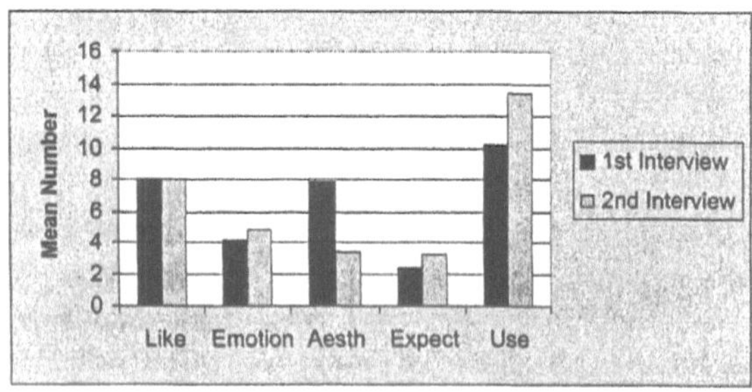

Figure 6. Mean number of all types of statements.

In the second interview subjects tended to say less about aesthetics ($t(19)=4.57$, $p<.001$) and more about usability ($t(19)=-2.77$, $p<.01$). There were no difference the numbers of likeability, emotion and expectation statements ($p>.05$). This is not surprising. One would expect that participants already said what they wanted in the first interview, and there is no reason to think that they would repeat themselves a second time. The larger number of usability statements can be attributed to a greater awareness of usability issues resulting from the task requirements.

A comparison of the proportion of positive statements in the two interviews shows that there was no overall decline in the user experience from one interview to the next in terms of aesthetics ($p>.05$), as shown in Figure 7. Thus, although subjects had less to say about aesthetics in the second interview than in the first, they did not find the site uglier after the usability test.

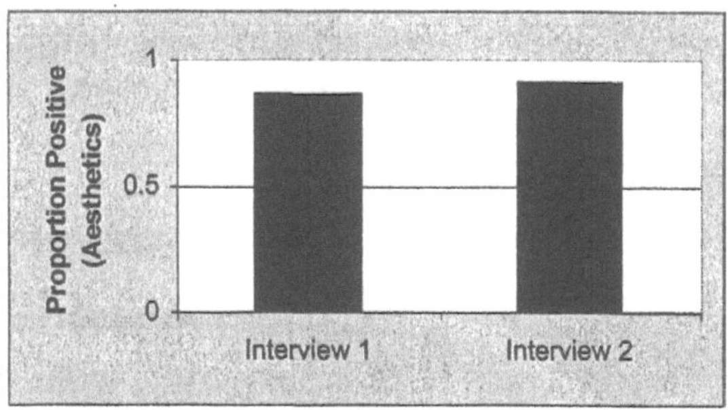

Figure 7. Proportion of positive aesthetics statements.

The pattern of results for the other categories are shown in Figures 8-11. For likeability (Figure 8) and expectation (Figure 9) the overall number of positive statements remained similar ($p>.05$).

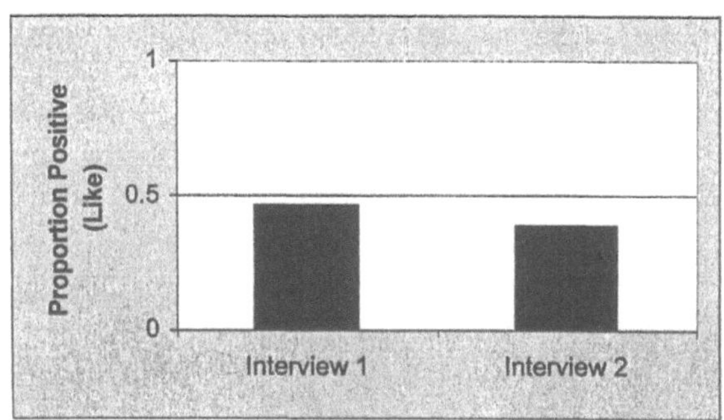

Figure 8. Proportion of positive likeability statements.

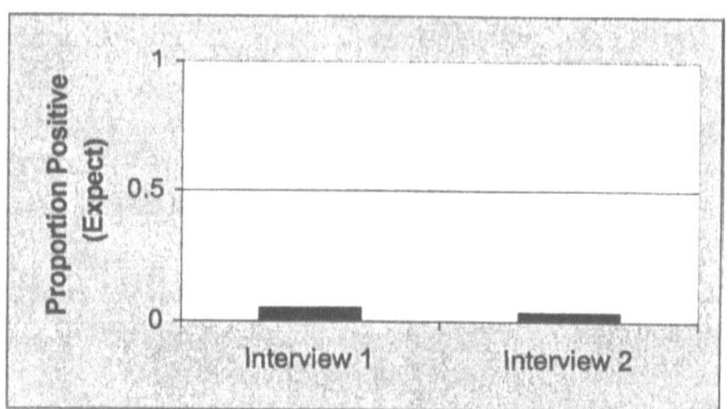

Figure 9. Proportion of positive expectation statements.

For emotion (Figure 10), a two tailed t-test ($t(18)=4.17$, $p<.001$) showed that significantly fewer positive emotions were expressed in the second interview than the first. It appears that participants changed their minds about their experience after encountering usability problems.

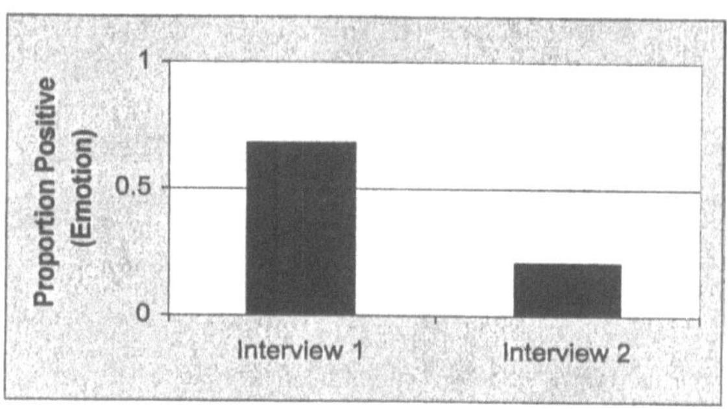

Figure 10. Proportion of positive emotion statements.

For usability statements, there was also a difference. As shown previously in Figure 5, there were more usability statements made in the second interview than there were in the first. However, looking at the proportions of positive and negative statements shows that they changed their minds about their experience regarding usability as well, as shown in Figure 11. A two-tailed t-test for paired samples showed that there were significantly fewer positive usability statements made during the second interview than the first ($t(19)=2.98$, $p<.001$). Thus, although subjects did identify numerous negative usability issues before they completed the usability tasks, these assumed more prominence during the usability test and in the subsequent interview.

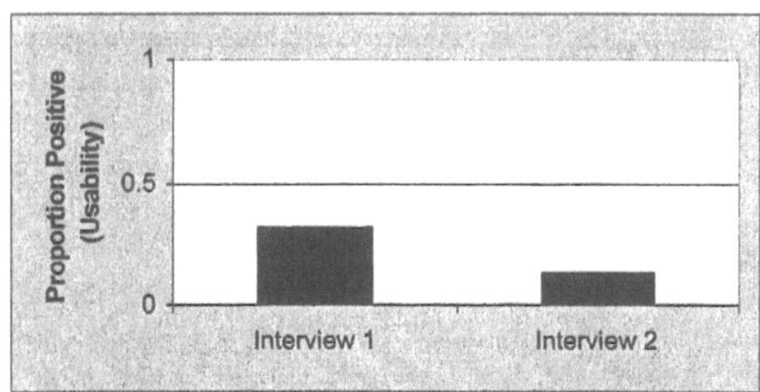

Figure 11. Proportion of positive usability statements.

4. DISCUSSION

Considering first the notion of aesthetics, our results appear, on the surface, to agree with Tractinsky et al.'s (2000) findings in the sense that subjects did not consider the user interface uglier after completing usability tasks than before. However, Tractinsky and his colleagues use the term 'aesthetics' interchangeably with 'affect'. They appear to believe that aesthetics ratings are indicative of user satisfaction. Their subjects rated three aspects of the user interfaces, namely aesthetics, ease of use, and amount of information on the screen. Yet, the authors argue that "there are strong correlations between users' satisfaction from using the system and their perception of its aesthetics and usability" (p. 141). By contrast, our results suggest that the interactive experience comprises at least the five dimensions discussed here, including perceived aesthetics and usability. This repeated finding leads us to argue that usability rightfully belongs under the umbrella of satisfaction and that the notion of user satisfaction is more complex than a correlation between aesthetics and usability. Indeed, our results suggest that the two are not correlated at all: perceived usability is likely to change after encountering usability problems whereas perceived aesthetics is not.

A closer look at Tractinsky et al.'s (2000) findings suggests that the usability problems they introduced did not seriously hamper subjects' performance. The authors describe three usability problems, all of which delayed performance, for example, introducing a delay of nine seconds on average per task. However, all subjects completed all the 11 tasks successfully. By contrast, our subjects completed roughly one half of the eight tasks successfully, as discussed earlier. Our subjects liked the site less overall after experiencing serious usability problems, and the proportion of negative usability comments increased in the before-after comparison of usability statements. The problem seems to be in the definition of 'aesthetics'. Tractinsky et al. (2000) uses it interchangeably with 'appeal', and 'beauty'. Our results have consistently shown that 'appeal' or what we call 'user satisfaction' comprises more than 'beauty', which by our definition is taken to equate 'aesthetics'. More research is needed to clarify these issues and sharpen the terminology we use to capture and describe the user experience.

With respect to the strength of the first impression, our results suggest that subjects who knew they would be performing usability tasks liked the site less on first encounter than subjects who were 'just browsing'. Thus, the different task demands resulted in different browsing patterns that called more attention to usability. Subjects who knew that they would be asked to complete usability tasks browsed the site in a systematic, goal-oriented fashion, whereas those who were 'just browsing' let themselves be carried away by the show unfolding before their eyes. This raises the issue of site design vis à vis the purpose a given site is intended to fulfil. Because the pen site did not allow users to select and buy items, we believe it was designed to yield a pleasant, but passive experience. In contrast, shopping sites aim to engage users actively and guide them effortlessly through a purchasing transaction. Usability was clearly not a major design objective. However, our usability task demands led subjects to focus on usability. Consequently, the first impression suffered. The first impression would thus appear to depend upon the user's goal: if seeking an obligation-free entertaining experience, subjects pay more attention to the experiential aspects than to usability factors, but when visiting a site to buy goods, the reverse seems to be the case. Thus, user satisfaction seems to be driven by the users' motivation for visiting the site and cannot be reduced to a by-product of aesthetics, usability or even a combination of both.

5. CONCLUSION

The present study suggests that goals determine the users' frame of mind, within which the site is perceived and interpreted, and that this first impression may change as a consequence of facing serious usability problems. While subjects are aware of usability problems even when they are 'just browsing' these affect their opinion of the site less. Finally, the results suggest that concern for traditional usability issues is an integral part of the interactive user experience, however, user satisfaction is a complex construct involving more than an impression of 'aesthetics' or 'usability' alone. The relationship between appeal and user satisfaction, and between perceived/actual usability remain evasive and need much more research to be clearly understood. While the first impression may be strong and may relate to the immediate appeal of the web site, satisfaction may change as a function of encountering serious usability problems in the context of accomplishing a specific goal. Thus, if it is true, that the first impression is based on immediate appeal, UI designers would be well advised to create aesthetically appealing sites that clearly and immediately reflect its purpose.

6. REFERENCES

Anderson, N.H. (1981), *Foundations of information integration theory*, Academic Press, London.

Anderson, N.H. (1982), *Methods of information integration theory*, Academic Press, London.

Bornstein, R. (1992), *Subliminal Mere Exposure Effect, Perception Without Awareness: Cognitive, Clinical, and Social Perspectives*, Bornstein, F. and Pittman, T. (eds) The Guilford Press: New York.

Edwardson, M. (1998), Measuring Consumer Emotions in Service Encounters: An Exploratory Analysis, *Australian Journal of Market Research*, 6, 2, July, p. 34-48.

Hassenzahl, M., Beau, A., & Burmester, M., Engineering Joy, (2001), *IEEE Software*, January-February.

ISO (1997), ISO/DIS 9241-11. Ergonomic requirements for office work with visual display terminals (VDTs): Guidance on usability.

Jones, T. & Sasser, E. Jr. (1995), Why Satisfied Customers Defect, *Harvard Business Review*, November - December.

Kim, J. & Moon, J. (1998), Designing towards emotional usability in customer interfaces-trustworthiness of cyber-banking system interfaces, *Interacting with Computers*, 10, 1-29.

Kirakowski, J. (1996), The software usability measurement inventory: Background and usage, in P. Jordan, B. Thomas & B. Weerdmeester (Eds), *Usability evaluation in industry*, Taylor & Francis, London.

Lindgaard, G. (1985), Weighting of individuating information elements and base rate in a nursing decision making task involving non-diagnostic case information, Unpublished Masters Thesis, Department of Psychology Monash University, Clayton, Australia.

Lindgaard, G. & Dudek, C. (2002), What is this beast we call user satisfaction?, submitted to *Interacting with Computers*.

Macleod, M., Bowden, R., Bevan, N., & Curson, I. (1997), The MUSiC performance measurement method, *Behaviour and Information Technology*, 16, 1-27.

Mynatt, C.R., Doherty, M.E. & Tweney, R.D. (1977), Confirmation bias in a simulated research environment: An experimental study of scientific inference, *Quarterly Journal of Experimental Psychology*, 29, 85-95.

Russell, J. A. (1980), A Circumplex Model of Affect. *Journal of Personality and Social Psychology, 39*, 6, 1161 - 1178.

Slovic, P. & Lichtenstein, S. (1971), Comparison of Bayesian and regression approaches to the study of information processing in judgment, *Organizational Behaviour & Human Performance*, 6, 649-744.

Tractinsky, N., Katz, A. & Ikar, D. (2000), What is Beautiful is Usable, *Interacting with Computers*, 13, p.127-145.

Zajonc, R. (1980), Feeling and Thinking: Preferences need no References, *American Psychologist*, February, p.151.

Usability: Gaining a Competitive Edge
IFIP World Computer Congress 2002
J. Hammond, T. Gross, J. Wesson (Eds)
Published by Kluwer Academic Publishers

Evaluating Security Tools towards Usable Security

A Usability Taxonomy for the Evaluation of Security Tools based on a Categorization of User Errors

Johannes Kaiser and Martin Reichenbach
Institute for Computer Science and Social Studies, University of Freiburg, Germany.

Abstract: The main success of the internet is its openness. To guarantee security in the internet - for example to protect the user's privacy - the use of security tools is essential. Because today's internet users cover almost all educational levels and professional groups, we assume that in most cases they will be security novices. Unfortunately, the usage of today's security tools is mostly too complex and incomprehensible, thus opening security leaks caused by incorrect usage. In order to identify security leaks arising from the user interface, an *objective* measure for the usability of security tools is necessary. At present, such a measure does not exist. This paper develops such a measure for the usability of security tools. We propose problem categories for errors in security tools. Based on this categorization, we propose a taxonomy for the usability of security functions. Applying this taxonomy, security functions may be ranked according to the user's ability to avoid self-induced, security-critical user errors. Additionally, the taxonomy may explain possible causes of errors, introducing design alternatives to avoid these errors.

Key words: usability, multilateral security, security-critical user errors, usability evaluation

1. INTRODUCTION

Beyond doubt the main success of the internet is its openness. In order to protect the user's privacy or the security of online transactions, internet users have to be aware of security. Thus, the average user is confronted with security tools and embedded security functions in internet applications and therefore with the necessity to understand the underlying security concepts. In the following, the term security tool also implies embedded security functions in internet applications.

In (Whitten, 1999), it is shown that the underlying security concepts are mostly unfamiliar and incomprehensible to the security novice user and hence the security tool is not usable.

For evaluating the usability of security tools and for developing criteria for the design of usable security tools, it is necessary to establish an objective measure. Unfortunately, such an objective measure for the usability of security tools does not yet exist.

In the following, we present the concept of multilateral security. By applying this concept, the relevance of usability problems for security may be identified.

1.1 Multilateral security and its basic functions

The protection goals of multilateral security were proposed to guarantee secure communication (Rannenberg, 1999). These are confidentiality, integrity, availability and accountability. The protection goals will be fulfilled directly by security functions (see figure 1) (Rannenberg, 1998).

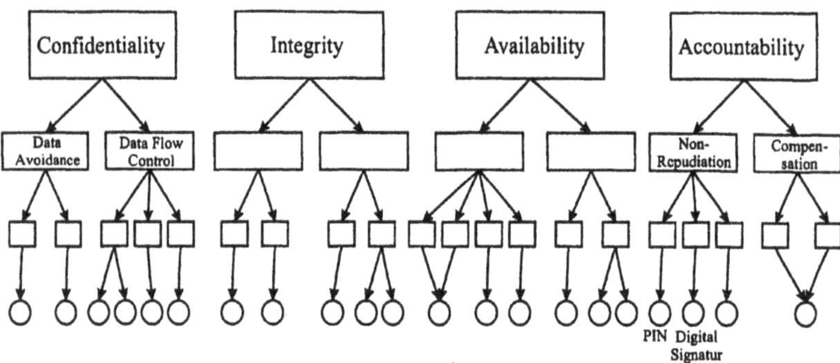

Figure 1: The hierarchy of protection goals, protection principles, functional building blocks and security functions.

These security functions can be controlled partly by the system, so the user is not burdened with having to deal with this. In most cases, however, security functions with their underlying security concepts stand directly in dialog with the users. Hence, user errors through an incorrect handling of the security functions are possible. Such a user error is critical for security, if at least one protection goal of multilateral security is threatened. These security-critical user errors are the main subject of this article. We are using the terms security critical user error and security critical usability problem synonymously.

In the following section, we propose an essential assumption about the average user of security tools and discuss the meaning of the usability of security. In Section 2, we derive a taxonomy based on security-critical user errors as an objective measure for evaluating the usability of security tools. Section 3 describes an error database for the design of usable security, realized by collecting security-critical user errors and adequate design alternatives for avoiding these errors.

1.2 User profiles of security tools

In order to design usable security tools, the system's developer needs an idea of the user's understanding of underlying security concepts. The more the system design takes into account the user's security competence, the more securely the user is able to handle the security tool. Thus, the system design must adapt to the user's security competence.

As system design based on automatic recognition of an individual user's competence is too complex and the results are mostly unsatisfactory, it seems reasonable to design security tools for user profiles according to their security competence. Examples for profiles based on the security competence are security novices, security interested persons and security experts.

Considering the demographic development of internet users, today's internet users cover almost all educational levels and professional groups. We assume, therefore, that today's average internet users are not internet experts, much less security experts. In consequence, we propose the following assumption of the user's security competence: In most cases, the average user of the internet will remain a security novice.

Based on this assumption, it is important to develop security tools according to the user's low security competence without reduction or abandonment of security functionality. This assumption also implies that a security tool will be widely used if it can be used securely by users with little security knowledge and little security experience.

It is important to take user profiles into account in the design of security systems because the design may be completely different for security experts than for security novices.

For these reasons, we consider the average user as being a security novice. After all, security is usable even if the average user as security novice is able to use the security tool in a secure way, i.e. without producing security-critical errors.

In the following, we define and categorize security-critical user errors, resulting in a taxonomy that enables system developers and system administrators to evaluate the usability of security tools.

2. CATEGORIZATION OF USABILITY AND SECURITY PROBLEMS

2.1 Sets of usability and security problems

Security systems may be considered to be secure if they fulfil, for example, the Common Criteria for Information Technology Security Evaluation (CCITSE, 2000). By certifying security systems according to the CCITSE, security problems on the technical layer can be avoided.

Security problems can also stem from the user interface, however. Usability problems can be divided into the following two sets:

- Security-non-critical usability problems;
- Security-critical usability problems.

Assuming security-non-critical usability problems are avoidable by ergonomic guidelines for software design as stated in (ISO 9241, 1996), these problems may be ignored.

Usability problems, on the other hand, are security-critical if at least one protection goal of multilateral security (Rannenberg, 1999) is threatened. In the following we discuss whether security-critical usability problems exist in security tools, despite certified security (CCITSE, 2000) and despite common usability guidelines.

Considering usability guidelines, we point out that security aspects are not yet considered. This is illustrated below by two examples of security-critical user errors occurring in security systems certified by the CCITSE, and that are not addressed by present usability guidelines:

1. The user wants to send an encrypted e-mail. He encrypts the e-mail correctly for the receiver. Because the e-mail tool is using the S/MIME standard, the security concept behind the e-mail tool means that the header of the e-mail with the subject is not encrypted. So it is security-critical if the user reveals information in the subject about the possible confidential content of the encrypted e-mail. The protection goal confidentiality is threatened.
2. For authentication by digital signature, a password is frequently used to activate the private key. Due to so-called PIN inflation, the user writes down his PIN or password on a paper list. So attackers on the digital signature can steal or copy this list. This user error is security-critical because if the attacker has also stolen the private

key, he can take the identity of the attacked person in the internet. The protection goal accountability is threatened.

According to the above mentioned assumption that users will be mostly security novices, these security-critical user errors are real.

Altogether, three essential sets of problems in security applications could be identified (see figure 2):

- Usability problems which are not security-critical;
- Security-critical usability problems;
- Security problems (on the technical layer) which do not arise from user interactions.

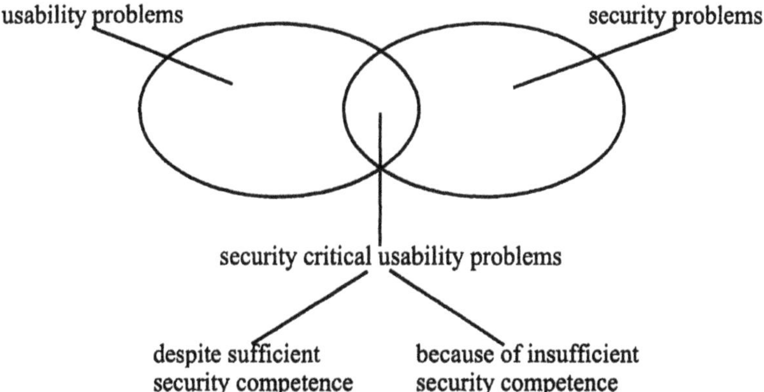

Figure 2: Three essential sets of problems in security applications.

2.2 Problem categories

Usability problems which are not security-critical are represented in the following by problem category I. Security problems which do not arise from user interactions are represented in the following by problem category IV.

According to the user's competence, it is important to divide security-critical usability problems into two further sub-categories. These sub-categories are presented by problem categories II and III (see Figure 2):

Problem category I

Usability problems which are non-critical to security.

Problem category II

Usability problems which are critical to security and arise despite the user's sufficient security competence.

Problem category III

Usability problems which are critical to security and arise from the user's insufficient security competence.

Problem category IV

Security problems which do not arise from user interactions.

This differentiation of security-critical usability problems in problem categories II and III is important for the design or redesign of security tools. A redesign based on problem category II will be extremely different from a redesign based on problem category III. For instance, user errors of problem category II can more likely be avoided by emphasising the underlying security concept. The redesign aiming at avoiding category III errors, however, would more likely succeed by concealing the underlying security concept and searching for an adequate comprehensible security concept as a substitute.

The cause of category III errors is the user's insufficient security experience. In order to detect the causes of category II errors, further investigations of security-critical usability problems are necessary as discussed in the next section.

At this point, user errors act as indicators for the conformance between the real world as perceived by the user, and the system world (Prabhu et al, 1997). That is, if a security concept is not well known to the user, he may still be able to handle the dialog correctly if he knows an adequate rule or analogy from the real world. The real world as perceived by the user is conform to the system world.

On the other hand, if the user is familiar with the underlying security concept, we can also talk about a conformity of the real world perceived by the user and the system world. For the design of security tools, it is important to know if the real world perceived by the user conforms with the world mapped by the system.

2.3 Familiarity with security concepts

Category II errors strongly depend on the degree of the user's familiarity with the underlying security concept. With a higher familiarity with system dialogs, less errors will be made by users in everyday use. Therefore, the degree of familiarity of security concepts may show how well the user is able to avoid category II errors by himself.

A first approach for identifying the user's familiarity with the underlying security concept is the subdivision of errors into slips and mistakes (Prabhu et al, 1997):

- Slips: The plan of the action may be correct but the action does not go as planned.
- Mistakes: The action may go as planned but the plan itself is wrong.

If a security concept is very familiar to the user, a probable error cause might be a slip, i.e. the action does not go as planned. If the security concept is known without sufficient familiarity to the user, a probable cause of the user error might be a wrong plan (mistake).

Slips occur on an action level (skill-based level), whereas mistakes occur on a plan level (Rasmussen, 1986). This plan level is differentiated by Rasmussen into two further levels: the rule-based level and the knowledge-based level (Rasmussen, 1998). If a user is not able to solve the problem on the rule-based level, he might change to the knowledge-based level. The mental effort or cognition complexity on the knowledge-based level is higher than on the rule-based level. The higher the cognition complexity, the more likely user errors become (Reason, 1990).

Generally, in order to recognize the user's familiarity with a security concept, the deployment of usability tests is recommended (Nielsen, 1993).

The following section uses the above-mentioned categorization of security-critical usability problems to rank security tools according to their usability.

2.4 Usability taxonomy of security tools

By the differentiation of security-critical usability problems into problem categories II and III, user errors may be ranked according to the user's ability to avoid errors by himself. If a security tool's user interface presents the user with an unfamiliar security concept (problem category III errors), the ability of the user to avoid errors is lower. On the other hand, with a security tool's user interface reflecting familiar security concepts (problem category II errors), user-driven error prevention is more likely.

This is illustrated by the following inequality:

$$\text{user error}_{\text{problem category II}} < \text{user error}_{\text{problem category III}},$$

where "<" means "… is easier to avoid by the user than …"

If the user error belongs to problem category II, the error arises in spite of the user's familiarity with the security concept. The three performance levels (skill-based, rule-based and knowledge-based level) suggest a ranking of category II errors by their inherent cognitive familiarity (Reason, 1990).

Errors on the skill-based level occur in a familiar environment, while errors on the rule-based level occur in a somewhat familiar environment and errors on the knowledge-based level occur in a unfamiliar environment (Rasmussen, 1986).

This is reflected by the following inequality:

$$\text{user error}_{\text{problem category II, skill-based}} < \text{user error}_{\text{problem category II, rule-based}} < \\ < \text{user error}_{\text{problem category II, knowledge-based}}$$

According to transitivity, we are proposing the following taxonomy of user errors in security tools:

$$\text{user error}_{\text{problem category II, skill-based}} < \text{user error}_{\text{problem category II, rule-based}} < \\ < \text{user error}_{\text{problem category II, knowledge-based}} < \text{user error}_{\text{problem category III}}$$

For detecting user errors in security tools, either the cognitive walkthrough or the heuristic evaluation method may be used (Nielson, 1993). User errors may be identified as critical for security by simply examining whether at least one protection goal is threatened.

Hence, user errors and their security relevance are objectively measurable. This taxonomy can, therefore, supply an objective measure for the usability of security tools.

3. IDENTIFYING USER ERRORS BASED ON THE CONCEPTS OF MULTILATERAL SECURITY

An important aim of research into usable security must be to investigate the usability of security functions of multilateral security. If security-critical user errors are possible, the introduced taxonomy shows how well the user may avoid the errors by applying his security competence. Based on these results, design alternatives for avoiding security-critical user errors have to be found.

In accordance with the threatened protection goals of multilateral security, the design alternatives and the alternative security functions will lead us to a collection of usable security functions. An alternative security function on the one hand substitutes the entire security function. A design alternative on the other hand avoids the security-critical user error through better design of the original security function (see Figure 3).

This collection of user errors will be realized as a publicly available database in order to support the work of designers of security tools, for example, to implement usable tools for novice users. The database can also support system administrators or system officers to find out how secure a security system really is during use. Additionally, a user may use this database to find security tools which can be easily and securely used with his degree of security competence.

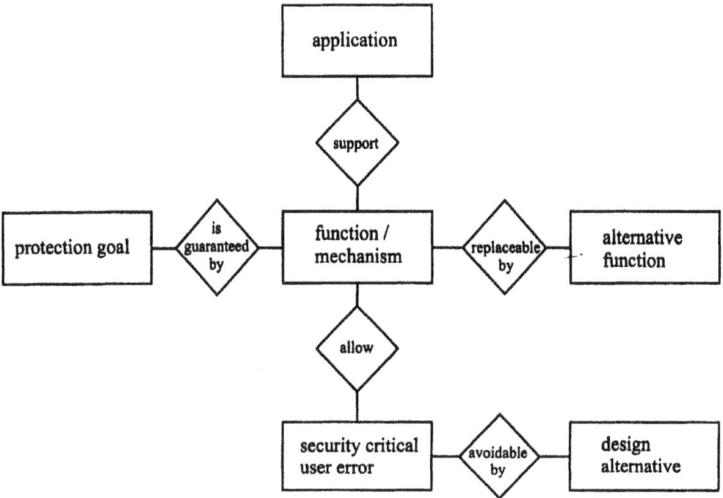

Figure 3: Entity-relationship-model of the error-database.

4. CONCLUSION

This paper puts forth a taxonomy for a usability evaluation of security tools. In further work, currently deployed security functions in security tools will be evaluated according to the taxonomy introduced. According to the results of usability tests, these concepts will be improved in order to avoid further security-critical user errors.

Avoiding security-critical errors in spite of the user's low security competence may finally lead to an increased acceptance of security tools.

5. REFERENCES

CCITSE - The Common Criteria for Information Technology Security Evaluation (2000): Common Criteria Version 2.1 / ISO IS 15408.

Common Criteria for Information Technology Security Evaluation V 2.1, Version 2.1.

ISO-Standard, no. 9241-part 10 (1996): Guidlines for dialogue design.

Nielsen, J. (1993), *Usability Engineering*, Academic Press.

Prabhu, P.V. & Prabhu G.V. (1997), *Human Error and User-Interface Design*, in Helander, M., Landauer, T.K. & Prabhu, P.V., *Handbook of Human-Computer Interaction*.

Rannenberg, K., *Zertifizierung mehrseitiger IT-Sicherheit – Kriterien und organisatorische Rahmenbedingungen* (1998); Reihe DuD-Fachbeiträge im Verlag Vieweg, Braunschweig u.a.

Rannenberg, K., Pfitzmann, A., & Müller, G. (1999), *IT Security and Multilateral Security*. In Müller, G. & Rannenberg, K. (Eds.), Technology, Infrastructure, Economy, Volume 3 of *Mulitlateral Security in Communications*, pages 21-29, Addison Wesley Longman Verlag GmbH.

Rasmussen, J. (1986), *Information Processing and Human-Machine Interaction*, Amsterdam: North Holland.

Reason, J. (1990), *Human Error*, Cambridge University Press.

Whitten, A. & Tygar, J.D. (1999), Why Johnny Can't Encrypt: A Usability Evaluation of PGP 5.0, in *Proceedings of the 8th USENIX Security Symposium*.

Usability: Gaining a Competitive Edge
IFIP World Computer Congress 2002
J. Hammond, T. Gross, J. Wesson (Eds)
Published by Kluwer Academic Publishers

Improving Usability in Decision Support Systems:
Practical Use of the Decision Enquiry Approach for Requirements Analysis

Caroline Parker
Centre for Research in Systems and People (CRSP), Computing Department, Glasgow Caledonian University, Cowcaddens Road, Glasgow, G4 0BA c.g.parker@gcal.ac.uk

Abstract: The function of Decision Support Systems (DSS) is to help their users to make more effective decisions by providing information in a way that actively assists the decision process. However despite widespread development and investment very few agricultural DSS in the UK have been taken up by end users. This paper describes the use of a method for requirements analysis based on Arinze's (1992) Decision Enquiry approach and on the use of workshops, in three agriculturally based DSS developments[1]. It concludes that the method provides a cost-effective and practical means of gathering information about the task of decision making, organising it and using it as the basis for design decisions and could usefully be applied in other sectors beyond agriculture. The approach is being widely used in UK agricultural DSS production and the next stage in the development of the methodology is the specification of design and evaluation procedures.

Key words: usability, decision support, decision enquiry, workshop, method

1. INTRODUCTION

'Usability is critical to the success of computer systems and products. Too many systems exist which are difficult to learn, complicated to operate, and are often under-used or misused.' Maguire (1997).

Decision Support Systems (DSS) are a branch of the Information Technology software family whose particular purpose is to offer aid to those making decisions. DSS are intended to help users to make more effective decisions by providing information in a way that actively assists the decision process. Unlike expert systems, which are usually designed to supplant some aspect of an expert's role, DSS exist to complement and 'support' decision-makers rather than to replace them. DSS have been developed on many platforms in many industries and for a wide variety of uses, for example medicine (Plougmann et al., 2001) utilities (Lindquist et al, 1996), transport (Zografos et al., 2002), financial services (Zhou et al., 2001), and agriculture (Wong et al., 2001). They are usually based around a spreadsheet or simulation model, or a rule-base, or a combination of all three.

In UK agriculture, as in other countries, DSS have been promoted as a means of revitalising the knowledge transfer process in the wake of the removal of state funded advisory services. They seem to have plenty to offer to an industry that is desperately trying to make more cost effective and more environmentally sensitive decisions in the face of information overload. However, despite the potential and the investment very few systems in the UK have been taken up by end users. A previous paper has argued that the underlying reason for the lack of uptake is the absence of users in the design and development process (Parker & Sinclair, 2002).

Most professionals interested in the delivery of useful and usable systems believe the starting point has to be the user and that some form of user-centred design methodology should be employed in the development process. User-centred design is taken to be the involvement of users at all stages of system development from initial planning, through requirements analysis, into development and evaluation. This approach however has not been easy for DSS developers in agriculture to adopt, largely because of a lack of appropriate and practical methods. The author has argued (op cit.) that to produce usable and marketable DSS, small scale developers, like those in agriculture, need prescriptive, user-centred and DSS applicable methods that are easy and relatively inexpensive to adopt.

This paper describes the practical use of the requirements capture component of one such approach. Previous papers have described the development of the method within a UK agricultural project called DESSAC (Parker, 2001). The method worked well in DESSAC and the user interface developed as a result generated good usability feedback in pre-release user trials. DESSAC was however a well-funded project which ran over five years and there was no evidence that the approach would work in the smaller, shorter and resource restricted projects which are more characteristic of the industry. This paper therefore describes the practical application of the method within three current agricultural projects: PASSWORD, a DSS for pest and disease management in Oilseed Rape,

WMSS, weed management DSS and Slugs, a DSS for slug management in brassica and salad crops.

2. USER REQUIREMENTS ANALYSIS FOR AGRICULTURAL DSS

The method described in the paper is part of a suite of related approaches to the user-centred design and development of agricultural DSS (Parker, 1999). It is a method for the initial identification of user requirements for DSS and is based on two foundations, the Decision Enquiry approach to requirements capture developed by Arinze (1992) and the use of workshops as a cost-effective means of involving users in the design process. These will be discussed in brief before the method itself is outlined.

2.1 Decision enquiry or question-based approach

Arinze reasoned that the key information flow between the DSS and the user is the stream of requests from the user, i.e. the questions that the user asks of the system when using it to support decision making, and that these should therefore be the key determinant of the shape and form of the DSS. The data from the DESSAC project suggested that much of the crop protection decision task was indeed concerned with getting answers to questions about the weather, disease levels, product effectiveness etc. The focus on user questions, both from the observations of system failure and the observations of the decision making process, seemed therefore to support the Arinze argument.

Where Arinze's work is particularly useful to task analysis and requirements specification is the division of these questions or 'decision enquiries' (Arinze's term) into a functional taxonomy (op cit.). He argues that when decision-makers interact with a DSS they will invariably make an enquiry of one of three main types, labelled: state, action and projection enquiries.

State enquiries are made when the user is seeking information about the state of the world (or a model of it), i.e. enquiries about:

- entities (e.g. products, diseases)
- processes (e.g. pest and disease lifecycles, market behaviour)
- attitudes (e.g. buyer attitudes, consumer attitudes)
- policies (e.g. legislation, buyer policies)
- people (e.g. staff, customers, suppliers)

Action enquiries are requests for a plan of action to achieve a specified end state. This is a reverse 'what if' question, i.e. instead of what will happen if I do this, an action enquiry asks how do I get to this pre-specified end-state. In this type of query, it is the function of the DSS to generate actions in response to the user's goal setting.

Projection enquiries are more commonly known as 'what if' enquiries. They are requests for an indication of outcome given a set of defined conditions e.g. 'How much will I lose if I delay the application of this spray for three days?'. The importance of this taxonomy is that it provides a direct link to specification. The identification of State enquiries tells the developer what data the user needs to have at hand, in DSS databases, linked programs or encyclopaedia, identification of action and projection enquiries provide a definition of the models that will be needed to support the user.

2,2 Workshops

What is the best and most cost effective method of involving users in design? Workshops, or focus groups, were adopted within the case study project for a number of reasons: their relative cheapness compared to interviews and co-opting methods, their use in human factors research and usability evaluations. Jordon (1998), and a history of successful use within agriculture (Norton & Mumford, 1993). Another reason for the use of workshop or focus groups is that the workshop participants "stimulate and encourage one another" (Bruseberg & McDonagh-Philip, 2002) and a short workshop can generate a wealth of information and consensus on issues of importance. Consensus on the most important issues is particularly useful to highly-cost restricted projects where hard decisions have to be made about priorities for research and development.

3. USER-CENTRED USER REQUIREMENTS METHOD FOR DSS

This section of the paper outlines the method used in the three agricultural DSS projects, WMSS, PASSWORD and Slugs. WMSS and Password are DSS for arable farmers and Slugs is a DSS for horticultural brassica and salad growers. The main distinction between the user groups for these systems is that arable farmers tend to focus on yield and gross margin while horticultural growers are forced by the nature of their product and their markets to focus on quality.

Each of these projects is LINK funded, i.e. partly government and partly industry funded, with a consortium made up of research and commercial partners, and has a heavy emphasis on basic biological research in addition to DSS development. All three projects were in the first year of their three-four year life span at the time of the requirement's analysis and the funds available for the identification of user requirements were very limited in all three cases. While each of the three projects felt that the product they were developing was solidly based in a real need, expressed by the industry and supported by the industrial partners on the team, none had previously carried out any form of detailed requirements analysis. In all cases therefore there was an urgent need to identify a clear set of requirements to inform the biological and technological development, in as cost effective way as possible.

The workshops took place at different times but all within the 'slack' period for crop producers i.e. mid-November to mid-March. WMSS workshops took place in December 2000, PASSWORD in February 2001 and Slugs in March 2001. In each case the lead partner in the project arranged for invitations to take part to be sent to a large mailing list of appropriate producers, both farmers and those who provide advice to them on agronomic matters i.e. independent and distributor based consultants. Workshops for each project were planned to take place over two days, with two workshops per day, one in the morning and one in the afternoon. Separate sessions were held for farmers and consultants as previous experience suggested that these groups talked more freely in the company of their peers, without the complication of a commercial relationship.

The aim of these sessions were: to identify the sub-tasks or stages within the decision process, the questions asked within them and the sources of information currently used to inform the questions. Additional aims were to prioritise requirements and to provide answers to specific questions raised by the technical partners in the projects.

Topic	WMSS	PASSWORD	SLUGS	Mins (approx)
Introduction	✓	✓	✓	5
Aspects of decision making.				
Whether to act	✓	✓	✓	20
What type of action to take	✓			20
When to act	✓	✓	✓	20
What to apply	✓	✓	✓	20
Coffee break	✓	✓	✓	5
Additional support	✓	✓	✓	30
Most important problems	✓	✓		10
Availability of data	✓	✓	✓	20
Delivery mechanisms	✓	✓	✓	20
Questionnaire	✓	✓	✓	10
			Total	180

Table 1. Format of workshops

All of the workshops followed the same basic structure and took between 2 and 3 hours to run, flip charts and tape recordings were used to record the data. The structure and approximate timing of each is represented in Table 1. Eleven of the twelve planned sessions went ahead with 70 people in total taking part, roughly one-third farmers and two-thirds consultants. The Slug project workshops were less well attended because they were unavoidably delayed until late March when spring activities begin to demand attention.

After the participants had settled and the aims of the project and of the workshop were explained to them they were taken through the main stages or sub-tasks in the decision process. These sub-tasks were identified by the author prior to the workshops, on the basis of past experience. The subtasks are almost identical in the three groups and problem management can be said in all cases to include the decisions: whether to act, when to take action and what type of chemical to apply if action is needed and chemicals have been chosen. Only in the case of weed decision making (where cultivation is also an option) is there any real choice between chemicals and other options in intensive crop production.

The participants were asked to list the questions or issues that were most important at each stage i.e. what questions did they ask before they felt able to take the decision. Their answers were recorded on flip-charts and were visible during the discussions. After the questions were exhausted the participants were asked where they obtained the information to answer their queries. The aim of this section was to identify decision enquiries which could be translated via the Arinze taxonomy into concrete requirements for model and database components.

While the issues were fresh in their minds the participants were asked to split up into groups of two or three with a cup of coffee and identify areas in which they felt more support would be useful i.e. where information was either not readily available to answer their questions or was of poor quality. After about twenty minutes they were asked to re-convene and to report back to the group. Once again their suggestions were recorded on a flip-chart in plain view. The final part of this exercise was the ranking of the items in order of importance i.e. very important, important, useful or nice to have. The aim of this section was to identify the areas that the user group considered to be most important and therefore provide a concrete means of prioritising the work of the project.

In a related exercise the WMSS and PASSWORD groups were asked to identify the weeds or pests or diseases that they felt were most important to them, this was not seen as relevant to the Slug groups as few people are actually capable of distinguishing between slug species.

DSS are highly data driven and in order to identify the limitations under which the software would have to operate each group was asked the degree of access they had to observation and weather data. At the time of the workshops there was serious debate in all projects about the potential use of the Internet as a means of delivering DSS. The participants were asked what type of delivery mechanisms they might prefer for different elements of the support package they had defined. Finally participants were asked to complete a short questionnaire which contained specific questions raised by the technical partners and which obtained a more personal view of users willingness to invest in additional data gathering equipment or conduct more field level observations.

4. DATA ANALYSIS

The questions and issues generated in the decision-making session were divided into the three Arinze (1992) taxonomies, State, Action and Projection on the basis of best fit. The questions were placed in a table alongside the information used to answer them and the groups that suggested it as important. An example of this layout, showing a single decision element, taken from the WMSS weeds project, is provided in Table 2.

Decision element :	*Do I need to act?*				
Enquiry category :	*State:*	*Groups*			
Question	Information sources	1	2	3	4
What are the levels/population in the crop? E.g. good, bad, horrific; low, moderate, severe	Crop walking/observation Weed map, black-grass map Distribution Field history	✓		✓	✓

Table 2. Example of table for decision element data

In this example three of the WMSS groups said that when making the decision about whether to act against weeds they needed to find out what the levels were in the crop. One group did not specifically mention this question. The question is of the type 'state' because it relates to the current state of the 'system'. The information currently used to answer the question is listed in the second column. Of the data outlined only field history is available in digital format.

The collation of the questions relating to the different decision elements and the enquiry categories provided information about the broad task approach. The data from the next phase provided a starting point for the projects by identifying the perceived support needs of the users. The areas suggested by the groups as requiring more support were collated by the author under headings selected on the basis of a perceived natural grouping. The raw data was made available to project partners to allow alternative groupings to be selected if necessary. In the event none of the groupings was changed. These headings were also tabulated and the ranking provided by each group listed. An averaging of these ranks provided a means to sort the suggestions in order of priority. Table 3 provides an example of the format used from the weeds project.

Need	Questions/notes	Groups 1	2	3	4	Rank Σ
Dose response information	Size, timing and weather? (In quarter doses is fine.) When can get away with 1/2 dose? How much will do the job? Consequences if wrong? Circumstances of trials data (to compare)? Impact on resistance? More info on broad leaf weeds	H	H	H	H	20
Adjuvants	Are any worth paying for? Impact of pH of water?		M	M		6
Support for impact of product on specific weeds	What is the impact of dose on weed size? When might a weed not be killed? What does moderate mean? 75%? What are scenarios when it works and when it doesn't work?			H		5

Table 3: Example of format used to summarise and rank support requirements

Other results e.g. those relating to availability of weather and observation data, the acceptability of web and PC delivery formats and other project specific questions were summarised and reported back to the projects in tabular and textual form.

5. CONCLUSIONS

The approach described above has been used in three different projects and performed equally well in all of them. It was simple to organise and run, the participants enjoyed taking part and, despite disappointing numbers in some cases, generated a wealth of information. Asking users to think in terms of questions is a useful way to encourage them to think about the decision task. The responses are not however always phased in pure question format require some interpretation. Subsequent checking with those involved in the workshops described here did support the author's analysis. While the method is still not entirely free from this type of subjectivity it does provide a relatively formal and practical means of gathering information.

The approach is also easy to run. Two of the workshops sessions, in the PASSWORD project, were managed by non-human factors specialists. The general scope of the data resulting from these sessions matched that of the previous two sessions run by the author, however they were a little less detailed. This suggests that some workshop or meeting management skills are required to encourage discussion and elaboration.

In summary the decision enquiry/workshop approach provides a means of describing the task of decision making, of organising that description and using it as the basis for design decisions; and it can be used to ensure that tasks and functions are appropriately allocated within a decision support system. It is also widely applicable. There is nothing specific to agriculture about the approach, indeed the Arinze (1992) taxonomy originated in a mainstream business sector, and the author therefore believes its employment as described in this paper has general utility. By identifying the 'enquiries' or questions inherent in a decision making process, it becomes possible to state the users' requirements for data and for mathematical models, two key components of DSS. Because the designer knows that the system has to support the posing and answering of specific questions, this knowledge also guides the development of the interface. The collated set of user questions provides a ready source of evaluation criteria available from the design stage onwards.

This approach to requirements capture and specification is being promoted widely within UK agricultural DSS projects and will hopefully contribute to a big increase in the usability of the next generation of software. The next stage in the development of the methodology is the specification of design and evaluation procedures. Rapid prototype based activities in the context of workshops are likely to form the basis of this phase.

6. ACKNOWLEDGEMENTS

The author would like to acknowledge the essential funding provided by DEFRA, HGCA and HDC, and the ADAS and HRI subcontracts that made this work possible.

7. REFERENCES

Arinze, B. (1992), A user enquiry model for DSS requirements analysis: a framework and case study. *International Journal of Man-Machine Studies,* **37,** 241-264.

Bruseberg, A. and McDonagh-Philip,D. (2002), Focus groups to support the industrial/product designer: a review based on current literature and designer's feedback. *International Journal of Human-Computer Studies.* **55** (4): 435-452.

Jordon, PW (1998), *An Introduction to Usability.* Taylor & Francis.

Lindquist, K., McGee, M. & Cole, L. (1996), TVA-EPRI River Resource Aid (TERRA) - reservoir and power operations decision-support system. *Water Air And Soil Pollution,* **90** (1-2), 143-150.

Maguire, M. (1997), Usability Matters. Web source.

http://www.lboro.ac.uk/research/husat/inuse/usabilitymatters.html Last updated 15.5.97.

Norton, G.A. & Mumford, J.D. (1993), *Decision Tools for Pest Management.* CAB International, Wallingford, UK.

Parker, C.G. (1999), A user-centred design method for agricultural DSS. In U. Rickert (ed.) *EFITA-99: Proceedings of the Second European Conference for Information Technology in Agriculture.* Bonn, Germany. 27-30th September 1999, Bonn: Universität Bonn-ILB. Vol A. pp. 395-404.

Parker, C.G. (2001), An approach to requirements analysis for decision support systems. *International Journal of Human-Computer Studies,* **55,** 423-434.

Parker, C.G. & Sinclair, M. (2002), "Why user-centred design works: the case of decision support systems in crop production". *Behaviour and Information Technology,* **20** (6) 449-460.

Plougmann S, Hejlesen OK, Cavan DA (2001), DiasNet - a diabetes advisory system for communication and education via the internet. *International Journal of Medical Informatics.* 319-330, Special Issue December 2001. **64** (2-3)

Wong MTF, Corner RJ, Cook SE (2001), A decision support system for mapping the site-specific potassium requirement of wheat in the field. *Australian Journal Of Experimental Agriculture.* **41** (5): 655-661.

Zhou ZY, Cheng SW, Hua B, Zeng MG & Yin QH (2001), An investment decision support system for process industries. *Chinese Journal of Chemical Engineering .* **9** (4): 402-406.

Zografos KG, Androutsopoulos KN, & Vasilakis GM (2002), A real-time decision support system for roadway network incident response logistics. *Transportation Research Part C-Emerging Technologies .* **10** (1): 1-18.

Usability: Gaining a Competitive Edge
IFIP World Computer Congress 2002
J. Hammond, T. Gross, J. Wesson (Eds)
Published by Kluwer Academic Publishers

TEACHING HUMAN-COMPUTER INTERACTION

Qualitative Support for an Alternative Approach

Paula Kotzé[1] and Lars Oestreicher[2]

[1] *Department of Computer Science and Information Systems, University of South Africa*
[2] *Department of Information Science, Uppsala University, Sweden*

Abstract: Traditional methods of teaching HCI and usability are not as successful and easy as is generally thought. Methods based on traditional software engineering teaching approaches have not provided the answer. This paper suggests an alternative way to approach the teaching of HCI. The method involves what we call the 'establishment of an HCI mindset within the student'. To successfully implement the approach would require a resource base of suitable HCI material and examples that can be drawn upon. The second half of the paper addresses the issues involved in setting up and developing such a resource base.

Key words: Human-computer interaction, usability, teaching, resource base, information quality, credibility, trust.

1. INTRODUCTION

Teaching human-computer interaction (HCI) is sometimes regarded as an easy task and it has occasionally even been regarded as something that can simply be tacked onto a general course in software engineering. The focus in this case is usually on teaching a few simple rules, usability guidelines, and some information relating to methods for task analysis, usability engineering, and conceptual modelling. Although HCI is now a more established discipline in itself, this perspective on teaching HCI is unfortunately still quite common, and is linked to several proposed curricula (for example Computing Curricula 2001 (Joint Task Force on Computing Curricula Association for Computing Machinery & IEEE Computer Society, 2001). Furthermore, in many cases HCI textbooks are based on the information/lecturing sequence of psychology, interface aspects, methods for HCI, and possibly evaluation. Although this approach may work for introductory undergraduate studies, it only provides for a small part of the knowledge that a practitioner in HCI might need. This problem becomes even more pressing at postgraduate level, where the existing books are clearly insufficient to provide effective course material.

To 'practise' HCI basically means to apply the knowledge one has about HCI to design situations, using rules and methods, at best with relevant background knowledge from, for example, computer science, psychology, sociology, and linguistics. On a more problem-oriented level, practising HCI means knowing the solution to a problem once it is apparent, which of course is very useful in itself.

'Understanding' HCI, on the other hand, means that the professional will not only know the solution (or where and how to find it), but even more importantly, s/he will know when a problematic situation will arise in the first place. Usability professionals must not only know how to do things the HCI way, but also why a situation constitutes an HCI problem and how this affects the general design/evaluation process. S/he must therefore know when and why HCI problems may or will occur, and make sure that proper steps are taken to avert them.

In this paper we argue that HCI education needs to embrace the more holistic view of both practising and understanding HCI. From this perspective, HCI education needs educational tools that will enable teachers to equip students with a good theoretical understanding of the problem situation, as well as a good knowledge of the practical application of HCI knowledge in everyday design situations. The paper proposes an alternative way of teaching HCI and usability based on this premise, and proposes the development of an HCI resource base to support this approach.

1.1 History of the Project

The origins of this paper stemmed from a number of HCI education workshops that took place between 1999 and 2001. Although many of the ideas and much of the supporting content reported upon here was put together by the authors, it is important to recognise and acknowledge the ideas of and contributions made by other workshop participants.

The first of these workshops (Cox et al., 1999) at the INTERACT '99 Conference in Edinburgh, discussed topics linked to HCI teaching material and good textbooks (or the lack of them). The majority of the existing HCI textbooks in use were found to be too broad in scope, too unspecific, or not suitable for a complete course in HCI. The need for material that supported the inculcation of an HCI mindset in the student, something that the traditional textbooks do not do, was also emphasised. It was suggested that an example database with good or useful examples of teaching materials should be constructed.

The aim of the second workshop on the development of educational material for HCI (Kotzé et al., 2000; Oestreicher et al., 2000), at the NordiCHI 2000 Conference in Stockholm, was to investigate alternative possibilities for providing the HCI community with a qualitative resource base of educational material. This material had to be useful, accessible, and affordable. Issues considered included the identification of resources to support educators and learners, and how to make resources accessible to educators around the world.

The third workshop in the sequence (Kotzé et al., 2001), held at the INTERACT '01 Conference in Tokyo, focussed on specific topics and appropriate types of material that would be suitable for contributions to the data resource, and on how to implement the results practically. Possible quality control measures and validation procedures that could be applied to the materials published in the resource base, were also addressed.

After these three workshops the results were consolidated and supplemented by additional material, to form the basis of this paper.

1.2 Layout of the Paper

Following this introduction, a proposed alternative method for the teaching of HCI and usability is introduced. This method requires the development of additional educational resources, which forms the basis of Section 3. Section 3 consists of a discussion of the development of a reusable HCI educational resource base. Issues focused upon include the kind of resources that are required to equip teachers and learners properly; the topics to be covered in such a resource base; what is required to make these resources useful; and how to make the contents of such a resource base credible.

2. AN ALTERNATIVE APPROACH TO THE TEACHING OF HCI AND USABILITY

In this section we propose an alternative to the traditional classroom method for the teaching of HCI. This involves allowing the student to experience HCI in addition to learning the theory related to HCI and its practical applications. The method, dubbed the 'Six Golden Rules to Shake the Student's Mind' by the participants of the 1999 Workshop (Oestreicher, 2000), consists of the following steps:

1. Read thought-provoking literature: The first step is to lay the mental foundation for the learning experience. This is done by giving the students literature to read that will broaden their horizons. Examples of such resources are the books by Norman (1992; 1993; 1998) and good books on industrial and/or graphic design (such as Spalter (1999)), i.e. not the traditional set of HCI textbooks.
2. Observe real users using real tools: One way of raising students' level of consciousness concerning HCI problems is to make them go out into the real world and observe people using real artefacts (such as vending machines, doors, copiers, parking ticket machines, and video cassette recorders), and to note the problems being experienced. Reflection on these experiences in the steps that follow may kindle in the student a mental mindset of continuous awareness and observation of the usability of common artefacts.
3. Analyse the findings in the observation: By analysing and documenting the information gathered during the observation step, the students will be forced to try to understand and rationalise the reasons behind the problem situation. This would form the first step in the process of redesign and also increase the aspect of awareness. The analysis can start from their gained understanding, combined with ideas from the literature in step 1.
4. Mix the results from the analysis with theory: The observations then need to be pursued and anchored in a proper theoretical foundation. By adding theory after (or in parallel with) the observation studies, a student should be able to form a better conceptual basis, retain the theory better, and connect the theoretical knowledge to practical experience.
5. Redesign the artefact: By redesigning the artefact the student is required not only to criticise a design, but also to make constructive suggestions for improving the design based on aspects relating to improved usability, but also other relevant properties of the artefact, such as ergonomic design. The use of prototypes or storyboard walkthroughs is suggested to overcome the practical problems of redesigning a real-world artefact.
6. Iterate the observation phase: When the redesign is completed, the students needs to get feedback on their own designs and/or prototypes. This can be done by iterating the observation, analysis, and redesign phases. One important part of the iteration process is that the students are encouraged to assess their own ideas in relation to the initial product. It is a very important part of HCI education to make the students realise that their solutions are not necessarily the best or optimum solutions, but that it may raise new problems in the interface.

These six rules are intended neither as a new curriculum in HCI, nor the sole educational tool in an introductory HCI course. They should rather be seen as a means of raising students' awareness of HCI issues and making them see and understand the traps in everyday design. If the students' awareness level is raised, they will be more open to the general content of HCI education, rather than only to the specific details that are taught in textbooks. The application of the six rules can be done in a variety of ways, incorporating some or all of them, depending on the purpose and the situation.

The mixing of theory and practice does, however, require a good knowledge source, where the knowledge in the theory is suitable for mixing with the practical experiences. The use of a good HCI textbook, such as for example Dix et al. (1998) and Preece et al. (2001) will have to be augmented by an additional resource in which HCI teachers and usability trainers can find good examples of supporting material (such as real world artefacts, case studies, and examples from software illustrating both good and bad design practices). For this purpose we propose the development of an HCI resource base (not to be confused with an HCI bibliography) that would contain such material. The sections that follow will address issues involved in the development of such a resource base.

3. HCI RESOURCE BASE

The underlying belief in the development of a reusable resource base of HCI educational material, is that the reuse of existing tried-and-tested resources or knowledge to create new educational resources will lead to improvements in both product and process, i.e. better HCI educational resources, and better teaching and learning. These assumptions echo similar goals for shared resource collections in both the business world and the software engineering community (Sumner et al., 2001). It is true that the software engineering community has been vigorously promoting software reuse for years to ensure programmer productivity and software quality, and that the business world has recently started to focus on using shared repositories to support knowledge management and best practices to improve organizational efficiency. Nevertheless, until now very little research has been done to determine the effects of reuse on teaching and learning.

The development of an HCI resource base aimed at providing the HCI community with a qualitative reserve of educational material, which is useful and accessible, sets a number of challenges and raises a number of questions.

In the first place, the development of an HCI resource base is based on the assumption that providing an HCI educational resource will:

- improve the quality of HCI education by promoting the reuse of educational resources that have already proved to be effective;

- improve the productivity of HCI teachers through the reuse and sharing of resources; and
- serve in the establishment of an active HCI community of learning innovation, where best practices and resources are developed and shared (Marchionini, 1995).

It is clear that many questions and issues will arise when considering a resource base of this nature. Not all of them can be addressed in a single paper, and many would call for a major research effort on their own. In order to give some idea of what is involved, we have identified a number of issues we consider as being of primary importance. The remainder of the discussion will primarily focus on four of these: required resources and content, conceptual framework, credibility of the resource base, and the handling of cultural issues.

Before we attempt to identify possible resources that are required for successfully supporting the teaching of HCI, we have to look at why such a resource base is actually needed. One of the main issues that can be raised relates to the shortcomings of existing HCI textbooks, and refers to features that are missing or not very well treated in the current textbooks. Many of these problems are linked to the nature of the print medium, which confirms the call for an additional HCI resource base as valid. The following are some of the shortcomings of these textbooks that have been identified. The textbooks:

- are mostly oriented towards an Anglo-American reader, largely neglecting the situation and practices in the rest of the world;
- have little coverage of multicultural issues (or limited to only a short discussion on multilingual aspects);
- are predominantly centred on direct manipulation or graphical user interfaces;
- lacking a firm interdisciplinary perspective;
- focus on essential topics but miss out on lateral thinking;
- provide ineffective connections between theory and practice;
- have little or no coverage of issues relating to physical ergonomics;
- lack references to further and updated information;
- are mostly a step behind new technological developments; and
- have illustrative material that is limited to text, still graphics, and pictures.

Bearing these shortcomings in mind, the consensus is that the material to be collected, developed, and recorded in an HCI resource base should focus on topics that are not exactly textbook topics, and should not duplicate the material generally found in HCI textbooks. Instead, the material should support the theory provided in the textbooks. Each example should be explained and linked to associated theoretical issues. In cases where the theory is incomplete or absent from available textbooks, the associated theoretical background should be provided as explanatory text, or as appropriate references to assessable sources.

3.1 Content of the Resource Base

Several types of material were identified that would be both valuable and useful to all parties concerned. Several issues need to be addressed when considering the actual content of the resources base, ranging from the people involved in using the resource base, the teaching and learning context in which the resource items can be used, to specific topics that should be included. We elaborate on these in these in this section.

The first issue addresses the target market of the resource base. Is the resource base aimed at teachers or learners, or both? Will the focus be on users from a single subject, or will it be multidisciplinary? Is the focus on both novices and individuals with prior experience? The target market will largely determine how the resource base should be structured and the type of user interfaces that should be provided.

The teaching and learning context focuses on didactic issues and the perspective from which the database items should be described, for example:

- What will the format of the material be – formal lectures, experiential, through to project-based?
- Will the tuition be face-to-face, distance (including online), or global?
- Will it be focused on individual or group work, or independent of class size?
- What will the focus of the organizational context be – private, public?

The typical content items that should be considered for the resource base need to fit in with the target group, but can be classified under three headings:

1. HCI curriculum issues, including examples of desirable, achievable and essential curricula; structure, content, objectives and principles; various perspectives for each item (for example computing-related, software engineering, ergonomics, human factors, multicultural, tools, and skills).
2. Theories from various disciplines, including the social sciences (such as psychology, linguistics, and sociology); engineering sciences (such as computing, mathematics, and electronics); education (such as learning theories, and cognitive issues); design (such as art, system, and industrial and technical design).
3. A variety of application domains, including real-time, CSCW, mobile applications, text-based, multimedia, multimodal, web-based, e-commerce, e-learning, hardware design, and non-desktop applications.

Typical items for inclusion in the resource base to support the above classifications include both low-tech and high-tech solutions to problems; cartoons and stories focusing on interactive issues; material related to country-specific cultural issues as well as globalisation; annotated 'Interface Hall of Shame' (Iarchitect, 2001) type of examples backed by sound theoretical motivations and ways to correct the problems; annotated standards, guidelines and patterns; lists of research topics; 'textbook chapters' on material not found in textbooks; lecture notes and teaching methods related to a specific theme; assignments, examinations, laboratory exercises; and collaborative links.

3.2 Conceptual Framework for Resource Base Structure

In order to be successful, this kind of resource base requires an accessible and sound infrastructure. The creation of an educational framework, with a set of dimensions that will describe the items in terms of didactic issues, educational objectives, point of view, and use, is important and necessary. It is essential that the HCI topics to be covered should form the guideline for the categorization of items in the database. During the workshop discussions it was also emphasized that users of the resource base should be made aware of the fact that the items in the database and their use are people's suggestions, and that theirs might not be the one and only way of using such items. The possibility of annotating an item with additional uses should therefore be an option.

If needed, an item needs to be accompanied by a description of the 'afterprocessing' or how to proceed after the effect has been achieved. In other words it should indicate solutions to a problematic example or confirmatory material in the case of positive engagements – in other words how to pick up the teaching principles from the example. The 'afterprocessing' might be even more important for the success than the item, or the topic, itself.

Therefore, each item should be considered with regard to:

- the purpose of the item (why you are doing it);
- the conten*t* of the item (what is going into it);
- the process of using the item (how to use it); and
- the intended outcomes when using the item (what the result will be).

Based on this, a basic framework, as illustrated in Figure 1, is proposed as a conceptual structure for organizing and recording items in the envisaged resource base. The framework essentially consists of nine components, namely:

1. a set of keywords, selected from a central dictionary of technical terms with definitions and a set of associate synonyms;

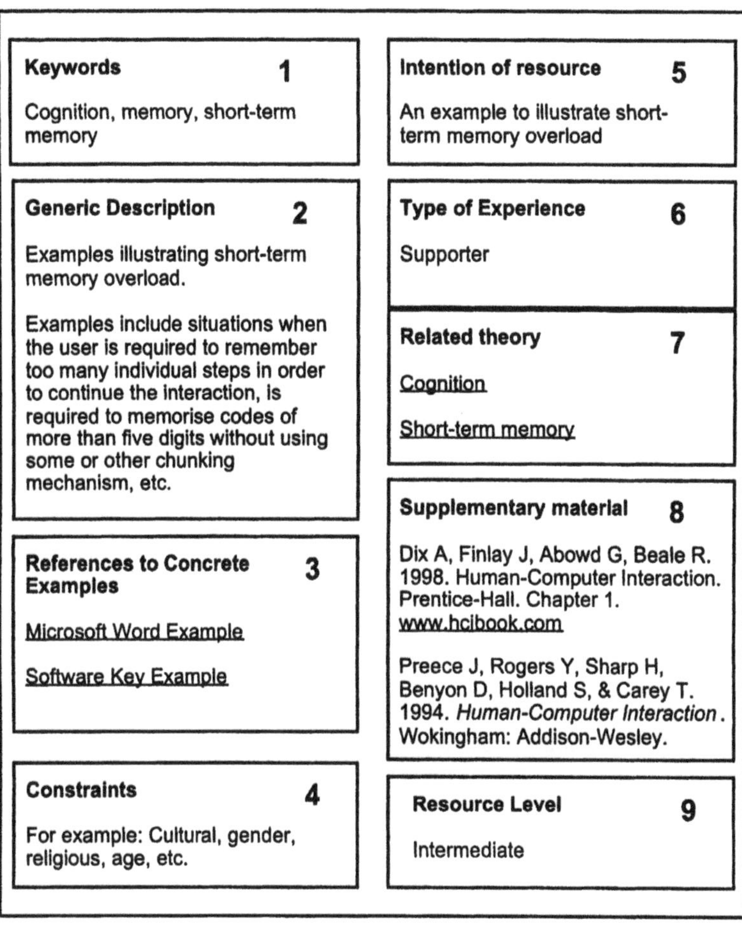

Figure 1. Conceptual framework for resource base structure

2. a generic description of the resource base item;
3. references to concrete examples (within the resource base or external);
4. constraints on the use and applicability of the resource item;
5. the intention behind the resource (why the item is there and suggestions for its use);
6. the type of experience or effect expected from using the item in the teaching or learning process (mind shaker, explainer, supporter);
7. links to relevant or associated theory stored within the resource base;
8. links to external supplementary material supporting the resource item; and
9. the resource item level (basic, elementary, advanced).

3.3 Credibility of the Resource Base

The envisaged resource base will only be successful if it is based on successful collaboration of high quality and is perceived to be credible. The key to this includes (Collings, 2001):
- commitment and mutual trust;
- acknowledgement that the work involved in undertaking collaborative work is valid academic work, in the same way as for research collaborations;
- finding ways of successfully addressing issues of intellectual property;
- avoidance of any sense of 'commoditisation' of HCI teaching materials;
- working in pairs or small groups (collaborative development); and
- quality of resource and learning outcomes for students.

3.3.1 Credibility and Trustworthiness

Credibility matters a great deal when computer products act as knowledge resources, instruct or tutor users, or act as decision aids (Fogg et al., 1999), as is the case with the proposed HCI resource base. 'Credibility' can be defined as having the properties of being believable and worthy, and has two key components:
1. trustworthiness, defined by terms such 'well-intentioned', 'unbiased', 'truthful', capturing the perceived 'goodness' or morality of the resource; and
2. expertise, defined by terms such as 'knowledgeable', 'experienced', 'competent', capturing the perceived knowledge and skill of the resource.

A credible resource base will have high levels of both trustworthiness and expertise (Fogg et al., 2001). Building and using the HCI resource base would require both elements. Collaboration is most effective and rewarding when all the parties trust each other. In the absence of trust, transactions would require negotiated formal rules and regulations, which are legislated and enforced (Fukuyama, 1995). To communicate successfully and efficiently, people must assume common ground in respect of world knowledge and intentions (Greenspan et al., 2000). Establishing common ground when participants are not together may cause problems (Health et al., 1997). Trust is more easily established if face-to-face communication can take place (or has taken place prior to the collaboration) (Rocco, 1998). This might pose a challenge for the establishment of the HCI resource base, and the trust users have in the resource afterwards.

3.3.2 Quality of the resource

Credibility of an electronic or web-based resource can be made to depend on several quality factors. These quality factors can be divided into two broad categories: information-related and site-related.

'Information-related' (content) factors refer to aspects such as the 'correctness' of information, and how the contained information can be validated. Several categories of information quality can be identified and should be considered in setting up and maintaining the resource base, including (Huang et al., 1999; Katerattanakul et al.; 1999; Rieh et al., 1998; Wilson, 1983; Zhu, 2000):

- intrinsic information quality, denoting the fact that information has quality in its own right. The two main dimensions of intrinsic information quality are the accuracy of the information content and the accuracy of the navigation. Inaccuracy in the information leads to concerns about believability or reliability of information. Comprehension is affected by layout, navigation and orientation.
- contextual information quality, highlighting the requirement that information must be considered within the context of the task at hand. The information must be informative, relevant and complete.
- currency, measured by the time stamp of the last modification of the source; and
- source authority, generally considered a key aspect for judging the perceived quality of information and for filtering the information. Studies have shown that people depend more on the authority and credibility of sources in the online environment than on the print-based environment.

The main forms of validation of information content suggested for the HCI resource base are the use of editors, peer-review, reader voting (grading or validation of readers), as well as certification of the developers, users and the resource. The latter also relate to the issue of intellectual property rights. If we have copyrighted material, we have to make sure that both the teachers and the students are registered to have access rights for this purpose.

'Site-related' (form) factors include aspects related to the design and user interface, site navigation, searchability, aesthetics, levels of site consistency, the potential to print, copy, and the worldwide accessibility of the site. Two important issues central to site-related information quality are (Huang et al., 1999; Katerattanakul et al., 1999; Rose et al., 1998; Zhang, 2000).:

- representational quality, referring to the format of the information. The information must be presented in a concise, clear and consistent way, must be aesthetically appealing, and must keep typographical issues (such as background, colour, text, font, and images), and the amount of information displayed, in mind. The meaning of information is affected

by layout, navigation and orientation, interpretability, and ease of understanding – all of which are affected by the representation.
- accessibility quality, emphasising the fact that the system must be accessible but secure. It is affected by navigation efficiency (consistency, quantity, functionality and relevance of links), technical accessibility of the system, suitable and alternative search strategies, and privacy or confidentiality of the information.

3.3.3 Handling of Cultural Issues

Cultural factors, such as common knowledge shared within a culture, cultural differences in information processing, the hierarchical structure of society and workplace, and culture-specific rhetorical strategies, are major variables that would determine the usability and acceptability of the resource base. To be successful, subtle cultural nuances and cross-cultural communication issues must be addressed. Addressing issues of culture in the resource base could influence it in two ways, namely by:
1. providing examples which illustrate cultural biases and conventions; and
2. customising the resource base, based on the preferences of the user and cultural markers.

Cultural markers (Barber, 1998) refer to interface elements that are preferred by, and prevalent within, a particular cultural group. Specific cultural markers signify a cultural affiliation and are used to denote a convention in the use of a system feature. Since the envisaged resource base would be an international resource, the use of cultural marking will have to be investigated.

The major categories of cultural markers that have to be considered are:
- language, denoting the local language for the target audience;
- visuals (pictures and graphics), related to the local culture, including different categories of metaphors, icons, flags, geography, shapes, and architecture in order to make examples familiar;
- colour conventions and uses; and
- page layout, directing the scanning of information and mirroring the logical flow of the task.

Language addresses localisation on a surface level, while the last three are more closely related to the cultural level.

3.3.4 Further Research

Many of the issues discussed above would require intensive additional research in order to ensure the success of the resource base. The following are some specific issues that can be identified as still open and unanswered, and requiring further research:

- Who would manage the resource and who would be responsible for entering the information into the resource base and maintaining the information and resource integrity (person efforts)? Collecting, cataloguing, and indexing is a very time-consuming process.
- How will copyrights and trademarks be handled?
- How would contributions to the resource base be recognised?
- How to build trust across cultures, space and conventions?
- How to manage access to the resource base?

4. CONCLUSION

This paper has presented the basis for an alternative approach to the teaching of HCI and usability. It also proposed a framework for the development of a resource base of material that will be essential for the success of the proposed alternative teaching approach.

The foundations for the first steps in this alternative approach to the teaching of HCI and usability have been laid in the ideas developed as a result of the three workshops. The second step is already halfway fulfilled in that a large number of exercises and examples have already been gathered by various HCI teachers around the world. The challenge lies in bringing these together in a coherent and motivated way.

To collect this source of knowledge would require a major effort, and in order to make this manageable we can foresee the need for the implementation of a simple classification scheme that will have to be standardised – the third step. The final step will therefore consist of the gathering of data in connection with the implementation of the above-mentioned classification system. It is envisaged that over time the system will evolve and expand to include a wider classification of topics and representation.

5. ACKNOWLEDGMENTS

We would like to acknowledge the contributions of the following people during the HCI Education Workshops (in alpabetical order): Julio Abascal (Spain), John Cass (Ireland), Penny Collings (Australia), Daphne Econonomou (Greece), Judy Hammond (Australia), Adrian Houtsma (Netherlands), Maddy Janse (Netherlands), Jésus Lores (Spain), Lydia

Palmer (South Africa), Matthias Rauterberg (Netherlands), Markus Stolze (Switzerland), and Mark Toleman (Australia).

6. REFERENCES

Joint Task Force on Computing Curricula Association for Computing Machinery & IEEE Computer Society, (2001). *Computing Curricula 2001 – Steelman Draft (August 1, 2001)*, www.computer.org/education/-cc2001/steelman/cc2001/index.htm.

Barber, W. & Badre, A. (1998), Culturability: the merging of culture and usability, in *Proceedings of the 4th Conference on Human Factors and the Web*, www.research.microsoft.com/users/marycz/hfweb98/barber/index.htm.

Collings, P. (2001), Position Paper. INTERACT '01 HCI Education Workshop.

Cox, M., Oestreicher, L., Quinn, M., Rauterberg, M. & Stolze, M. (1999), HCI in Education, Theory or Practise, in *Human-Computer Interaction - INTERACT '99: Proceedings of the seventh IFIP Conference on Human-Computer Interaction*, IOS Press.

Dix, A., Finlay, J., Abowd, G. & Beale, R. (1998), *Human-Computer Interaction*. Prentice Hall.

Fogg, B. J. & Tseng, H. (1999), The elements of computer credibility, in *Proceedings of CHI '99*, ACM, pp. 80 – 87.

Fogg, B.J., Marshall, J., Laraki, O., Osipovich, A., Varma, C., Fang, N., Paul, J., Rangnekar, A., Shon, J., Swani, P. & Treinen, M. (2001), What makes web sites credible? A report on a large quantitative study, in *Anyone. Anywhere. Proceedings of CHI 2001*, ACM, pp. 61 – 68.

Fukuyama, F. (1995), *Trust: the Social Virtues and the Creation and Prosperity*, Simon & Schuster.

Greenspan, S., Goldberg, D., Wiemer, D. & Basso, A. (2000), Interpersonal trust and common ground in electronically mediated communication, in *Proceedings of the Computer supported Cooperative Work 2000 Conference*, ACM, pp. 251 – 259.

Health, C., Luff, P. & Sellen, A.J. (1997), Reconfiguring media space: supporting collaborative work, in K.E. Finn, A.J. Sellen, & S.B. Wilbur (eds.), *Voice-mediated Communication*, LEA, pp. 323 – 348.

Huang, K., Lee, Y.W. & Wang R.Y. (1999), *Quality Information and Knowledge*. Prentice Hall.

Iarchitect. (2001), *The Interface Hall of Shame*, www.iarchitect.com/mshame.htm.

Katerattanakul, P. & Siau, K. (1999), Measuring information quality of websites: development of an instrument, in *Proceedings of the 20th International Conference on Information Systems*, pp. 279 – 285.

Kotzé, P., Lorés, J., Oestreicher, L. & Palmer, L. (2000), *A Framework for the Development of a Database of Educational Material for Human-Computer Interaction*, www.dis.uu.se/eduworkshop/nordichiWS2000.pdf/.

Kotze, P., Oestreicher, L., Rauterberg, M. & Toleman, M. (2001) Workshop on Developing Educational Material for HCI: Validation and Quality Control Issues, in M Hirose (ed.), *Human-Computer Interaction - INTERACT '01: Proceedings IFIP 13.1 International Conference*, Kluver, p. 840.

Marchionini, G. & Maurer, H. (1995), The roles of digital libraries in teaching and learning, *Communications of the ACM*, 38(4), pp. 67 – 75.

Norman, D.A. (1992), *Turn Signals are the Facial Expressions of Automobiles*, Addison-Wesley.

Norman, D. A. (1993), *Things that Make Us Smart: Defending Human Attributes in the Age of the Machine*, Addison-Wesley.

Norman, D.A. (1998), *The Design of Everyday Things*. MIT Press.

Oestreicher, L. (ed.) (2000), *The six golden rules to shake the student's mind*, www.dis.uu.se/~larsoe/eduworkshop/.

Oestreicher, L. & Kotzé, P.(2000), Workshop on Developing Educational Material for HCI, in *NordiCHI 2000 – Design vs. Design, Proceedings from the 1st Nordic Conference on Computer-Human Interaction.*

Preece, J., Rogers, Y., & Sharp, H. (2001), *Interaction Design: Beyond Human-Computer,* Interaction, Wiley.

Rieh, S.Y. & Belkin, N.J. (1998), Understanding judgement of information quality and cognitive authority in the WWW, in *Proceedings of the ASIS Annual Meeting*, ASIS, pp. 279 – 289.

Rocco, E. (1998), Trust breaks down in electronic contexts but can be repaired by some initial face-to-face contact, *in Proceedings of CHI '98*, ACM, pp. 496 – 502.

Rose, A., Wei, D., Marchionini, G., Beale, J. & Nolet, V. (1998), Building and electronic learning community: from design to implementation, in *Proceedings of CHI '98 Conference*, ACM, pp. 203 – 210.

Spalter, A.M. (1999), *The Computer in the Visual Arts*, Addison-Wesley.

Sumner, T. & Dawe, M. (2001), Looking at digital library usability from a reuse perspective, in *Proceedings of the Joint ACM/IEEE-CS Conference on Digital Libraries (JCDL '01)*, ACM, pp. 416 – 425.

Wilson, P. (1983), *Second-hand Knowledge: an Inquiry into Cognitive Authority*, Greenwood Press.

Zhang, X., Keeling, K.B. & Pavur, R.J. (2000), Information quality of commercial web site home pages: and explorative analysis, in *Proceedings of the 21st International Conference on Information Systems*, pp. 164 – 175.

Zhu, X. (2000), Incorporating quality metrics in centralized/distributed information retrieval on the world wide web, in *Proceedings of the 23rd Annual International SIGIR Conference on Research Development in Information Retrieval*, ACM, pp. 288 – 295.

Usability: Gaining a Competitive Edge
IFIP World Computer Congress 2002
J. Hammond, T. Gross, J. Wesson (Eds)
Published by Kluwer Academic Publishers

Usability: Who Cares?

An Analysis of Indifference Towards Usability Within the IT Industry

Thomas McCoy
Department of Defence, Canberra, Australia

Abstract: For decades, usability professionals have been seeking to convince the IT industry of the value of their work. However, in the twenty-first century we still find countless application development projects in which usability is ignored. This paper attempts to understand why the situation exists, from economic, psychological and organisational perspectives, and suggests ways of moving forward.

Key words: Usability, human-computer interaction, organisation, cost-benefit

1. INTRODUCTION

As information technology professionals, our primary mission, above all else, is to create systems that help people to carry out their tasks in an effective and enjoyable way. In other words, to build systems high on usability. Yet, despite the fact that the discipline of human factors has existed since the 1940s, our twenty-first century software development practices still largely ignore the real end-user of the systems we create (Shneiderman & Gehl, 2000).

The aim of this paper is to examine why this situation exists and to suggest a way forward.

2. ORGANISATIONAL CONTEXT

Software development teams create software either for organisations whose core business is software development (e.g. Microsoft, Oracle,

Adobe) or organisations with another core business (e.g. Coca-Cola, Panasonic, the Department of Defence).

Organisations that develop software for sale on the open market have made some progress towards usability through the establishment of usability testing facilities and laboratories and the engagement of usability professionals (Tremaine, 2001). With the growth in consumer awareness of "ease-of-use", several software development companies now promote their products as being user friendly. Even though the market sectors for many types of software product feature minimal competition, usability will be driven forward by the desire of companies to have their existing user base upgrade to newer versions of their software. Therefore, for software development companies, there will be a natural push towards increasing levels of usability.

The same is not true of organisations whose core business does not involve developing software for the open market. This is the context in which the majority of the world's software development takes place: systems are custom developed to support organisations whose core business is not IT. The systems may be created in-house by the organisation's own staff, or through a contractual relationship with an IT services company. In general, these organisations have not adopted usability practices to any large degree (Catarci et al, 2000) and they are the primary focus of this paper.

3. BARRIERS TO THE ADOPTION OF USABILITY

It would be most unusual today to expect a software development team to function without a business or systems analyst (or without people who possess analysis skills), yet most teams develop software in ignorance of usability principles. This is despite ongoing attempts by the usability community to promote its value. Much effort has been expended by usability specialists (Berry, 2001; Bias & Mayhew, 1994) in targeting the "bottom line" (i.e. trying to demonstrate a return on investment for usability activities) but this has been largely ineffectual (Lund, 1997). What are the factors that have led to something whose value should be beyond question to be ignored?

3.1 Economic Factors

3.1.1 Cost

To maximise profitability and sharemarket value, companies try to keep costs down. There is no question that doing usability properly (i.e. having it integrated into the entire system development life cycle rather than just doing a few tests at the end) is expensive, in the same way as doing anything well is more expensive than mediocrity. Although usability makes promises of cost savings, it requires an up-front investment that is tied to uncertain returns. This makes it unattractive to many managers as shown by the fact that the global amount of money devoted to improving application usability is still only a fraction of what is required (Catarci et al, 2000).

3.1.2 Time

Doing usability takes time. Throwing together an application with minimal user involvement, featuring semi-random screen designs that work most of the time, is faster than designing properly. In particular, with today's rapid development environments an application can be an idea at breakfast and implemented after lunch (Spencer, 2000). This relentless time pressure is illustrated in a classic cartoon that shows a project manager leaving his team with the words "I'll go and find out what the users want, the rest of you start coding". While that attitude prevails, there will not be sufficient time allocated to do serious usability work.

3.2 Psychological Factors

3.2.1 Mistrust of IT Promises

The IT industry is often big on promises and small on results (Harvard Business Review, 1999). The entire usability argument is based on promises: if you use these techniques, you will save X dollars or gain Y hours of added productivity or reduce Help Desk calls by Z. Managers who have been burnt by vendor promises in the past are unlikely to be receptive to these claims and there is often no follow-up to compare promises with results.

3.2.2 Glorification of Technology

The glorification of technology and the worshipping of complexity are further barriers to the widespread adoption of usability techniques. The implicit message here is that machines are clever and humans are stupid. This particularly applies to the many over-engineered user interfaces available today, where even a word processing screen contains more controls than the flight deck of a 767. The inadequacy most people have been taught to feel when confronted with an overly complex user interface compels them to keep quiet. For that reason users often prefer to seek assistance from co-workers rather than from IT staff (Shneiderman & Gehl, 2000) and the reticence of users to express their frustrations openly is a major barrier to usability.

3.2.3 Separation Between Developers and Users

The people who develop software are often physically removed from the real end users, and may never meet them or see them operate in their working environment. At design meetings, end users are often represented by their managers, who are generally not the people who will use the application on a day-to-day basis. It has been suggested that substantial "psychological separation" intrinsically exists between software developers and users (Wiebe, 2000) and augmenting this with physical separation means the developers often fail to take account of the concerns of the users. Furthermore, once applications are released, it is rare for developers to see users working with the applications in-situ for any significant period so they remain blind to the effects their work has on others. This leads to an absence of concern for the user.

3.2.4 Dislike of Usability Professionals

Most people dislike having their work criticised. The way usability professionals have been used so far (being brought in at the last minute and focusing almost exclusively on usability testing and evaluation) has created resentment among application developers (Dougherty, 2001). The developers generally work under substantial pressure with complex technologies and invest vast amounts of effort into getting applications to work (more or less) correctly. When outsiders, who may not have spent the last month working 100-hour weeks to finish the project on time, are brought in at the end to pass judgement on the work of the developers, the resentment is understandable. In particular, usability professionals often recommend changes that would involve massive re-engineering of the application. The dislike of usability professionals when operating in the "usability police" role does little to advance adoption of usability techniques in organisations.

3.3 Organisational Factors

3.3.1 Powerlessness of End-Users

The end users of many applications often hold no power in organisations and it is usually their managers who are involved in IT projects. This is even truer when the application will serve users outside the organisation (e.g. a job search kiosk application provided by the Department of Employment). After implementation there is generally no significant feedback from end users to project managers. Furthermore, there is often no effective way for users to report their frustrations.

Since the majority of users in organisations work at the clerical level, there tends to be a lack of interest in user difficulties as long as they can "muddle their way through". Only when IT processing comes to a standstill or when deficiencies directly frustrate a senior executive is action usually taken.

3.3.2 Distribution of Rewards and Punishments

Software developers are taught, very early in their careers, that the most important factor in climbing the career ladder is to deliver systems on time and within budget (Bloomer & Croft, 1997). Almost nothing else matters. Rewards are not given for application aspects that are hard to assess, such as quality, reliability, or usability and attention to these aspects by concerned developers could, in fact, jeopardise timely delivery.

Furthermore, in the complex world of software development, staff quickly learn that they have dozens of available excuses for usability deficiencies: "the user is stupid", "that was the only way it could be done", "it will be fixed in the next release", "training will look after it", etc. With powerful structures in place that fail to reward usability and savagely punish late delivery (often against arbitrarily determined deadlines) a major barrier to usability exists in most organisations.

3.3.3 Separate Budgets for Development and Support

Companies generally maintain separate budgets for development and support. Understandably, the people running software development will want to minimise their costs, and will be unconcerned if deficiencies in application design result in vastly increased expenditure on support (Norman & Rohn, 2000) through Help Desk calls, training needs and system fixes.

With nobody keeping an eye on the whole-of-life (i.e. creation to retirement) cost of an application, the real expense of poor usability remains hidden, making companies reluctant to invest in usability expertise.

3.4 Other Factors

3.4.1 Captive Users

In general, users have little choice over whether they wish to use a given application. The workplace provides applications and expects staff to use them. Outside their working lives people must interact with a range of applications, such as automatic teller machines, telephone bill-pay services, touch screen kiosks, etc. of which they are "captive users". Where people will be captive users of applications there is little incentive for developers to worry too much about usability.

3.4.2 Lack of Usability Expertise

Many organisations would not consider maintaining an in-house usability group or hiring external usability consultants. Even if they did, there is a shortage of usability professionals in many parts of the world. Instead, organisations expect their software developers to look after all aspects of the application (including usability) but most have received no training in this area (Tremaine, 2001), have only the vaguest conception of what usability involves, do not know where to find usability information, and have no incentive to seek it out.

3.4.3 The Systems Development Life Cycle in Practice

The systems development life cycle as described in textbooks would have us believe that there is an orderly and steady progression from project inception to completion. In practice, there is a prolonged period of confusion at the start followed by a frantic scramble to finish on time at the end (Wiebe, 2000). This usually results in all "non-essential" activities being jettisoned and, like proper documentation and comprehensive system testing, usability concerns are quickly cast aside in the massive effort to get the application up and running.

4. SO WHO CARES?

While many people might care about usability, the factors described above generally prevent them from taking action. The person who would care the most is the end user because, similar to a chef who is asked to work with a blunt knife, the user suffers the frustration and stress of trying to achieve a task with inadequate tools.

As IT toolmakers we should also care. Apart from having pride in our work, the Codes of Ethics of professional computer societies bind us to ensuring that the systems we build serve our users well.

5. WHERE TO FROM HERE?

Translating concern into action in such a multi-faceted problem is difficult and there are no easy answers. However, it is clear that focusing predominantly on cost-benefits is not enough.

The push to have usability incorporated into all systems development life cycles must come from IT professionals. Unlike usability staff, who are often regarded as "outsiders", we are central to the development process and have access and influence within organisations. However, we cannot do this alone. We need assistance from our usability colleagues to provide expertise and from a number of other sources, as shown below.

5.1 IT Professionals

Measures that could be taken by us, as IT professionals, include the following.

- **Speak out against arbitrary and unrealistic deadlines.** Every time project managers acquiesce to these without challenge, usability, along with any "soft" aspect of application development (such as documentation or training), suffers. In the same way as a surgeon asked to perform a triple bypass operation in ten minutes would explain the risks and refuse, IT professionals need to subtly resist being forced into timeframes that would substantially lower quality and usability.
- **Request usability expertise within project teams.** When assembling teams, project managers should request that somebody with usability expertise be included. This expertise must be readily available for the life of the project (not just at the end) and the usability person would ideally be a permanent team member (and carry the same accountability for project success as the technical staff).
- **Acquire knowledge of usability techniques.** Many excellent books (Constantine & Lockwood, 1999; Nielsen, 1993; Shneiderman, 1998; Tognazzini, 1996) and web sites (www.asktog.com, www.nngroup.com, www.useit.com) are available that describe usability in practical terms and do not require specialist human factors knowledge to be understood. As part of their continuing education IT professionals would benefit from learning about usability, thereby being able to build applications that meet with greater user acceptance.

- **Involve project team closely with the end user.** Ideally, the project team should be collocated with the end user. If this is not practical they should at least visit the users regularly in their workplace and perhaps even socialise with them. This would help IT people to understand the world of the user. It would be especially useful, upon project implementation, for application developers to "floor walk" the users' workplace and actively look for difficulties.
- **Promote the value of usability.** This can be done through formal presentations to staff or informally (and perhaps more effectively) via water cooler, corridor and coffee room conversations. Project managers could encourage a usability focus among their staff.
- **Empower the users.** IT professionals need to treat users with respect and courtesy at all times (even when apparently "stupid" questions are asked). In particular, they need to avoid "defending" applications from criticism and be willing to accept that if a feature caused confusion, a design improvement might be necessary.

5.2 Organisations

Senior executives of organisations could, under encouragement from their IT staff, implement these changes.

- **Modify reward structures to increase emphasis on quality and usability.** The present obsession with "time and budget" encourages the sacrifice of quality and usability for short development cycles. Qualitative aspects of applications should be assessed, valued, and rewarded no less than rapid development. If organisations fail to demonstrate a commitment to quality and usability they risk losing these attributes in their applications.
- **Monitor application support costs.** The enormous costs of help desks, training and ongoing application maintenance are too often accepted as the inevitable cost of running a computer application. However, many support costs are the result of poor design during application development, particularly in the usability area. Rather than having separate development and support budgets, organisations should consider tracking total costs (development and support) per application. This approach should encourage usability improvements, as the costs of poor usability were made visible.
- **Consider establishing a usability group.** This would not suit all organisations, but if such a group were established it should be corporately funded (to provide independence from the IT division) and its members should be seconded onto projects as required. The group could become a "centre of excellence" for usability techniques and provide

regular training for developers and users. There is an increasing tendency these days to subsume usability staff into broader quality assurance groups. Unfortunately, because usability is already such a broad, multi-disciplinary area, this carries the risk of de-skilling staff (as their work becomes too broad to manage) and usability can become sidelined. It also diminishes the collegiate atmosphere present in a team of usability professionals.

- **Continuously assess user satisfaction with applications.** Many organisations use surveys to do this but people soon suffer "survey fatigue", so face-to-face techniques (particularly in the person's working environment) may be more effective. However, it is important that somebody skilled in interviewing techniques gathers this information and to avoid contaminating the results it should not be the interviewee's supervisor or the application developer. A usability professional would be ideal.
- **Provide responsive and friendly reporting mechanisms for problems.** Users should be encouraged to report problems and difficulties. In particular, help desk staff should be trained in customer relations to reduce the inadequacy users feel when struggling with applications and dealing with support staff who speak fluent techno-babble.
- **Ensure that software development contracts with external suppliers contain detailed usability specifications.** Specialist usability advice would be necessary to do this. In particular, there must be a precise specification of how compliance would be assessed. Too often vague requirements such as "the application must be highly usable" are made and these help neither the supplier nor the client.

5.3 Usability Professionals

Our colleagues working in usability could take these measures.

- **Follow through on promises of usability benefits.** Where promises of usability benefits are made, usability professionals could encourage a post implementation review that verifies promises made against results. In the absence of verification promises lose credibility and executives need to be shown what metrics could be used to verify claims.
- **Refuse "usability police" roles.** If possible, these roles should never be undertaken. Where the usability staff have not worked with and guided the development team throughout the project, the team should not then be subject to external judgement. Usability staff placed in this role (unintentionally) antagonise developers and this may be part of the reason why some are calling for the abolition of the term "usability".

- **Discourage the test/retest strategy.** Many IT people view usability as no more than usability testing. However, it must be continually emphasised that starting usability at the final testing stage before implementation is almost always too late. Furthermore, people need to be taught that "one cannot test one's way to good usability" and that usability techniques are of most value during initial design.
- **Learn more about software development.** Usability professionals can enhance their skills greatly by learning about software development (preferably with some hands-on experience) so they can appreciate the pressures, skills and tradeoffs of a development environment. Without this knowledge they may appear insensitive to the enormous intellectual effort developers invested in creating an application.

5.4 Educational Institutions

Educational institutions (universities, colleges and private providers) have an enormous part to play in promoting usability.

- **Make usability courses a compulsory part of the computing curriculum.** Too many IT professionals receive no training in usability or human factors in their formal qualifications. Educational institutions need to respond to this by including compulsory usability courses in current IT-oriented degrees and diplomas and by offering these to past graduates.
- **Increase usability course offerings.** There are still not enough courses available for usability professionals and these need to be increased, both to attract people into the profession and to allow usability practitioners to upgrade their skills.

5.5 Professional Computer Societies

Professional computer societies all over the world are responsible for continuously improving the state of professional IT practice and with their access to members they make valuable allies and could help in the following ways.

- **Promote the value of usability to the membership.** Computer societies are well placed to promote usability, particularly since it ties in closely with their codes of ethics. This can be done through professional development sessions and through their publications (which have traditionally featured a dearth of usability related articles).
- **Include usability in software engineering certifications.** People who wish to certify as software engineers or developers should be required to demonstrate competence in usability knowledge and techniques. Current

certifications, such as the one proposed by the IEEE Computer Society, have not yet included this.

6. CONCLUSION

The reasons why few people involved in software development appear to care about usability are many and extend beyond simple cost considerations. To address this problem a prolonged, multi-faceted approach is needed that must be driven "from the inside" by the software developers and by managers.

All of us are, on many occasions, computer users and with the enormous pace of technology uptake, computerisation will touch our lives in ways we cannot imagine. If not for our fellow human beings, we need to take usability seriously for our own sake. I will always remember an executive I worked for who steadfastly refused to invest any time or money in usability activities while cursing out loud whenever he was unable to operate our cantankerous in-house applications.

The fundamental objective of usability is to "match design with need", and when people ask "if your computer were a person, how long till you punch it in the nose?" (John & Bass, 2001) it is apparent that there is still much work to be done in making usability a central part of the systems development life cycle.

7. REFERENCES

Berry, J. (2001), Site usability must enter ROI calculus, *InternetWeek*, March 2001, p. 69.

Bias R.G. & Mayhew D.J. (1994), *Cost-Justifying Usability*, London: Academic Press.

Bloomer, S. & Croft, C. (1997), Pitching usability to your organisation, *Interactions*, Nov./Dec. 1997, pp. 18-26.

Catarci, T., Giacinto, M. & Raiss, G. (2000), Usability and public administration: experiences of a difficult marriage, *Proceedings of the Conference on Universal Usability*, Arlington, Virginia, USA, pp. 24-31.

Constantine, L. & Lockwood, L. (1999), *Software for Use – A Practical Guide to the Models and Methods of Usage-Centred Design*, New York: ACM Press.

Dougherty, D. (2001), Invasion of the usability experts, *Web Techniques*, 6(2), pp. 90-91.

Harvard Business Review (1999), *The Business Value of IT*, Boston: Harvard Business Review.

John, B.E. & Bass, L. (2001), Usability and software architecture, *Behaviour and Information Technology*, 20(5), pp. 329-338.

Lund, A.M. (1997), Another approach to justifying the cost of usability, *Interactions*, May/June 1997, pp. 48-56.

Nielsen, J. (1993), *Usability Engineering*, Boston: Academic Press.

Norman, D. & Rohn, J. (2000), Organisational limits to HCI, *Interactions*, May/June 2000, pp. 36-60.

Shneiderman, B. (1998), *Designing the User Interface: Strategies for Human-Computer Interaction*, Reading, MA: Addison-Wesley.

Shneiderman, B. & Gehl, J. (2000), Credit for computer crashes, *Ubiquity* 1(31).

Spencer, R. (2000), The streamlined cognitive walkthrough method, working around social constraints encountered in a software development company, *CHI Letters*, 2(1), pp. 353-359.

Tognazzini, B. (1996), *Tog on Software Design*, Reading, MA: Addison-Wesley.

Tremaine, M. (2001), Business: Where do I start, *Interactions*, Sept./Oct. 2001, pp. 25-28.

Wiebe, R. (2000), Deep realities: the fit of usability in business, *ACM Journal of Computer Documentation*, 24(4), pp. 220-226.

AUTHOR INDEX

KEYWORD INDEX

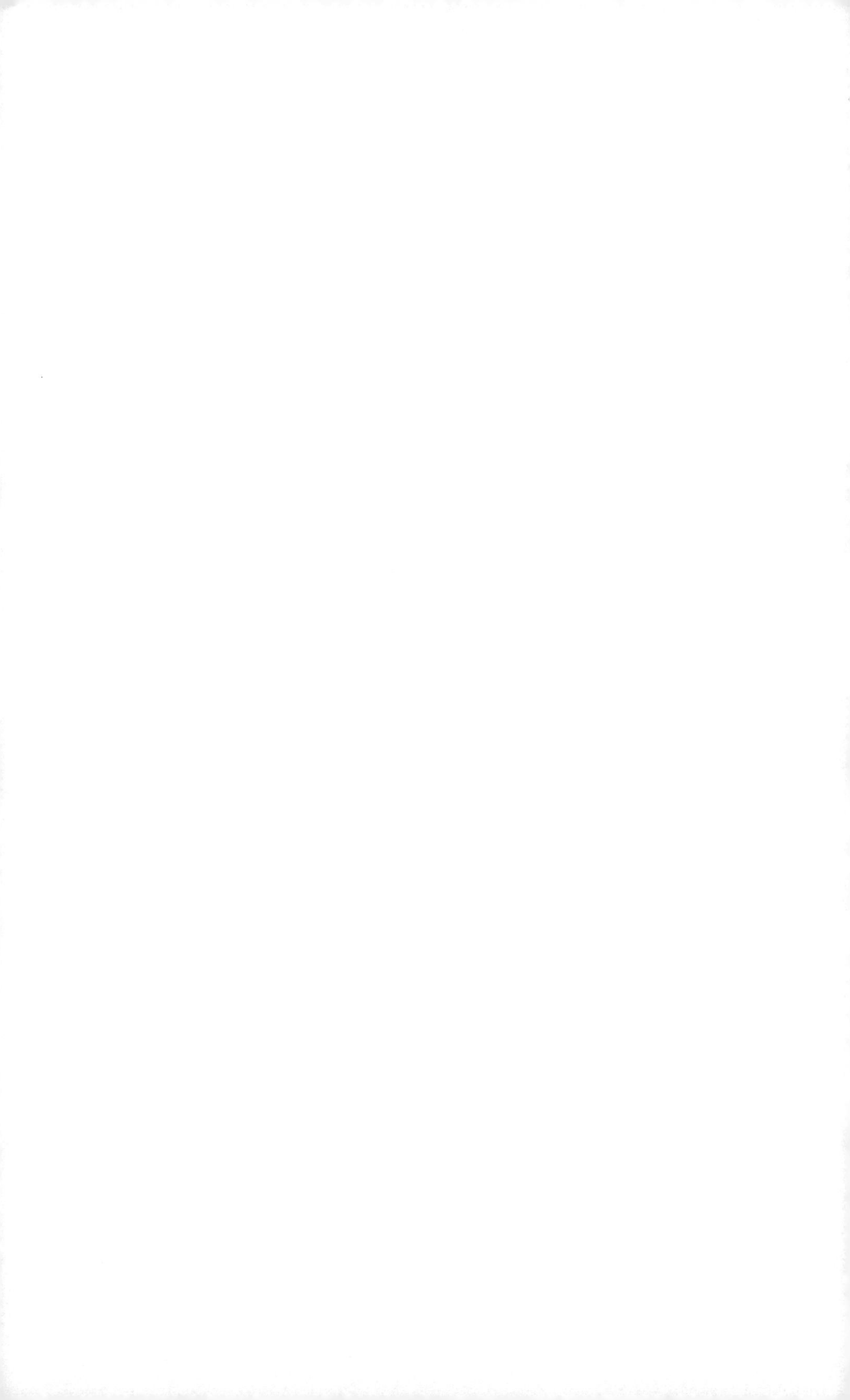

www.ingramcontent.com/pod-product-compliance
Ingram Content Group UK Ltd.
Pitfield, Milton Keynes, MK11 3LW, UK
UKHW041858190726
13854UKWH00002B/968

* 9 7 8 1 4 7 5 7 6 9 0 9 8 *